85¢

Feb '67

Dizziness and Vertigo

Diagnosis and Treatment

Dizziness and Vertigo

Diagnosis and Treatment

Edited by

MARTIN SPECTOR, M.D.

Associate Professor of Otorhinology, Temple University School of Medicine and Hospital; Chief of Otorhinology, Kensington Hospital; Consultant in Otology, St. Mary's Hospital, Philadelphia, Pennsylvania

91 illustrations

GRUNE & STRATTON New York • London

Library of Congress Catalog Card No. 66-19230

381 Park Avenue South
New York, N. Y. 10016

Printed in U.S.A. (K-A)

Contributors

OWEN BELMONT, M.D.
Senior Assistant Surgeon, Wills Eye Hospital; Instructor in Ophthalmology, University of Pennsylvania Graduate School of Medicine; Associate in Ophthalmology, Albert Einstein Medical Center, Philadelphia, Pa.

LYCURGUS M. DAVEY, M.D.
Assistant Clinical Professor of Neurosurgery, Yale University School of Medicine, New Haven, Conn.

DAVID A. DOLOWITZ, M.D.
Associate Professor of Surgery and Chairman, Division of Otorhinolaryngology, University of Utah College of Medicine; Staff, Holy Cross Hospital, Salt Lake City, Utah

ALBERT J. FINESTONE, M.D., M.SC.
Clinical Professor of Medicine, Temple University School of Medicine and Hospital; Chief, Diabetic Service, Episcopal Hospital, Philadelphia, Pa.

JOSEPH A. FUREY, M.D.
Chief of Otolaryngology, Burdette Tomlin Memorial Hospital, Wildwood, N.J.; Chief of E.N.T., Mercy Hospital at Sea Isle City, N. J.; Associate, Vertigo Clinic, Temple University School of Medicine and Hospital, Philadelphia, Pa.

HERBERT B. GOLDMAN, M.D.
Chief of Otology, Hempstead General Hospital, Rockville Center, N. Y.

DAVID J. GOODFRIEND, D.D.S.
Fellow, Section of Otolaryngology, American Medical Association; Past President, American Equilibration Society; Life Member, American Dental Association; Life Member, Pennsylvania State Dental Society; Member, New York Academy of Sciences

DUNCAN HATTON, M.D.
Otologist, Crozier-Chester Medical Center, Chester, Pa.; Associate, Vertigo Clinic, Temple University School of Medicine and Hospital, Philadelphia, Pa.

MARC S. LAPAYOWKER, M.D.
Associate Professor of Radiology, Temple University School of Medicine and Hospital, Philadelphia, Pa.

JOHN R. LINDSAY, M.D.
Professor and Chairman, Department of Otolaryngology, University of Chicago School of Medicine, Chicago, Ill.

GUNNAR O. PROUD, M.D.
Professor and Chairman, Department of Otorhinolaryngology, University of Kansas Medical Center, Kansas City, Kan.

PHILIP E. ROSENBERG, PH.D.
Associate Professor and Director, Section of Audiology, Temple University School of Medicine and Hospital, Philadelphia, Pa.

MAURICE SALTZMAN, M.D.
Assistant Professor of Otorhinology, Emeritus, Temple University School of Medicine and Hospital; Consultant in Otolaryngology, Albert Einstein Medical Center, Philadelphia, Pa.

BERNARD SANDLER, M.D.
Professor and Chairman, Department of Physical Medicine and Rehabilitation, Temple University School of Medicine and Hospital, Philadelphia, Pa.

PAUL SLOANE, M.D.
Associate Professor of Clinical Psychiatry, University of Pennsylvania School of Medicine; Chairman, Department of Psychiatry, Albert Einstein Medical Center; Training Analyst, Institute of the Philadelphia Association for Psychoanalysis, Philadelphia, Pa.

Martin Spector, M.D.
Associate Professor of Otorhinology, Temple University School of Medicine and Hospital; Chief of Otorhinology, Kensington Hospital; Consultant in Otology, St. Mary's Hospital, Philadelphia, Pa.

Ernest Spiegel, M.D.
Professor and Head, Department of Experimental Neurology, Temple University School of Medicine and Hospital, Philadelphia, Pa.

Joseph U. Toglia, M.D.
Associate Professor of Neurology and Otorhinolaryngology, Temple University School of Medicine and Hospital, Philadelphia, Pa.

Henry L. Williams, M.D., M.S. (Otolaryng.)
Chief, Otolaryngology Service, U. S. Veterans Administration Hospital; Professor of Otolaryngology, School of Medical Sciences, University of Minnesota; Emeritus Professor of Otorhinology and Laryngology, Mayo Foundation Graduate School, University of Minnesota; Former Head of Section of Otorhinology and Laryngology, Mayo Clinic, Minneapolis, Minn.

William H. Wilson, M.D., M.Sc. (Otolaryng.)
Assistant Professor of Otolaryngology, University of Colorado School of Medicine, Denver, Colo.

Henry J. Woloshin, M.D.
Professor of Radiology, Temple University School of Medicine and Hospital, Philadelphia, Pa.

Contents

Part II. Clinical Syndromes of Otologic Origin

Part III. Clinical Syndromes of Nonotologic Origin

Preface

The complaint of vertigo or dizziness may arise from many sources in the body. Dizziness is a symptom which is encountered in all fields of medicine. Books and monographs heretofore have been presented from the narrow viewpoint of one specialty, such as otolaryngology or neurology. It is considered worthwhile to survey and classify our present state of knowledge and to bring together in one book the knowledge from various fields—i.e., otolaryngology, neurosurgery, neurology, psychiatry, internal medicine, dentistry, allergy, ophthalmology, physiatry, etc. Each aspect will be covered by a specialist experienced in that specific field. The choice of material has been guided by a desire to present the facts useful to the reader. The content reflects the experiences and prejudices of the contributors. A searching, even partisan, approach has been stressed in order to avoid a book which merely culls and polls the literature. No attempt has been made to stifle contributors or to overemphasize one aspect.

We have attempted to present a systematic scheme for the proper recognition of the symptom, elucidation of salient points in the history, details of the special vestibular tests, and radiology. The significance of the various findings will be assayed and their relative importance will be evaluated. A classification of the causes on a clinical and anatomical basis will be presented. Treatment, both medical and surgical, will be reviewed.

We hope that this book will enable the practitioner to decide in which category each case belongs. Many of the vertiginous patients can be completely handled by the general practitioner. A minority of the patients will require hospitalization. This book is designed for the general practitioner and the many various specialists who encounter dizziness. The student and the resident should find the book useful as a reference. Bibliographic citations are placed at the end of each section.

The editor appreciates the cooperation of the contributors who consented to write special sections for the book. The drawings and content obtained from other authors and publishers are acknowledged under the appropriate figures. The editor wishes to express his appreciation for the use of this material and the generous way in which the requests were met.

Part I. Anatomy and Physiology, History, Examinations

CHAPTER 1

Outline of the Anatomy and Physiology of the Nonacoustic or Statokinetic Labyrinth

E. A. SPIEGEL

ANATOMY

The internal ear consists of the cochlea, the vestibule, and semicircular canals. Many authors designate the entire internal ear as labyrinth; the semicircular canals and the vestibule, lying in back and above, are called the pars superior labyrinthi, or nonacoustic or static labyrinth; some (like Alexander) designate the pars superior only as the labyrinth. In clinical usage the term "peripheral vestibular" refers to the vestibule and semicircular canals and their first sensory neuron, and "central vestibular" refers to the respective rhombencephalic nuclei, their axons and and central projections. The whole system is frequently designated as labyrinthine or vestibular apparatus.

From the middle ear the oval window leads into the osseous vestibule; into the posterior part of the latter open the semicircular canals, and into its anterior and lower part the osseous cochlea opens; the entrance of the aquaeductus vestibuli lies on the medial wall of the vestibule. The anterior part of this wall is a shallow little groove, the recessus sphaericus (sacculi); above this, separated by a ledge, is the recessus ellipticus (utriculi).

The osseous semicircular canals comprise a superior (anterior), an inferior (posterior), and an external (lateral or so-called horizontal) semicircular canal. The superior canal forms an angle of about 45° open anteriorly with the sagittal plane; the posterior canal has a similar angle open posteriorly with this plane (Fig. 1). Thus, the terms frontal and sagittal for the superior and inferior canals, respectively, should be avoided. When the head is erect, the horizontal semicircular canal deviates downward and backward and forms an angle of from 20° to 30° with the horizontal plane. According to Perez, and according to Girard, however, in all mammals the external semicircular canal lies in the horizontal plane in the resting state. In the human, the influence of the position of the eyeballs may be an additional factor.

In general, the horizontal semicircular canals of both sides are parallel to each other, and the superior semicircular canal of one side is parallel to the opposite inferior canal. Starting from and returning to the vestibule, these canals pursue a semicircular course. One end of each semicircular canal shows an expansion, the so-called ampullar end; the other end is simple (smooth or sinus end). Although each ampulla opens separately into the vestibule, so that there are three ampullae on each side—those of the superior, of the horizontal, and of the inferior semicircular canal—there are only two smooth ends on each side, since the smooth ends of the su-

Dr. M. Spector's help in collecting part of the recent literature is gratefully acknowledged.

perior and inferior canal join in the crus commune.

The endosteum lining the osseous labyrinth encloses the perilymphatic space with the perilymph. Attached to the endosteum of the vestibule is the membranous vestibule, consisting of the utriculus and the sacculus (Fig. 2). The membranous vestibule is lined with epithelium and filled with the endolymph. The upper of the two sacs, the utricle, lies in the recessus ellipticus and contains the opening of the membranous semicircular canals. The lower sac, lying in the recessus sphaericus, is the saccule; it communicates with the utricle by the narrow ductus utriculosaccularis, and with the ductus cochlearis by the canalis reuniens.

The ductus endolymphaticus communicates with the saccule and with the ductus utriculosaccularis; it is located in the aquaeductus vestibuli and ends on the posterior surface of the petrous bone in the saccus endolymphaticus. This canal is important for the regulation of endolymphatic pressure; increased endolymphatic pressure may cause dilatation of the saccus endolymphaticus and thus become reduced, while increased intracranial pressure, by compressing the saccus endolymphaticus, may cause increased pressure in the internal ear.

The utricle and the saccule contain receptors, the so-called maculae, flat thickenings of their walls, toward which nerve fibers course through the perilymphatic space. The longitudinal axes of the utricular and saccular maculae are approximately perpendicular to each other; when the head is held erect, the longitudinal axis of the macula sacculi is about vertical, the axis of the macula utriculi about horizontal. The plane of the macula utriculi is parallel to that of the clivus. According to Burlet, the planes of the two sacculi cross each other at an angle of from 50° to 70°.

The maculae exhibit two kinds of cylindric epithelial cells, supporting cells and hair cells (sensory cells); the nerves form a plexus at the base of the maculae. A gelatinous membrane, the so-called statolith membrane, in which are embedded crystals called otoliths or statoliths, rests on these cells. Into this membrane the hairs of the sensory cells protrude.

In the osseous semicircular canals lie the membranous canals, which are also lined with epithelium and filled with endolymph. The

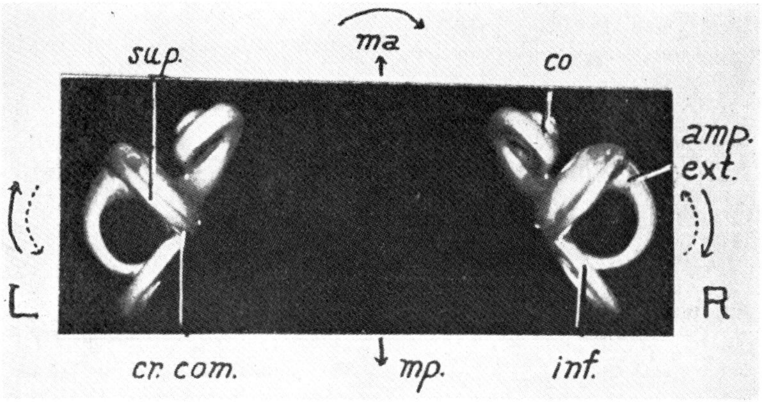

FIG. 1. Models of left (L) and right (R) labyrinths seen from above. amp ext = ampulla of external semicircular canal. co = cochlea. cr com = crus commune. inf = inferior semicircular canal. sup = superior semicircular canal. m a↑= anterior end, m p = posterior end of midline (↓). ↕ indicates endolymph movement in horizontal canals on acceleration of clockwise rotation around vertical axis. ⌒ indicates endolymph movement when this rotation is stopped or decelerated. (From Spiegel and Sommer.)

membranous ampulla of each canal nearly fills the osseous ampulla; the rest of each membranous canal is narrow, oval in cross section, and is attached to the greater circumference of the osseous canal, filling about one-fifth of its lumen.

In the ampulla of each semicircular canal lies the crista ampullaris, the nerve end organ. The crista protrudes like a ledge toward the lumen, its longitudinal axis being perpendicular to the longitudinal course of the semicircular canal. The histologic structure of the neuroepithelium of the crista resembles that of the macula (Fig. 3). The nerve plexus lies toward the periosteum, while the epithelial layer, with the supporting cells and the sensory cells (hair cells), faces toward the lumen of the canal. The hairs of the hair cells extend into canals (Kolmer) of the so-called cupula, a gelatinous structure lying upon the crista. Like the statolith membrane, it represents a cuticular body, both being analogous to the membrana Corti of the cochlea.

Using observations based on electron microscopic studies, Wersäll described two types of vestibular hair cells (Fig. 3): (1) Flask-shaped cells (type I) that he considered phylogenetically higher developed, but not essential for the basic function of the labyrinth, since they are absent in the ray. They lie chiefly at the summit of the cristae and in the center of the maculae. Around each type

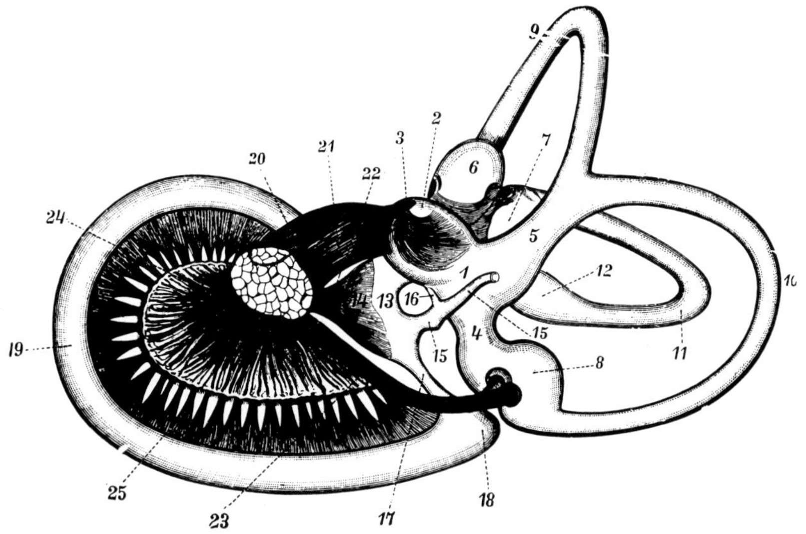

FIG. 2. Membranous labyrinth of a human fetus. (After Retzius, modified by Rauber and Kopsch.)

1-5	Utricle
2	Recessus utriculi
3	Macula utriculi
4	Posterior sinus
5	Superior sinus
6	Membranous superior ampulla
7	Membranous lateral ampulla
8	Membranous posterior ampulla
9	Upper
10	Posterior
11	External semicircular canal
12	Dilated entrance of the crus simplex of the external semicircular canal in the utricle
13	Saccule
14	Macula sacculi
15	Ductus endolymphaticus
16	Ductus utriculosaccularis
17	Ductus reuniens
18	Utricular end of the ductus cochlearis
19	Ductus cochlearis
20	N. facialis
21-24	N. acusticus
21	N. ampullaris superior
22	N. saccularis
23	N. ampullaris posterior
24	N. cochlearis
25	Its endings on the lamina spiralis ossea

I cell a chalice is formed by branches of relatively thick nerve fibers, each thick nerve fiber innervating only a few chalices within a small area. (2) Cylindrical cells (type II), located chiefly at the periphery of the cristae and of the maculae. On their base, branches of thin nerve fibers end, forming a plexus; it seems that the thin nerve fibers often innervate a larger number of cells within a considerable area.

The nervus vestibularis (labyrinthicus) occupies the posterior part of the internal audi-

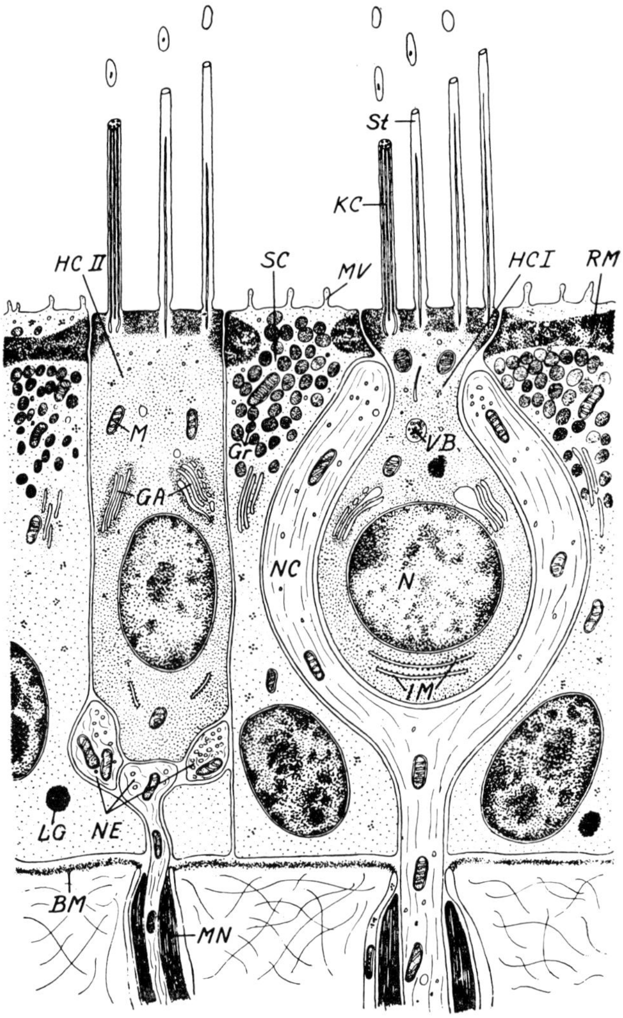

FIG. 3. Sensory epithelium of the crista ampullaris. (Schematic drawing. After Wersäll: Acta Otolaryngol. Suppl. 126: 1-85, 1956.)

BM	basal membrane	MV	microvilli
GA	Golgi apparatus	N	nucleus
HC.I	and HC.II (hair cells, type I and II)	NC	nerve calyx
IM	intracellular membranes	NE	nerve endings
KC	kinocilia	RM	reticular membrane
LG	lipid granule	SC	supporting cell
M	mitochondrium	ST	stereocilia
MN	myelinated nerve	VB	vesicular body

tory canal. Here the nerve divides into a superior and an inferior branch. The upper branch (ramus superior) sends fibers toward the macula utriculi, the superior and the horizontal crista ampullaris, and to the macula sacculi. The lower branch (ramus inferior) sends fibers to the crista ampullaris inferior and also to the macula sacculi. In the internal auditory canal lies also the trophic center of the peripheral neuron, the ganglion vestibulare Scarpae (superius and inferius) in which each part of the labyrinth has its definite localization (Lorente de Nó). It corresponds to the spinal ganglia; its bipolar cells send their peripheral fiber to the sensory epithelium of the maculae and cristae, where they form nongranulated nerve endings, and their central fiber to the rhombencephalon, where they synapse around cells of the vestibular nuclei.

After the union of its branches, the nerve courses in the internal auditory canal in a frontal direction toward the rhombencephalon and enters the latter medially and cephalad to the cochlear nerve.

In the internal auditory canal anastomoses are often found not only between the superior and inferior vestibular ganglia, but also between the superior vestibular ganglion and the geniculate ganglion of the facial nerve, and between the inferior vestibular ganglion and the ganglion spirale cochleae. Poljak and also Lorente de Nó deny the existence of true anastomoses between the cochlear and the vestibular nerve and consider such connections as apparent only. Oort described a vestibulocochlear anastomosis from the inferior vestibular ganglion to the ganglion spirale cochleae. Lorente de Nó considers this anastomosis an aberrant cochlear branch; Weston, however, believes that it contains fibers originating from cells of the vestibular ganglion. Hardy discovered a ramus cochleosaccularis and designated it as a true branch of the cochlear nerve. According to Weston, a part of this ramus, in some mammals at least, is made up of dendrites of vestibular ganglion cells lying in close relation to the cochlear ganglion.

Efferent fibers in the vestibular nerve were demonstrated by Petroff and by Rasmussen and Gacek; further degeneration studies by Gacek suggest that these fibers originate in the lateral vestibular nucleus. Special granulated nerve endings in the vestibular epithelium are considered by Engström as presynaptic terminals of efferent fibers.

In experiments on cats, Sala found that repetitive electrical stimulation of the area of the nucleus Deiters at frequencies of 12/sec. inhibited the spontaneous electrical activity of the opposite vestibular nerve; stimulation with single pulses, however, induced the appearance of afferent activity in the contralateral vestibular nerve. In view of the long latent period (22-32 msec.), the author considered this as a rebound effect. Following midline section of the floor of the fourth ventricle, this phenomenon disappeared. Stimulation of a labyrinth with hot water in decerebrate cats produced a depolarization of this labyrinth and hyperpolarization of the contralateral labyrinth; cold water stimulation had the reverse effect. These experiments suggested a feedback system between both labyrinths. The author inferred that the efferent vestibular fibers have a modifying influence upon vestibular impulses, which is inhibitory or excitatory depending on the functional state of the receptors.

Dohlman's histochemical studies suggest that butyrylcholine may be the chemical mediator for the receptor system, and acetylcholine for the efferent nerve endings in the labyrinth.

FUNCTION OF THE NONACOUSTIC INNER EAR

In general, it may be stated that the cristae contain receptors for angular acceleration and the macula utriculi gravitational receptors. The macula sacculi seems to react chiefly to sound and vibrational stimuli (Frisch and Stretter on fishes; Ashcroft and Hallpike on frogs), and its elimination does not produce definite disturbances of equilibrium (McNally and Tait on frogs; Versteegh on rabbits). In the elasmobranch, however, the posterior part of the saccular macula yields positional responses (Löwenstein).

A sharp distinction between the functions of the cristae and of the macula utriculi has also become doubtful. At least at high degrees of angular acceleration, the utricular macula may be stimulated (McNally and Tait; dampening of the cristae according to these authors, in contrast to Maxwell's opinion of a synergistic action). X-ray pictures of decapitated sharks showed that on rotation around a transverse axis the otolithic membrane lags behind by about 2°; this movement takes place between otolith and sensory cells (Vilstrup and Vilstrup). Conversely, at least the vertical canals of pigeons may respond with righting reflexes (Groebbels). Lorente de Nó assumed that the nerve endings of the cristae may be excited on changes of position due to displacement of the membranous semicircular canals. With these exceptions in mind, one may regard the utricular macula as reacting chiefly to gravitational or centrifugal forces (position of the head, changes of its position) and the cristae to angular acceleration.

Progressive movements (linear accelerated movements) may also induce reactions by stimulating labryinthine receptors—for example, lifting of the head and downward extension of the arms occurring in infants held at the pelvis and moved downward, lowering of the head at the beginning of upward movements (Schaltenbrand). Similar reactions still appear in guinea pigs after the otoliths have been separated from the maculae by centrifugation (Magnus and de Kleijn; disputed by Hasegawa), so that it is uncertain to which extent endolymph flow in the semicircular canals (Ornstein and Burger) and to which extent macular stimulation (Breuer) causes these reactions. In rabbits, destruction of the sacculus induced only a diminution of the reactions induced by linear acceleration from one ear to the other (Jongkees).

As long as the otoliths are in contact with the maculae, it seems justified to assume that the bending of the hairs of their receptor cells by gliding of the otoliths (Breuer) and/or the pull of the otoliths on these hairs (Magnus and de Kleijn) represent the stimuli for the macula utriculi. According to the latter authors, there is maximum excitation of the macula utriculi if the otolith lies below the macula and pulls on its hairs, and a minimum excitation if the otolith lies above the macula and presses on it. One has to bear in mind, however, that de Kleijn and Versteegh and also Hasegawa still observed positional reflexes after throwing off the otoliths by centrifugation, in contrast to Magnus and de Kleijn's earlier experiments.

The equation of the motion of an otolith is probably that of a harmonic oscillator (DeVries). The macula utriculi can record the position relative to the vertical, as well as oscillations. Electrographic recordings from single nerve fibers of the isolated labryrinth of Raja clavata (elasmobranch fish) have shown that the utricular macula is not a uniform structure (Löwenstein). Its main portion responds to tilting. It reacts also to linear acceleration, while some units discharge steadily, unaffected by changes of position, furnishing continuous, tonic impulses.

The reactions induced by the macula utriculi are chiefly tonic (static) reflexes that have been carefully analyzed by Magnus and de Kleijn. These authors distinguished (1) compensatory deviations of the eyes, serving the maintenance of the point of fixation of the eye in space; (2) tonic labyrinthine reflexes upon the body musculature and the extremities seen particularly in decerebrate animals (maximum extensor tonus with the otoliths below, minimum tonus with the otoliths above the macula utriculi). While these latter reflexes are centered in the rhombencephalon, the midbrain (probably its reticular formation) is necessary for (3) the labyrinthine righting reflexes that bring the head from an abnormal to the normal erect position, also after exclusion of retinal influences and irrespective of the body's position when it is held in the air.

The adequate stimulus for the cristae of the *semicircular canals* is rotatory movement of the head with positive or negative angular acceleration; it induces a movement of the endolymph resulting in deviation of the cupula and bending of the hairs of the crista ampullaris. This so-called hydrodynamic theory (Breuer, Mach, Crum Brown, Ewald) has been experimentally proved by Steinhausen in the living pike for rotational as well as for caloric stimuli.

On rotation of the head, the endolymph flow occurs in those semicircular canals, the plane of which is most nearly perpendicular to the axis of rotation. Inertia causes the endolymph to lag in respect to the wall of the canal in the beginning of the rotation or on acceleration, so that the cupula deviates in a direction opposite to that of the rotation. On stopping the rotation or on deceleration, the endolymph continues to flow for some time interval, and the cupula deviates in the direction of rotation. For instance, on clockwise rotation (to the right) with the head in the optimum position for the horizontal canal —i.e., inclined 30° forward—the cupula of the horizontal canal deviates in counterclockwise direction—i.e., in ampullopetal direction in the right, in ampullofugal direction in the left horizontal canal (Fig. 1). On continued rotation, for instance to the right, without change of angular velocity, the endolymph will eventually flow in the direction of rotation (in this case clockwise), and on stopping of the rotation to the right, the clockwise flow in the horizontal canal will continue due to inertia (ampullopetal in the left, ampullofugal in the right horizontal canal due to inertia).

A parallelism of the direction of the reactive movements with the plane of the stimulated canal has been observed by Flourens. Particularly the experiments of Ewald on pigeons have shown that the slow conjugate deviation of both eyes (also of the head in these animals, but not in man) takes place in the direction of the endolymph flow in the horizontal canal (opposite to the direction of rotation on acceleration, in its direction on deceleration). There is also a tendency of the extremities to deviate in the direction of the slow component of the eye movements as manifested, for instance, by past pointing in man.

On strong stimulation this slow deviation is followed by a rhythmic reaction of the eyes (nystagmus). The slow component of the nystagmus corresponds to the slow deviation in the direction of the endolymph movement. The quick component takes place in the opposite direction. According to clinical usage, the direction of the nystagmus is designated according to that of the fast component.

On one side of the crista the deviation of the cupula causes a pressure upon the hairs lying in its canals; they will pull on the other side of the crista. This is the mechanical stimulus for the hair cells of the crista.

The problem of how the endolymph flow and resulting deviation of the cupula and bending of the cilia of the hair cells of the crista induce an excitation of these cells cannot be answered with certainty. There are, however, some intriguing observations and theories. Vilstrup and Jensen found in the endolymph of a fish (Acanthias) a substance resembling hyaluronic acid. In vitro experiments (Jensen, Koefoed, and Vilstrup) showed that movement of hyaluronate solutions in a glass tube produced flow potentials that showed opposite polarity, if the direction of the fluid movement was reversed. Such electrical changes may provide a stimulus to the receptor cells. In radioisotope studies, Dohlman found that labeled polysaccharid molecules may rapidly pass into the open tubes of the cupula that contain the hairs of the hair cells. He supposes that the large and highly negatively charged polysaccharides adhere to the surface of the hairs. Movements of the cupula may squeeze or relax the tubes around the hairs and induce here fluid movements that may cause "displacement potentials" building up a static electric discharge. The electric charge of the surface of the hairs might constitute the basis for changes in potential through displacement of the fluid around the hairs. Van Eyck suggests that the microphonic potential appearing following a mechanical stimulus is the excitatory agent inducing the response of the nerve endings of the sense organ. Trincker assumes that the utriculopetal deviation of the cilia in the horizontal canal causes a depolarization, that in the opposite direction a hyperpolarization, of the cell membrane. Further experiments will be needed to test the validity of these theories.

The rule that the reflex movements of the eyes occur in a direction parallel to that of the stimulated canal applies chiefly to the horizontal canal. Deviations from this rule were found on stimulation of the vertical canals (in rabbits, Lorente de Nó; nystagmus in all three directions was obtained in rabbits with only the horizontal and superior canals on one side intact, de Kleijn and Versteegh). Based on experiments in the dog fish, Ivy assumed that also in man rotation in the frontal plane of the head (with the patient's head inclined maximally forward on rotation on a Bárány chair), rotational nystagmus is produced by stimulation of only the anterior canal or by simultaneous stimulation of both anterior or both posterior ampullae. If the person sits in the Bárány chair with the head inclined to the right or left shoulder, so that rotation is performed in the sagittal plane of the head, vertical nystagmus is produced, supposedly by stimulation of both vertical ampullae of one side.

Rhythmic eye movements can also be produced on repetitive electric stimulation of the labyrinth at rates up to 27/sec. (Spiegel). On stimulation of the ampullary nerves from the semicircular canals in cats with trains of closely spaced square waves, eye movements characteristic for each canal nerve were observed (Cohen, Suzuki, and Bender; Suzuki, Cohen, and Bender), e.g., on stimulation of the left anterior canal nerve dissociated upward movement (↑ in the left, ↖ in the right eye), on stimulation of the left posterior canal ↗ in the left, ↓ in the right eye; on stimulation of the left horizontal canal conjugate movements of both eyes to the right; on stimulation of both anterior canals conjugate upward movements of both eyes, on stimulation of both posterior canals conjugate downward movements of both eyes; on stimulation of the left anterior and posterior canals conjugate counterclockwise rotation of both eyes. During stimulation of any single canal nerve, every eye muscle was either activated or inhibited, excitatory and inhibitory activities being summated in a predictable manner.

The persistence of the nystagmus for some time after the rotation has been stopped requires special consideration. Mowrer found that the action potentials of the vestibular nerve outlast the rotation only for fractions of a second; it has been assumed, therefore, that this phenomenon is due to an after discharge in the central part of the vestibular reflex arc. However, the impulses from the receptor due to the deviation of the cupula in the direction opposite to that on starting should not be neglected.

Steinhausen, whose experiments on the living pike have been mentioned above, considered the deviation of the cupula as that of a torsion pendulum. Using this premise, Van Egmond and his associates were able to compute the deviation of the cupula ξ on sudden arrest of the rotating chair from an angular velocity γ and to verify the computations experimentally (Van Egmond et al.; Groen et al.).

$$\xi = \gamma \frac{\theta}{\pi} \left(e^{-\Delta t/\pi} - e^{-\pi t/\theta}\right).$$

In this equation θ = moment of inertia of the endolymph, π = moment of friction at unit angular velocity; Δ = directional momentum at unit angle caused by the cupula.

Experimentally one can determine the duration of the after-sensation tu following interruption of rotation at various velocities. One may assume that this after-sensation terminates when a minimal perceptible deflection of the cupula ξ min. is attained. The formula

$$tu = \frac{\pi}{\Delta} \log \left(\frac{\theta\gamma}{\pi\,\xi \text{ min.}}\right)$$

gives the relationship between the duration of the after-sensation and the angular velocity at the moment of arrest of rotation. Thus, the duration of the reaction is proportional to the logarithm of the impulse. Accordingly Van Egmond et al. obtained a cupulogram by determining the length of the after-sensation after interruption of rotation at various velocities and plotting on logarithmic paper the angular velocity (degree/sec. abscissa) against the duration of after-sensation (ordinate in min.). A straight line results which indicates the constant π/Δ. Similarly, a cupulogram may be obtained by using the duration of the after-nystagmus instead of the after-sensation (Hulk and Jongkees). The differences in the slopes of the 2 curves suggest differences in the mechanism of the 2 phenomena, particularly complicating central factors. Hallpike and Hood have used the oculogyric illusion (sensation of movement of a light attached to the rotating chair and fixated by the subject) for measurement of the course of the cupular deflection and obtained values in good agreement with those reported by Van Egmond et al. For such studies, precision rotating chairs permitting a wide range of angular accelerations and durations are necessary, e.g., those used by Byford et al.; Arslan; Buys; Hallpike and Hood; Montandon; and Toennis.

Despite Dittrich and Exterman's objections that it is as yet impossible to measure in man in a directly reproducible manner the above-mentioned constants and factors, cupulometry has proved to be a valuable progress in studies of the labyrinth.

Ewald's experiments in pigeons, in which he produced artificially endolymph movements in some semicircular canals, require a more detailed discussion. In experiments on pigeons Ewald sealed the external horizontal canal in one place and inserted a pneumatic hammer (piston of a syringe) between the plug and the crista ampullaris. By increasing the pressure in the external canal he could induce an ampullopetal, by decreasing the pressure, an ampullofugal endolymph flow in the canal. He observed that the reflex responses to the ampullopetal endolymph flow exceeded those to the ampullofugal flow. This so-called Ewald's second law has been the subject of much experimentation and discussion at the International Symposium on Problems in Otoneurology, Basle, May 1960 (Acta Otolaryng. [Stockholm] Suppl. 159:7-71). It was pointed out by Hallpike (p. 7) and Aschan (p. 69) that on syringing the ear with cold water (30°C.) with the head in the usual position for this test (ampulla above the smooth part of the external canal that is in a vertical position) an ampullofugal endolymph flow is produced. According to Ewald's experiments, one should expect that the effect of the cold syringing should be weaker than that of hot syringing (at 44°C.), which induced an ampullopetal deviation of the cupula. However, the hot irrigation was less effective than the cold. Only in cases in which following unilateral (e.g., right-sided) labyrinthectomy, there existed a tendency to spontaneous nystagmus (e.g., to the left) the hot water effect on stimulation of the left ear (duration of the nystagmus to the left) exceeded the cold water effect (duration of the nystagmus to the right). In the intact human subject apparently the responses of the external canal did not show the inequality to be expected from Ewald's experiments. It was, therefore, concluded that Ewald had created abnormal conditions in the external canal by plugging it and had applied excessive stimuli. Some clinicians, however, support Ewald's observations also for relatively weak stimuli; e.g., Montandon, using a chair that permitted very weak angular acceleration (1°-6°/sec.^{2}) and recording the electronystagmogram, confirmed the theory of a unidirectional preponderance of the motor responses.

Attempts to explain the caloric nystagmus by a direct effect of the temperature changes upon nerve endings or by vasomotor changes have failed because such theories could not account for the fact that the vertical position of the external canal with its ampulla above the smooth part is the optimum position for eliciting this type of nystagmus to the opposite side. This does not exclude, however, an accessory role of direct thermal effects upon the receptors or of indirect vasomotor effects induced by thermal changes. Such accessory effects are indicated by experiments with prolonged calorization of the labyrinth in cats (Spiegel and Aronson) in which nystagmic jerks of the eyeballs appeared for hours in groups interrupted by short periods of rest and sometimes uninfluenced by changes in the position of the head. In further experiments a depressor effect of cold upon static receptors of the labyrinth could be demonstrated (Spiegel), resulting in abnormal posture of the head similar to that seen after unilateral labyrinth paralysis (rotation of the head about the oro-occipital axis with the affected ear lying lower).

One of the rather puzzling findings of Ewald and of later experimenters is the observation that in the vertical canals an ampullofugal endolymph flow induces stronger responses than an ampullopetal flow, in contrast to the reverse conditions in the external canal. Since a plausible explanation of these different conditions in the horizontal and in the vertical canals is lacking, Groen's hypothetical explanation deserves to be mentioned.

Groen points out that the sensory cells of the labyrinth have a common origin, the placode found in the embryo. He hypothesizes that in the placode the sensory cells have a common specific orientation, which later leads to a specific directional sensitivity. This original orientation of the sensory cells is supposed to be maintained during the differentiation of the various parts of the placode. Phylogenetically the external canal develops from the anterior vertical. Groen assumes, therefore, further that the orientation of the sensory cells is the same in the cristae of the external and anterior canals. If one projects these two canals upon one plane, one finds that the ampullopetal flow in the external canal corresponds to the ampullofugal flow in the anterior vertical canal; due to the identical orientation and same direction of optimal sensitivity of the anterior and external cristae these currents have the same stimulating effect upon both cristae, while the opposite current (ampullofugal in the lateral, ampullopetal in the anterior vertical canal) depresses the resting discharge of the cristae.

In recent years *electrophysiologic studies* have helped to deepen our knowledge of the receptor apparatus of the nonacoustic inner ear. Ewald's concept of a "tonic action" of the labyrinth in the resting state received a confirmation from Löwenstein and Sand's studies on the nerves of the semicircular canals of the dogfish and from Ledoux's in frogs, showing the existence of electrical discharges of low frequency in the nerves from the ampulla in the resting state. Hallpike postulates also a tonic action of the nerve fibers from the utricle and believes that their loss after labyrinthectomy is a factor in the appearance of the directional preponderance of nystagmus to the normal labyrinth on caloric stimulation of the latter.

Low frequency discharges were also found in the vestibular nuclei in the *resting state* (Adrian; Gernandt and Thulin; Eckel; Duensing and Schaefer; Pompeiano and Cotti). It should be emphasized, however, that labyrinthectomy does not prevent a "spontaneous" activity of the vestibular nuclei (Spiegel and Sato) that is probably due to impulses from supranuclear centers.

Ledoux's experiments demonstrated that ampullopetal endolymph flow increases the electrical resting activity of the ampullar nerve in the frog indicating an increase of the tonic activity of the receptors in the external canal and producing a nystagmus to the side of stimulation. In contrast, ampullofugal endolymph flow inhibits the activity of the receptors of the external canal, so that the tonic action of the opposite labyrinth prevails and nystagmus to the latter results. With stimuli of moderate intensity Ledoux found that the responses to ampullopetal and ampullofugal currents are equal. Only on application of intense stimuli was the effect of the ampullopetal flow more pronounced than that of the ampullofugal endolymph movement.

For the testing of Ewald's second law, electrophysiologic studies related to the so-called Tullio phenomenon are important. The ampulla of a semicircular canal of a pigeon can be excited by a sound stimulus (Tullio, Huizinga), resulting in a deviation of the head to the opposite side; this reaction is increased, if the respective osseous canal is fenestrated (Tullio); it persists after elimination of the cochlea (Huizinga). Under these conditions, sound stimuli of 100-3000 cycles/sec. produce microphonic potential waves in the respective crista (Bleeker and de Vries; van Eyck). Further studies by van Eyck showed that stimulation of the crista by a click induces first a microphonic effect, then a response that may be attributed to the endings of the ampullary nerve. The initial microphonic wave is negative and of maximum voltage, if the click induces a deviation of the cupula in the direction that is most efficient for the respective ampulla according to Ewald's law; deviation of the cupula in the opposite direction induces an initial positive wave of small voltage. Similarly, Trincker's studies of the potential changes on the crista on utriculopetal and -fugal deviation of the crista seemed to agree with Ewald's second law. However, he applied rather strong, unphysiological stimuli.

The complexity of these problems is demonstrated by Löwenstein's findings in the elasmobranch labyrinth, indicating the existence of 3 groups of receptors in the semicircular canals. The majority are bidirectional, showing an increase in discharge rate on ipsilateral and a decrease on contralateral acceleration. The second group is unidirectional, discharging only during ipsilateral and after contralateral rotation. These units are gradually recruited if the intensity of the stimulus increases. A third group is not influenced by rotation. Transitional stages between these 3 types of receptors have been found. Gernandt found in the vestibular nerve of the cat in 83 per cent of the units acceleration of the discharges by rotation to the side of the recording and inhibition by rotation in the opposite direction (type I); in addition, he found 2 types of units, 1 showing an excitatory and the other an inhibitory response to acceleration in both directions. The volleys recorded from the vestibular nerve in mammals at rest are decreased by ampullofugal and increased by ampullopetal endolymph flow (Boenninghaus).

Rhythmic oscillations could also be led off from the ventromedial wall of the tympanic cavity in the cat; their amplitude was increased by rotatory or caloric stimuli; this effect persisted after decerebration, curarization (Fig. 4), or destruction of the vestibular nuclei and disappeared after cocainization of the labyrinth (Spector, Szekely, and Spiegel). Continuing these experiments with similar electrode placements, Dr. Alfred Finck* is trying to estimate the total response voltage; his preliminary experiments show that this voltage obtained from ampullopetal flow exceeds that from ampullofugal flow and the latter the resting level.

Vertigo is often associated with vegetative symptoms that are the result of *vestibulovegetative reflexes* and represent the chief manifestations of the various forms of motion sickness (for details see reviews by Spiegel; Spiegel and Sommer; Montandon). Summation effects seem to play an important role, since in the study of experimental motion sickness repetition of the stimulus for some time is often required before subjective or objective symptoms appear. Symptoms of the gastrointestinal system (increased salivation,

*Personal communication.

nausea, vomiting) predominate. Often one finds also vasomotor symptoms (pallor of the face, cold, clammy extremities), shallow respiration, and prostration. Measurement of the skin resistance (Behr, Preber, and Silfverskiöld) is a very sensitive method, indicating the influence of the labyrinth upon the vegetative system. On thermal as well as on rotatory stimulation of the labyrinth a fall of the skin resistance could be recorded. Vomiting is a combined somatomotor and vegetative reaction (contraction of the diaphragm and abdominal muscles increasing the intra-abdominal pressure, relaxation of the stomach except its pyloric part, contraction of the duodenum (Byrne; Lebensohn; Hemingway).

Experimental studies (Spiegel and Démétriades; Oppenheimer and Spiegel) showed that in rabbits under urethan-ether anesthesia and in decerebrate or anaesthetized cats and dogs a fall of blood pressure or a multiphasic reaction predominates on labyrinthine stimulation by rotation (Fig. 5). This fall of blood pressure is due chiefly to dilatation of the vessels in the splanchnic area, depressor impulses being transmitted by way of the triangular vestibular nucleus to the rhombencephalic vasomotor center. In nonanaesthetized animals—e.g., under curare paralysis or in bulbocapnine catalepsy, with the diencephalon and prosencephalon preserved—the labyrinthine stimulation often results in vasoconstriction and rise of blood pressure, probably at least partly due to excitement. A further hypertensive factor is the increase of intra-abdominal pressure during retching and vomiting. By application of vasoconstrictor drugs the vasodepressor effect of labyrinthine stimulation could be changed into a pressor response (Oppenheimer and Spiegel).

In man an influence of the labyrinth upon the blood pressure could only rarely be studied by recording the intra-arterial pressure (e.g., Karbowski et al.). This may explain, at least partly, the contradictory observations reported in the literature. Some authors noted a diphasic reaction of the blood pressure (Wotzilka; Talpis and Wolfkowitch), others no or only minimal changes (Dalla Torre and Cantele) or a slight elevation (Rossberg). In this connection it is of interest that the mere proposition to repeat an examination of the labyrinth may raise the patient's blood pressure (Stein and Bénesi). On continuous recording of the intra-arterial pressure, Karbowski et al. observed during caloric stimulation a slight rise that they considered as due to extralabyrinthine factors;

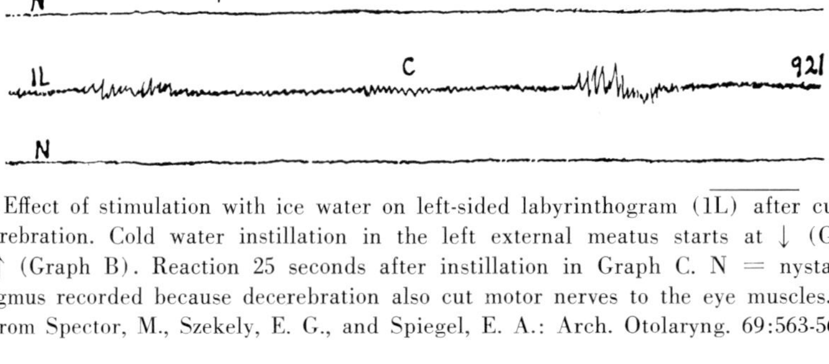

FIG. 4. Effect of stimulation with ice water on left-sided labyrinthogram (1L) after curarization and decerebration. Cold water instillation in the left external meatus starts at ↓ (Graph A), ends at ↑ (Graph B). Reaction 25 seconds after instillation in Graph C. N = nystagmogram. No nystagmus recorded because decerebration also cut motor nerves to the eye muscles. Time = 1 sec. (From Spector, M., Szekely, E. G., and Spiegel, E. A.: Arch. Otolaryng. 69:563-569, 1959.)

in the poststimulation phase there was an about 10 per cent depression of the systolic and diastolic pressure.

In seasickness a fall as well as a rise of blood pressure has been reported (Maitland; Geller; Sokalchuk). The depressor effect prevails, if one studies persons that have been subjected to a combination of rolling, pitching, and yawing movements for hours and days, as Sokalchuk did on a destroyer. Of 37 seasick crew members 30 showed a fall of the average systolic pressure (15 from 1-10 mm., 15 from 11 to 30 mm.), 5 rise or fall (from +4 to —11), 2 an increase from 1-10 mm.

The fluctuation of the blood pressure induced by labyrinthine stimulation secondarily affects the cerebral circulation as could be demonstrated in animal experiments (Spiegel and Démétriades; Spiegel, Henny and Wycis). Furthermore, Streiff, Montandon, and Monnier found in rabbits and cats that the fall of the general pressure recorded from the femoral artery was associated with a depressor reaction in the retinal artery, followed in the latter by a secondary hypertensive phase, chiefly on the side of the more stimulated labyrinth. In man a cerebral effect was suggested by Kramer's report of smallness of the diameter of the vessels of the retina and the paleness of the choroid. These changes of the cerebral circulation induced by labyrinthine stimulation may represent, at least in some instances, an accessory factor in the genesis of the vertigo syndrome, besides the disturbance of orientation.

Although a definite effect of labyrinthine stimulation upon the gastrointestinal system that is chiefly transmitted by way of the vagus could be observed, and although electrographically an influence of the vestibular nerve upon the homolateral vagus could be demonstrated (Akert and Gernandt; Gernandt), the effect of vestibular impulses upon the heart rate (bradycardia or tachycardia) as a rule is rather slight.

The labyrinthine reflexes upon the gastrointestinal and vasomotor system persist after decerebration by transection of the midbrain (Spiegel and Démétriades). An increase of frequency and amplitude of respiration could also be induced by rhythmic pitching movements after extirpation of the cerebral hemispheres and the diencephalon (Spiegel); thus,

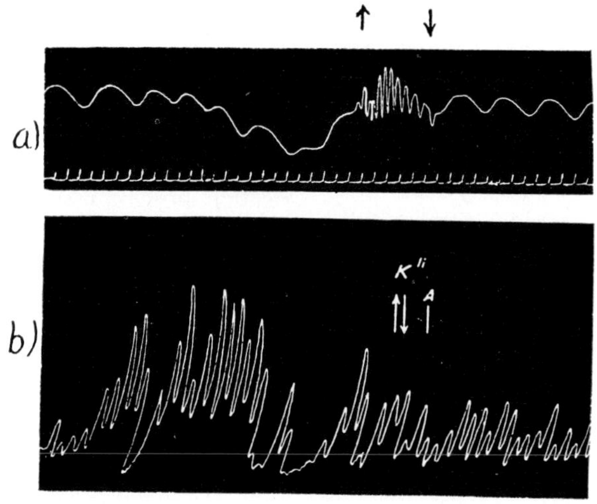

FIG. 5. (a) Effect of 10 rotations about longitudinal axis (from ↓ to ↑) upon blood pressure of rabbit under urethane-ether anesthesia. Blood pressure recorded from carotid artery. Severance of vagi and cervical sympathetics did not prevent reaction. Time in seconds. (b) Effect of cold water irrigation of left ear upon small intestine of decerebrate rabbit. At A, syringe is introduced. Syringing from ↓ to ↑. Read both curves from right to left. (From Spiegel and Démétriades.)

higher parts of the central nervous system are dispensable for these reactions.

The role of the cerebellum in the mechanism of vestibulo-vegetative reflexes seems to require further study. While Kreidl was able to induce seasickness in decerebellated dogs, Bard et al. reported that following ablation of parts of the vermis cerebelli (nodulus and uvula) motion sickness could no longer be elicited in their dogs. Spiegel and Démétriades still observed vestibulo-vasomotor reactions after nearly complete ablation of the cerebellum; this is in agreement with the experience of Magnus and de Kleijn that the tonic labyrinthine reflexes could be evoked in decerebellated animals.

It is an old experience that deaf mutes with unexcitable labyrinths (James) do not become seasick. Kreidl's experiments in dogs showed that elimination of the labyrinths prevents seasickness in dogs; similar experiments were made by Sjöberg in dogs when attempting to produce "elevator sickness" by vertical movements. In an attempt to localize the receptors for the vestibulo-vasomotor reactions it was found in guinea pigs that centrifugation at high speed did not prevent these reactions (Spiegel, Oppenheimer, and Wycis), although it could be demonstrated histologically (Lindsay, Oppenheimer, Wycis, and Spiegel) that in these experiments the otoliths were thrown off the maculae. Our further experiments showed that also puncture of the round window, following which procedure the reflex effect of the semicircular canals upon the eyes is abolished, does not prevent the vestibulo-vasomotor reaction. It was, therefore, concluded that the vestibulo-vasomotor reaction may be elicited from the maculae as well as from the cristae. In agreement with this conclusion are experiments by Graybiel demonstrating that "canal sickness" may be produced if the chief precipitating factor is an unusual stimulation of the semicircular canals and "otolith sickness," if abnormal stimuli act upon the otoliths and nonotolithic gravireceptors in the absence of a stimulation of the semicircular canals.

The threshold for vestibulo-vagal reflexes is only about one-third that for vestibulo-somatic reflexes (Gernandt). It has to be emphasized, however, that the central mechanisms of the vestibulo-vegetative reflexes and of the vestibular mechanisms inducing disturbances of orientation are rather independent of each other. Using a rotating chair that produced simultaneously with each rotation a head movement in a sagittal or frontal plane, Spiegel, Oppenheimer, Henny, and Wycis induced motion sickness in man; under certain experimental conditions (when the subjects watched stationary lights placed around the apparatus), there appeared only slight disturbances of orientation, but marked nausea; under other conditions (subjects watching a light participating in all head movements) illusions of swinging or rolling movements could be produced without vegetative symptoms.

Of practical importance is the phenomenon of *habituation*. It is well known that on a sea voyage many persons become accustomed after several days to the motion of the ship and are no longer disturbed by these abnormal movements, although there exist great individual variations, and some persons never lose their susceptibility to motion sickness. It should also be pointed out that adaptation to one type of motion does not prevent motion sickness produced by a different motion (Tyler and Bard). Experiments in dogs have shown that on repeated stimulation within short time intervals the amplitude and duration of the nystagmus decreased (Dodge). In the production of habituation, central factors seem to play a role. Experimentally it could be shown that the cerebellum (Pollock and Davis) and also parts of the reticular formation (Gernandt) have an inhibitory effect upon vestibular responses. In experiments by Spiegel, Szekely, and Gildenberg it was found that responses of higher parts of the central nervous system, particularly of the caudate nucleus, to vestibular impulses were increased after lesions affecting the dorsal part of the mesencephalic tegmentum.

A detailed description of the anatomy and physiology of the *vestibular nuclei* and of their fiber connections is beyond the scope of this chapter, and only a few facts will here be mentioned. (In this respect the reader is referred to the excellent monograph by Brodal, Pompeiano, and Walberg). The vestibulo-ocular reflex arc is rather simple, consisting chiefly of three groups of neurons: (1) an afferent represented by the bipolar cells of the ganglion vestibulare Scarpae and their peripheral and central branches; (2) an efferent to the eye muscle nuclei, represented by cells of the oculomotor, trochlear, and abducens nuclei; and (3) intercalated neurons, represented by cells of the vestibular nuclei, as has been reaffirmed by Szentágothai. In the vestibular nuclei one distinguishes the nucl. lateralis (Deiters), medialis or triangularis (Schwalbe), superior (Bechterew), and inferior or nucl. of the descending root. (Figs. 6 and 7).

According to Adrian's records of unit discharges in the vestibular nuclei, in the oral part of these nuclei are cells reacting to tilting of the head in the median plane and to horizontal rotation; the caudal part contains units reacting to tilting of the head in lateral direction and to rotation in the transverse plane. The microelectrode studies of Duensing and Schaefer showed that in some neurons of the vestibular nuclei of rabbits impulses from the cristae and from the maculae may converge. This may be the correlate of the finding that the position of the head may influence the plane of the nystagmus (Lorente de Nó; Koella).

Electrograms of the vestibular nuclei in rabbits (Eckel) showed Gernandt's reaction type I in three-fourths of the neurons, and bidirectional excitatory reactions (type II) in one-fourth of the neurons; only in a single

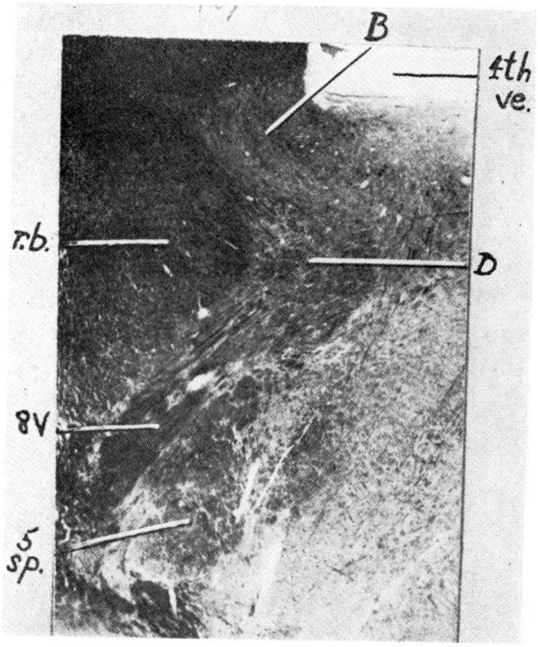

FIG. 6. Cross section through pons, with entrance of vestibular nerve. B = Bechterew's nucleus. D = Deiters' nucleus. r b = restiform body. 4th ve = fourth ventricle. 5 sp = spinal trigeminal root. 8 V = vestibular nerve. (From Spiegel and Sommer.)

instance, type III (bidirectional inhibition) was found.

Shimazu and Precht found neurons in the superior and medial vestibular nuclei primarily connected with receptors in the horizontal semicircular canal and activated by their excitation. They differentiated two types of such neurons: kinetic and tonic neurons; the former are characterized by lack of spontaneous discharge, high threshold for frequency increase, rapid time course of frequency changes, and steep gradient of acceleration-frequency relationship. The tonic neurons show opposite characteristics.

Dohlman points to phylogenetic differences in the ability of the vestibular nuclei to respond to changes in the resting frequency of the ampullar nerves. In all animals tested they can respond to an increase in the frequency of the potentials from the cristae. Lower animals, however, can not respond to a decrease, birds only to a certain extent, and man apparently equally well to an increase and decrease.

The extensor rigidity of the homolateral limbs in decerebrate cats is definitely decreased after unilateral lesions of the vestibular nuclei (Thiele). However, complete loss of muscle tonus in such decerebrate animals depends on additional lesions of the reticular formation (Bernis and Spiegel; Spiegel) indicating the importance of this latter area for the maintenance of the static innervation (Spiegel, 1927).

Regarding the quick phase of nystagmus, its central origin is indicated by the experience that both phases of nystagmus can be elicited by unilateral lesions of the vestibular nuclei in bilaterally labyrinthectomized dogs (Spiegel and Sato). Bárány's original concept that it is of cortical origin had to be abandoned, since both phases of nystagmus can still be elicited by labyrinthine stimulation after decerebration by a transverse section of the midbrain in front of the oculomotor nuclei (Magnus and de Kleijn). Bárány's second theory that the quick phase originates in the reticular formation of the rhombencephalon seemed to be supported by the experience that bilateral sectioning of the medial longitudinal fasciculus, the chief pathway connecting the vestibular and eye muscle nuclei, does not prevent the appearance of both components of labyrinthine nystagmus

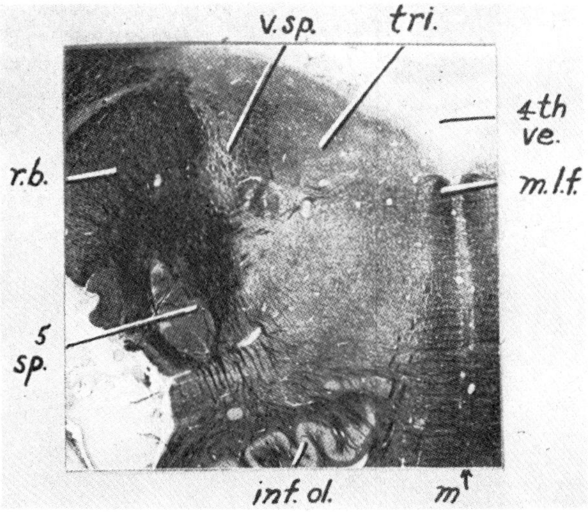

FIG. 7. Cross section of cranial part of medulla oblongata. inf ol = inferior olive. m = midline. m l f = medial longitudinal fasciculus, r b = restiform body. tri = triangular nucleus. v sp = spinal root of vestibular nerve. 4th ve = fourth ventricle. 5 sp = spinal trigeminal root. (From Spiegel and Sommer.)

(Lorente de Nó; Spiegel). However, further experiments by Spiegel demonstrated that rather extensive bilateral lesions of the reticular formation by a ventral approach did not abolish the fast component of nystagmus on labyrinthine stimulation, although the lesion reached quite close to the medial longitudinal fasciculus (Fig. 8). Spiegel inferred that there exists a double connection from the vestibular nuclei to the eye muscles: (1) by way of the medial longitudinal fasciculus and (2) by vestibulo-reticular pathways. This latter pathway, however, is dispensable in the genesis of the fast component of nystagmus. These conclusions were confirmed in further experiments by Spiegel and Price. They punctured the reticular formation through the floor of the fourth ventricle in the levels considered by Lorente de Nó as decisive (Figs. 9 and 10). If the animals were studied beyond the acute postoperative phase, rhythmic reactions with slow and quick components reappeared; de Nó's observation that after such operations labyrinthine stimulation elicited only tonic deviation of the eyeballs is apparently due to the fact that he limited his observations to the immediate postoperative period. Furthermore unilateral lesions of the reticular formation do not produce nystagmus, while this phenomenon can be easily produced by unilateral lesions of the vestibular nuclei. The origin of the quick phase was therefore ex-

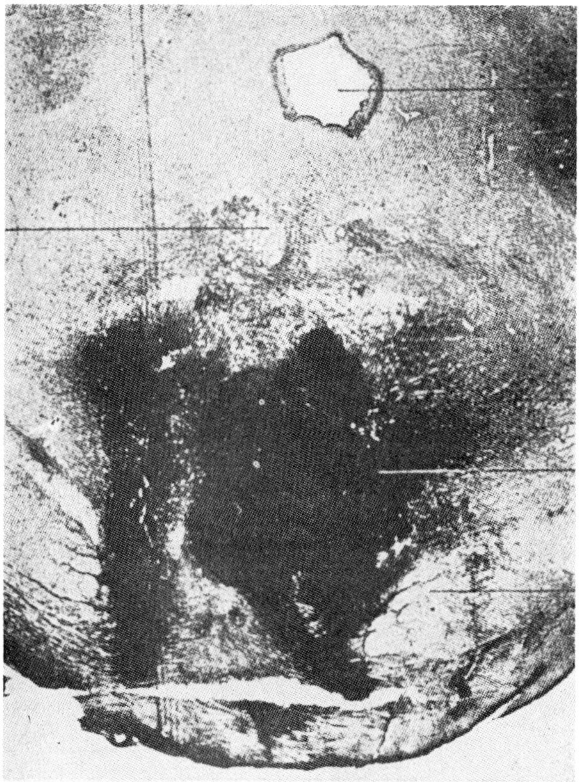

Fig. 8. Cat: Puncture of pons from ventrally produced large hemorrhages (L) in tegmentum in cranial parts of pons and caudal levels of midbrain. Hemorrhages reached close to medial (posterior) longitudinal fasciculus (F 1 p). Horizontal nystagmus in both directions, also vertical nystagmus, was still elicitable by rotation. Only definite anomaly was inverse direction of vertical nystagmus induced by rotation in some experiments (head in left side position: after 10 rotations to left, nystagmus ↑ instead of ↓). aq = aqueduct. py = pyramidal tract. (From Spiegel and Sommer.)

plained as due chiefly to rhythmic discharges of the vestibular nuclei (Spiegel), although a participation of the reticular formation in the genesis of the quick phase, with this region preserved, should not be denied, particularly in view of electrographic studies (Kirstein; Duensing and Schaefer). Authors still localizing the quick component exclusively in the reticular formation—e.g., Jung—simply disregard the above-mentioned experimental facts. Furthermore Eckel's microelectrode studies (interestingly from Jung's laboratory) revealed a rhythmic course of the frequency of the discharges recorded from these nuclei during their postrotatory activity. The duration of the single phases of this rhythm (steep rise, slow fall of the number of impulses) was somewhat over 1 sec., showing a rate similar to that of postrotatory nystagmus.

A nystagmogenic area at the mesodiencephalic level was found by Lachmann, Bergmann, and Monnier. On stimulation at 20-50

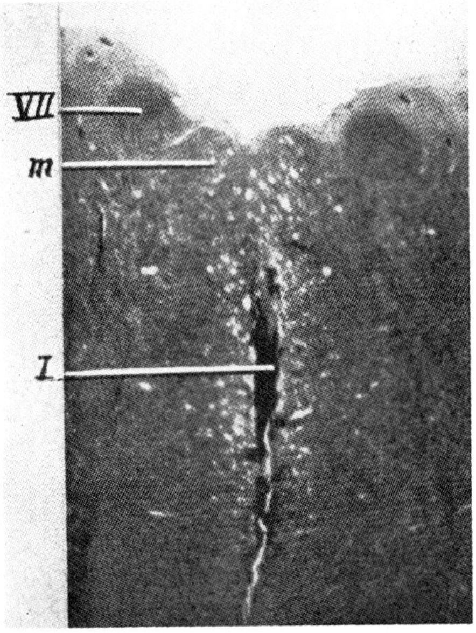

FIG. 9. Cat: Median incision (I) into pons. On first day after operation, rotation produced only tonic deviation of eyeballs; two days after operation, it produced vertical as well as horizontal nystagmus in either direction. m = medial longitudinal fasciculus. VII = knee of root of facial nerve. (After Spiegel and Price: Arch. Otolaryng. 30:586, 1939.)

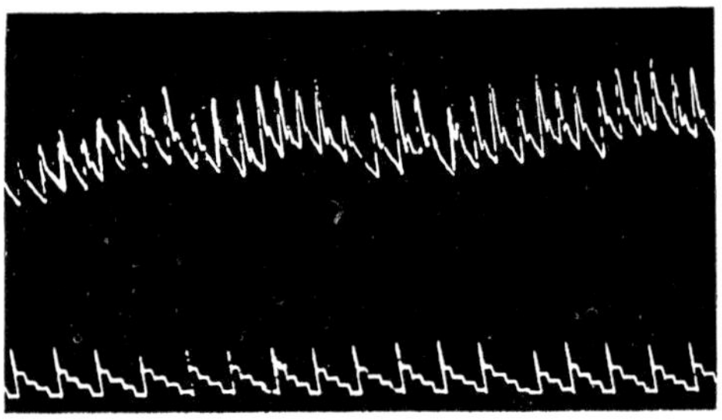

FIG. 10. Cat: Paramedian puncture of floor of fourth ventricle in front of right sixth nucleus, passing through right medial longitudinal fasciculus and reticular formation. Nystagmus elicited by galvanic stimulation one day following operation (anode in right, cathode in left external auditory canal). Upward lines represent ocular movements to left. Time in seconds. (After Spiegel and Price: Arch. Otolaryng. 30:581, 1939.)

cps they elicited in rabbits a nystagmus with its fast component usually directed to the opposite side. The most sensitive nystagmogenic area was located near the rostral end of the superior colliculus. Apparently this nystagmogenic area lies rostrally to the elementary three neuron reflex arc, connecting the labyrinth with the eye muscle nuclei. The authors assume that this stimulation starts the nystagmus by inhibiting the tonic innervation of the ipsilateral rectus internus and of the contralateral rectus externus. The reaction continues after cessation of the stimulation.

Nystagmus appearing after injection of stimulating substances—e.g., carbachol into the caudate nucleus, the lateral or third ventricle (Szekely and Spiegel)—seems to be due to excitation of diencephalic areas or oral parts of the mesencephalon related to the above-mentioned nystagmogenic area.

REFERENCES

1. Adrian, E. D.: Discharges from the vestibular receptors in the cat. J. Physiol. (London) 101:389-407, 1943
2. Akert, K., and Gernandt, B. E.: Neurophysiological study of vestibular and limbic influences upon vagal outflow. EEG. Clin. Neurophysiol. 14:904-914, 1962.
3. Alexander, G.: Makroskopische Anatomie der nervösen Anteile des Gehörorgans. Handb.

Neurol. Ohres 1:1, Vienna, Urban & Schwarzenberg, 1923.

4. Arslan, M.: Standardisation et simplification des techniques de l'examen de l'appareil vestibulaire. Rev. Laryng. (Bordeaux) Suppl. 72:290-310, 1951.
5. Arslan, M.: Physiologie de l'appareil vestibulaire. Encyclopédie Medicochir. Otorhinolaryngologie 200:37, 1963.
6. Ashcroft, D. W., and Hallpike, C. S.: On the function of the saccule. J. Laryngol. 44: 450-460, 1934.
7. Bárány, R.: Physiologie und Pathologie des Bogengangapparates, Wien, Deuticke, 1907.
8. Bárány, R.: Untersuchungen ueber den vom Vestibularapparat des Ohres reflektorisch ausgelösten rhythmischen Nystagmus und seine Begleiterscheinungen. Mschr. Ohrenheilk. 40:229, 1906.
9. Bárány, R.: Die nervösen Störungen des Cochlear u. Vestibularapparates in Handb.d. Neurologie (M. Lewandowsky, Ed.) I.1.p. 919, Berlin, Springer, 1910.
10. Bard, P., Woolsey, C. N., Snider, R. S. Mountcastle, V. B., and Bromiley, R. B.: Delimitation of central nervous mechanisms involved in motion sickness. Fed. Proc. 6:72, 1947.
11. Behr, K., Preber, L., and Silfverskiöld, B. P.: Recording of the skin resistance in thermal and rotatory stimulation of the labyrinth. Acta Psychiat. Scand. 30: 741-748, 1955.
12. Bernis, W. J., and Spiegel, E. A.: Die Zentren der statischen Innervation und ihre Beeinflussung durch Klein-und Grosshirn. Arb. Neurol. Inst. Univ. Wien 27:197-224, 1925.
13. Bleeker, E. D., and De Vries, H. L.: The microphonic activity of the labyrinth of the pigeon. Acta Otolaryng. 37:289, 1949.
14. Boenninghaus, H. T.: Tonic influence of peripheral vestibular organ on vestibular centers. Arch. Ohr. Nas. Kehlkopfheilk. 161: 405, 1952.
15. Breuer, J.: Ueber die Funktion der Bogengänge des Ohrlabyrinthes. Med. Jahrbuch (Wien), 4:72, 1874.
16. Breuer, J.: Neue Versuche an den Ohrbogengängen. Pflügers Arch. Ges. Physiol. 44: 135-152, 1889.
17. Brodal, A., Pompeiano, O., and Walberg, F.: The Vestibular Nuclei and Their Connections. Edinburgh-London, Oliver & Boyd, 1962.
18. Burlet, H. M. de: Die Stellung der Maculae acusticae. Morphol. Jahrb. 64: 377, 1930.
19. Buys, E., and Rijilant, P.: Le seuil d'excitation (accélération angulaire) des canaux semicirculaires. Arch. Int. Physiol. 49:101-112, 1939.
20. Byford, G. H., Hallpike, C. S., and Hood, J. D.: Design, construction and performance of new type of revolving chair. Acta. otolaryng. (Stockholm) 42:511, 1952.
21. Byrne, J.: Physiology of the Semicircular Canals and Their Relation to Seasickness. New York, Dougherty, 1912.
22. Cawthorne, T. E., Fitzgerald, G., and Hallpike, C. S.: Studies in human vestibular function. II. Observations on the directional preponderance of caloric nystagmus. (Nystagmusbereitschaft) resulting from unilateral labyrinthectomy. Brain 65:138-160, 1942.
23. Cohen, B., and Suzuki, J.: Eye movements induced by ampullary nerve stimulation. Amer. J. Physiol. 204:347-351, 1963.
24. Cohen, B., Suzuki, J., and Bender, M. B.: Eye movements from semicircular canal nerve stimulation in the cat. Ann. Otol. 73:153-169, 1964.
25. Crum Brown, A.: On the sense of rotation and the anatomy and physiology of the semicircular canals of the internal ear. J. Anat. Physiol. 8:327, 1874.
26. Dalla Torre, G., and Cantele, P. G.: Sui riflessi vestibolo-vegetativi. I. Riflessi Vestibolo-sfigmico e vestibolo-cardiaco. Osservazioni cliniche sperimentali. Riv. Otoneurooftal. 14:1-19, 1937.
27. de Kleijn, A., and Versteegh, C.: Some remarks upon the present position of the physiology of the labyrinth. J. Laryng. 42:649-655, 1927.
28. DeVries, H.: Physical aspects of the sense organs. *In:* Progress in Biophysics and Biophysical Chemistry, Vol. 6. J. A. V. Butler, Ed. New York, Pergamon Press, 1956, pp. 207-248.
29. Dittrich, F. L., and Exterman, R. C.: Biophysics of the Ear. Springfield, Ill., Charles C Thomas, 1963.
30. Dodge, R.: Habituation to rotation. J. Exp. Psychol. 6:1, 1923.
31. Dohlman, G. F.: Histochemical studies of vestibular mechanisms. *In* Neural Mechanisms of the Auditory and Vestibular System. (G. I. Rasmussen and W. F. Windle, Eds.), pp. 258-275. Springfield, Ill., Thomas, 1960.
32. Duensing, F., and Schaefer, K. P.: Die Neuronenaktivität in der Formatio reticularis des Rhombencephalon beim vestibulären Nystagmus. Arch. Psychiat. Z. Ges Neurol. 196: 265-290, 1957.

33. Duensing, F., and Schaefer, K. P.: Die Aktivität einzelner Neurone im Bereich der Vestibulariskerne bei Horizontalbeschleunigungen unter besonderer Berücksichtigung des vestibulären Nystagmus. Arch. Psychiat. Nervenkr. 198:225-252, 1958.
34. Duensing, F., and Schaefer, K. P.: Über die Konvergenz verschiedener labyrinthärer Afferenzen auf einzelne Neurone des Vestibulariskerngebietes. Arch. Psychiat. Nervenkr. 199:345-371, 1959.
35. Eckel, W.: Elektrophysiologische Untersuchungen im Vestibulariskerngebiet bei Drehreizen. Arch. Ohr. Nas. Kehlkopfheilk. 164: 487-513, 1954.
36. Engström, H.: On the double innervation of the sensory epithelia of the inner ear. Acta Otolaryng. (Stockholm) 49:109-118, 1958.
37. Engström, H.: The innervation of the vestibular sensory cells. Acta Otolaryng. (Stockholm) Suppl. 163:30, 1961.
38. Ewald, J. R.: Physiologische Untersuchungen über das Endorgan des N. Oktavus. Wiesbaden, Bergmann, 1892.
39. Fischer, M. H.: Die Regulationsfunktionen des menschlichen Labyrinthes und die Zusammenhänge mit verwandten Funktionen. Ergebn. Physiol. 27:209-379, 1928.
40. Fischer, M. H.: Die Seekrankheit: in Handb. d. norm u. pathol. Physiologie 15:495-516, Berlin, Springer, 1930.
41. Flourens: Expériences sur les Canaux Sémicirculaires de l'oreille. Paris, 1828.
42. von Frisch, K., and Stretter, H.: Sitz d. Gehörsinnes bei d. Elritze. Z. vergl. Physiol. 17:686, 1932.
43. Gacek, R. C.: Efferent component of the vestibular nerve. *In* Neural Mechanisms of the Auditory and Vestibular Systems. G. I. Rasmussen and W. F. Windle, Eds. Springfield, Ill., Charles C Thomas, 1960, pp. 276-284.
44. Geller, W.: Seekrankheit und ihre Behandlung. Klin. Wschr. 19:1310, 1940.
45. Gernandt, B. E.: Response of mammalian vestibular neurons to horizontal rotation and caloric stimulation. J. Neurophysiol. 12: 173-184, 1949.
46. Omitted.
47. Gernandt, B. E.: Vestibular Mechanisms. Handbook of Physiology, Sect. I. Neurophysiology 1:549-564, a publication of the Amer. Physiol. Soc., Washington, D.C., 1959.
48. Gernandt, B. E.: Somatic and autonomic motor outflow to vestibular stimulation. *In:* Neurological Aspects of Auditory and Vestibular Disorders. W. S. Fields and B. R. Alford, Eds. Springfield, Illinois, Charles C Thomas, 1964, pp. 194-211.
49. Gernandt, B. E., and Gilman, S.: Descending vestibular activity and its modulation by proprioceptive, cerebellar and reticular influences. Exp. Neurol. 1:274-304, 1959.
50. Girard, L.: L'attitude normale de la tête déterminée par le labyrinthe de l'oreille. Otorhinolarng. Internat. 14:517, 1930.
51. Graybiel, A.: Orientation in space with particular reference to vestibular functions. *In:* Environmental Effects on Consciousness. E. Schaefer, Ed. New York, MacMillan Co., 1962, p. 64.
52. Graybiel, A.; Vestibular sickness and some of its implications for space flight. *In:* Neurological Aspects of Auditory and Vestibular Disorders. W. S. Fields and B. R. Alford, Eds. Springfield, Ill., Charles C Thomas, 1964, pp. 248-270.
53. Groen, J. J.: Problems of the semicircular canal from a mechanico-physiological point of view. Acta Otolaryng. (Stockholm) Suppl. 163:59-66, 1960.
54. Groen, J. J.: On the repeal of Ewald's second law. Acta Otolaryng. Suppl. 159:42-46, 1960.
55. Groen, J. J., and Jongkees, L. B. W.: The turning test with small regulable stimuli. The cupulogram obtained by subjective angle estimation. J. Larnygol. Otol. 62:236, 1948.
56. Groen, J. J., and Jongkees, L. B. W.: The threshold of angular acceleration perception. J. Physiol. 107:1, 1948.
57. Groen, J. J., Löwenstein, O., and Vendrick, A. J. M.: Mechanical analysis of the responses from the end organs of horizontal semicircular canal in the isolated Elasmobranch labyrinth. J. Physiol. (London) 117:329-346, 1952.
58. Gröbbels, F.: Die tierexperimentellen Grundlagen der Labyrinthphysiologie. Klin. Wschr. 7:1784, 1928.
59. Hallpike, C. S., and Hood, J. D.: Speed of slow component of ocular nystagmus. Proc. Roy. Soc. [Biol.] 141:216, 1953.
60. Hallpike, C. S., and Hood, J. D.: Fatigue and adaptation of the cupular mechanism of the human horizontal semicircular canal: an experimental investigation. Proc. Roy Soc. [Biol.] 141:542-561, 1953.
61. Hardy, M.: Observations on innervation of macula sacculi in man. Anat. Rec. 59:403, 1934.
62. Hartog, H.: Over de functie van de horizontale

booggang. Thesis. Utrecht, Schotanus and Jens, 1963, pp. 78.

63. Hasegawa, T.: Labyrinthreflexe nach Abschleuderung der Otolithenmembranen. Arch. Ges. Physiol. 229:205, 1931.

64. Hemingway, A.: Physiological changes during motion sickness. Fed. Proc. 4:33, 1945.

65. Henriksson, N. G.: Correlation between speed of eye in slow phase of nystagmus and vestibular stimulus. Acta Otolaryng. 45:120, 1955.

66. Hilding, A. C.: On the threshold of minimal perceptible angular acceleration. Acta Otorhinolaryngol. Belg. 62:462, 1953.

67. Hulk, J., and Jongkees, L. B. W.: Turning test with small regulable stimuli. II. The normal cupulogram. J. Laryng. Otol. 62:70, 1948.

68. Huizinga, E.: Weitere Untersuchungen über Tullio's Schallreflexe. Pflügers Arch. Ges. Physiol. 237:494, 1936.

69. Ivy, A. C.: Physiology of vestibular nystagmus. Arch. Otolaryng. 9:123, 1929.

70. James, W.: Sense of dizziness in deaf mutes. Amer. J. Otol. 4:239-254, 1882.

71. Jensen, C. E., Koefoed, J., and Vilstrup, T.: Flow potentials in hyaluronate solutions. Nature. (Lond.) 174:1101-1102, 1954.

72. Jongkees, L. B. W., and Groen, J. J.: Considerations regarding the secondary after-sensations caused by a stimulation of the semicircular canal system. J. Laryng. 61:241-244, 1946.

73. Jongkees, L. B. W.: On the function of the saccule. Acta Otolaryng. (Stockholm) 38: 18, 1950.

74. Jung, R.: Neurophysiologische Untersuchungsmethoden. *In* Handb. d. inner. Mediz. Vol. I. G. v. Bergmann et al., Eds. Berlin, Springer, 1953, p. 1343.

75. Karbowski, K., Moret, P. R., and Martin, F.: Étude de quelques effets de la stimulation labyrinthique sur la fonction cardio-pulmonaire et l'activité électrique cérébrale. Conf. Neurol. 23:227-244, 1963.

76. Kirstein, R.: Action currents in reticular substance in rabbits after caloric stimulation. Arch. Ohr. Nas. Kehlkopfheilk. 162:229, 1953.

76a. Kleijn, A. de, and Versteegh, C.: Present position of the physiology of the labyrinth. J. Laryngol. 42:649-655, 1927.

77. Koella, W.: Gleichgewichtsorgan u. Augenmuskelsystem im Lichte der Koordinationslehre. Vjschr. Nat. Ges. Zürich 95:1950, Suppl. I.

78. Kolmer, W.: Mikroskopische Anatomie des nervösen Apparates des Ohres. Handb. d. Neurol. d. Ohres. Alexander, G., and Marburg, O., Eds. Vienna, Urban & Schwarzenberg 1:101, 1923.

79. Kramer, L.: Ueber die Seekrankheit. Prager Mediz. Wochenschr. 17:465-477, 1892.

80. Kreidl, A.: Beiträge zur Physiologie des Ohrlabyrinthes. Sitzungsb. Akad. Wissensch. Wien. Math-Naturw. Cl. 101:469, 1893; 102: 149, 1893.

81. Kreidl, A.: quoted by M. H. Fischer. Die Seekrankheit. pp. 500 and 512. (see complete reference under *Fischer*).

82. Lachmann, J., Bergmann, F., and Monnier, M.: Central nystagmus elicited by stimulation of the meso-diencephalon in the rabbit. Amer. J. Physiol. 193:328-334, 1958.

83. Lebensohn, J. E.: Car sickness. Arch. Opthal. (Chicago) 4:342, 1930.

84. Ledoux, A.: Activité électrique des nerfs des canaux semicirculaires du saccule et de l'utricle chez la grenouille. Acta otorhinolaryng. Belg. 3:335-349, 1949.

85. Ledoux, A.: New technique for studying electric activity of labyrinth nerves. Rev. Larng. 72:265, (Suppl.) 1951.

86. Ledoux, A.: Les canaux semicirculaires. Thèse d'Agrégation de l'Enseignement Supérieur. Éditions Acta Medica Belgica, 1958.

87. Lindsay, J. R., Oppenheimer, M. J., Wycis, H. T. and Spiegel, E. A.: Receptor apparatus of the vestibulo-vasomotor reaction. Arch. Otol. 42:257, 1945.

88. Lorente de Nó, R.: Die Labyrinthreflexe auf die Augenmuskeln nach einseitiger Labyrinthexstirpation nebst einer kurzen Angabe über den Nervenmechanismus der vestibulären Augenbewegungen. Wien, Urban and Schwarzenberg, 1928.

89. Lorente de Nó, R.: Die Augenmuskelreflexe beim Kaninchen und ihre Grundlagen. Ergebn. Physiol. 32:73, 1931.

90. Lorente de Nó, R.: Anatomy of the eighth nerve. The central projection of the nerve endings of the internal ear. Laryngoscope. 43:1-38, 1933.

91. Lorente de Nó, R.: Vestibulo-ocular reflex arc. Arch. Neurol. Psychiat. 30:245-291, 1933.

92. Löwenstein, O.: Comparative physiology of otolith organs. Brit. M. Bull. 12:110-113, 1956.

93. Löwenstein, O.: Peripheral mechanisms of equilibrium. Brit. M. Bull. 12:114-118, 1956.

94. Löwenstein, O., and Sand, A.: The activity of

the horizontal semicircular canals of the dog fish. J. Exp. Biol. 13:416-428, 1936.

95. Löwenstein, O., and Sand, A.: The mechanism of the semicircular canal. A study of the responses of single-fibre preparations to angular accelerations and rotation at constant speed. Proc. Roy. Soc. [Biol.] 129: 256-275, 1940.

96. Mach, E.: Grundlinie der Lehre von den Bewegungsempfindungen. Leipzig, 1875.

97. Magnus, R.: Körperstellung. Berlin, Springer, 1924.

98. Magnus, R., and de Kleijn, A. Experimentelle Physiologie des Vestibularapparates bei Säugetieren mit Ausschluss des Menschen. *In* Handbuch der Neurologie des Ohres Alexander and Marburg, Eds. I. Wien, Urban and Schwarzenberg, 1923, pp. 465-552.

99. Maitland, T. G.: General observations of seasickness and the labyrinthine theory. Brit. Med. J. 1:171, 1931.

100. Maxwell, S. S.: Labyrinth and Equilibrium. Philadelphia, Lippincott, 1923.

101. McNally, W. J.: The otoliths and the part they play in man. Laryngoscope 54:304-323, 1944.

102. McNally, W. J., and Tait, J.: Ablation experiments on the labyrinth of the frog. Amer. J. Physiol. 75:155-179, 1925.

103. McNally, M. J., and Tait, J.: The function of the utricular macula of the frog. Acta Otolaryng. (Stockholm) 20:73-76, 1934.

104. Montandon, A.: Le labyrinthe et le système nerveux végétatif. Basel, S. Karger, 1946.

105. Montandon, A., Monnier, M., and Russbach, A.: A technique of vestibular rotatory stimulation and of electrical recording of nystagmus in man. Ann. Otol. 64:701-717, 1955.

106. Mower, O. H.: The electrical response of the vestibular nerve during adequate stimulation. Science 81:180-181, 1935.

107. Oort, H.: Über die Verästelung des Nervus octavus bei Säugetieren. Anat. Anz. 51: 11, 272, 1918.

108. Ornstein and Burger: cited by Magnus, R.: Körperstellung. Berlin, Springer, 1924.

109. Oppenheimer, M. J., and Spiegel, E. A. Effects of various drugs upon vestibulovasomotor reactions. Arch. Int. Pharmacodyn. 73: 344, 1947.

110. Perez: Studien über vergleichende Anatomie im Verhältnis zur Otologie. Monatschr. Ohr. 56:243, 1922.

111. Petroff, A. E.: An experimental investigation of the origin of efferent fiber projections to the vestibular neuroepithelium. Anat. Record 121:352-353, 1955.

112. Poljak, S.: Über die doppelte Innervation der Macula sacculi und über das cochleo-vestibuläre Bündel bei den Säugetieren. Z. Anat. Entwicklungsgesch 84:145-152, 1927.

113. Pollock, L. J., and Davis, L.: The influence of the cerebellum upon the reflex activities of the decerebrate animal. Brain 50:277-312, 1927.

114. Pompeiano, O., and Cotti, E.: Analisi microelectrodica delle proiezioni cerebello-deitersiane. Arch. Sci. Biol. 43:57-101, 1959.

115. Rasmussen, G. L., and Gacek, R. R.: Concerning the question of an efferent fiber component of the vestibular nerve of the cat. Anat. Rec. 130:361-362, 1958.

116. Rossberg, G.: Vestibularis und Kreislauf: Z. Laryng. Rhinol. Otol. 28:511-525, 1949.

117. Sala, O.: The efferent vestibular system. Acta Otolaryng. Suppl. 197:5-34, 1965.

118. Shimazu, H., and Precht, W.: Afferent excitation of vestibular neuron. J. Neurophysiol. 28:1014-1028, 1965.

119. Shimazu, H., and Precht, W.: Tonic and Kinetic Responses of Cats Vestibular Neurons to Horizontal Angular Acceleration. J. Neurophys. 28:991-1013, 1965.

120. Sjöberg, A.: Experimentelle Studien über den Auslösungsmechanismus der Seekrankheit. Acta Otolaryng. (Stockholm) Suppl. 14: 1931.

121. Sokalchuk, A.: Blood pressure in seasickness. Fed. Proc. 6:207, 1946.

122. Spector, M., Szekely, E., and Spiegel, E. A.: Electrolabyrinthogram. A.M.A. Arch. Otolaryng. 69:563-569, 1959.

123. Spiegel, E. A.: Der Tonus der Skelettmuskulatur. Monogr. aus dem Gesamtgeb. der Neurol. u. Psych. Heft 51, Berlin, Springer, 1927.

124. Spiegel, E. A.: Experimentalstudien am Nervensystem. XV. Der Mechanismus des labyrinthären Nystagmus. Z. Hals-Nas-Ohrenheilk. 25:200-217, 1929.

125. Spiegel, E. A.: Effect of labyrinthine reflexes on vegetative nervous system. Arch. Otolaryng. 44:61-72, 1946.

126. Spiegel, E. A.: Respiratory reactions upon vertical movements. Amer. J. Physiol. 117: 349-354, 1936.

127. Spiegel, E. A.: Rhythmic stimulation of the labyrinth. Arch. Otolaryng. 33:572-578, 1941.

128. Spiegel, E. A.: Depressor effect of cold upon

the static receptors of the labyrinth. Fed. Proc. 3 (1): 1944 and Amer. J. Physiol. 141:404, 1944.

129. Spiegel, E. A., and Aronson, L.: Continuous stimulation of the labyrinth with sustained nystagmus. Arch. Otolaryng. 17:311, 1933.

130. Spiegel, E. A., and Démétriades, D.: Einfluss d. Vestibularapparates auf d. Gefässystem. Beiträge z. Stud. d. vegetativ. Nervensystems. III. Pflügers Arch. Ges. Physiol. 196: 185-199, 1922.

131. Spiegel, E. A., and Démétriades, Th.D.: Beiträge zum Studium des vegetativen Nervensystems. VII. Der zentrale Mechanismus der vestibulären Blutdrucksenkung und ihre Bedeutung für die Entstehung des Labyrinthschwindels. Pflügers Arch. Ges. Physiol. 205:328-337, 1924.

132. Spiegel, E. A., Henny, G. C., and Wycis, H. T.: Changes of cerebral circulation induced by labyrinthine stimulation. Amer. J. Physiol. 142:589-593, 1944.

133. Spiegel, E. A.: Oppenheimer, M. J., Henny, G. C., and Wycis, H. T.: Experimental production of motion sickness. War Med. 6:283-290, 1944.

134. Spiegel, E. A., Oppenheimer, M. J., and Wycis, H. T.: Receptor mechanisms of vestibulo-vasomotor reactions induced by rotations. Fed. Proc. 3:44, 1944.

135. Spiegel, E. A., and Price, J. B.: Origin of the quick component of labyrinthine nystagmus. Arch. Otolaryng. (Chicago) 30:576-588, 1939.

136. Spiegel, E. A., and Sato, G.: Experimentalstudien am Nervensystem, V. Über den Erregungszustand der medullären Zentren nach doppelseitiger Labyrinthausschaltung. Pflügers Arch. Ges. Physiol. 215:106-119, 1926.

137. Spiegel, E. A., and Sokalchuck, A.: Influence of medication upon blood pressure in seasickness. Fed. Proc. 6:209, 1946.

138. Spiegel, E. A., and Sommer, I.: Neurology of the Eye, Ear, Nose and Throat. New York, Grune & Stratton, 1944.

139. Spiegel, E. A., Szekely, E. G., and Gildenberg, P. L.: Vestibular responses in midbrain, thalamus and basal ganglia. Arch. Neurol. 12:258-269, 1965.

140. Stein, C., and Bénesi, O.: Tierexperimentelle und klinische Untersuchungen über die Beziehungen des Blutdrucks zum statisschen Apparate. Monatschr. Ohrenhk. 58: 581-593, 1924.

141. Steinhausen, W.: Nachweis d. Bewegung der Cupula in der intakten Bogengangsampulle des Labyrinths bei der natürlichen rotatorischen u. calorischen Reizung. Pflügers Arch. Ges. Physiol. 228:322-328, 1931.

142. Steinhausen, W.: Ueber die Beobachtung der Cupula in den Bogengangsampullen des Labyrinths des lebenden Hechts. Pflügers Arch. Ges. Physiol. 232: 500-512, 1933.

143. Streiff, E. B., Montandon, A., and Monnier, M.: Variations simultanées des pressions artérielle retinienne et générale en fonction des excitations vestibulaires caloriques. Conf. Neurol. 4:347-355, 1942.

144. Suzuki, Jun-Ichi, Cohen, B., and Bender, M. B.: Compensatory eye movements induced by vertical semicircular canal stimulation. Exp. Neurol. 9:137-160, 1964.

145. Szekely, E. G., and Spiegel, E. A.: Vertical nystagmus induced by injection of stimulating substances into the striatum, third or lateral ventricle. Neurology 13:306-314, 1963.

146. Szentágothai, J.: The elementary vestibulo-ocular reflex arc. J. Neurophysiol. 13:395-407, 1950.

147. Szentágothai, J.: Die Rolle der einzelnen Labyrinthrezeptoren bei der Orientation von Augen und Kopf in Raume. Budapest, Akadémiai Kiado, 1952.

148. Talpis, L., and Wolfkowitch, M.: Zur Frage des vom Labyrinth ausgehenden Reflexes auf die Blutgefässe. Monatschr. Ohrenhk. 62: 1278-1289, 1928.

149. Thiele, F. H.: On the efferent relationship of the optic thalamus and Deiters' nucleus to the spinal cord with special reference to the cerebellar influx of Dr. Hughlings Jackson and the genesis of the decerebrate rigidity of Ord and Sherrington. J. Physiol. (Lond.) 32:358-384, 1950.

150. Tönnies, J. F.: Beschreibung eines Drehstuhls mit unterschwelliger Anlaufsbeschleunigung. J. Psychol. Neurol. (Leipzig) 44: 468, 1932.

151. Trincker, D.: Bestandspotentiale im Bogengangsystem des Meerschweinchens und ihre Änderungen bei experimentellen Cupulaablenkungen. Pflügers Arch. Ges. Physiol. 264:351, 1957.

152. Trincker, D.: L'éléctrophysiologie de l'appareil vestibulaire et le problème de la transformation du stimulus méchanique en l'excitation nerveuse. Conf. Neurol. 20: 187, 1960.

153. Trincker, D.: Neuere Aspekte des Mechanismus der Haarzellerregung. Acta Otol. Suppl. 163:67, 1961.

154. Tullio, P.: Das Ohr. u. die Enstehung der Sprache u. Schrift. Berlin-Wien, Urban and Schwarzenberg, 1929.

155. Tyler, D. B., and Bard, P.: Motion Sickness. Physiol. Rev. 29:311-369, 1949.

156. Van Egmond, A. A. J., Groen, J. J., and Jongkees, L. B. W.: Mechanics of the semicircular canal. J. Physiol. 110:1, 1949.

157. Van Egmond, A. A. J., and Groen, J. J.: Cupulometrie. Practica Otol. 17:206-223, 1955.

158. Van Egmond, A. A. J., Groen, J. J., and Jongkees, L. B. W.: The Function of the Vestibular Organ. Basel, S. Karger, 1952.

159. Van Egmond, A. A. J.: Standardization and simplification of examination of vestibular apparatus. Acta Otolaryng. 43:283, 1953.

160. Van Eyck, M.: Contribution a l'étude de l'éléctrophysiologie de l'appareil vestibulaire. Éditions Acta Medica Belgica, 1951.

161. Vilstrup, T., and Jensen, C. E.: Three reports on chemical composition of the fluids of the labyrinth. I. Determination of hyaluronic acid in the endolymph. Ann. Otol. Rhinol. Laryng. 63:151-156, 1954.

162. Vilstrup, G., and Vilstrup, T.: Does the utricular otolithic membrane move on postural changes of the head? Ann. Otol. Rhin. Laryng. 61:189, 1952.

163. Wersäll, J.: Studies on the structure and innervation of the sensory epithelium of the cristae ampullares in the guinea pig. A light and electron microscopic investigation. Acta Otolaryng. (Stockholm) Suppl. 126:1-85, 1956.

164. Wersäll, J.: Electronmicrographic Studies of Vestibular Hair Cell Innervation. In: Neural Mechanisms of the Auditory and Vestibular Systems. G. L. Rassmussen and W. F. Windle, Eds. Springfield, Ill., Charles C Thomas, 1960, pp. 247-257.

165. Weston, J. K.: Observation on the distribution of ganglion cells and fibers related to the saccule. Acta Morph. Neerl. Scand. 1:136, 1937.

166. Wotzilka, G.: Untersuchungen über den Einfluss der Labyrinthreizung auf den Blutdruck. Z. Hals-, Nasen Ohr. 10:127-132, 1924.

167. Wotzilka, G.: Einfluss der Labyrinthreizung auf den Blutdruck. Z. Hals-, Nasen Ohr. 12:649-654, 1925.

CHAPTER 2

Anatomy and Physiology of the Cortical Projections of the Labyrinth

E. A. SPIEGEL

While the cortical projection of the cochlear part of the inner ear has been extensively investigated anatomically as well as physiologically since the turn of the century, there is still little known regarding the corticopetal course of the impulses from the nonauditory part of the inner ear, the so-called labyrinth.

ANATOMICAL STUDIES

In Obersteiner's book (1912) one finds the statement that fibers from the triangular nucleus enter the *reticular formation* of the medulla oblongata, and Held described in 1923 a vestibulo-reticulothalamic system to the ventrolateral area of the thalamus. Furthermore, Godlowski described (1) laterodorsal vestibular systems (vestibulo-mesencephalic tract) sending fibers to the nuclei of the fourth and the third cranial nerve, the nuclei of the posterior commissure, the median center and internal nuclei of the thalamus; and (2) a ventral-ascending vestibular tract, reaching ventral parts of the reticular substance of the midbrain (nucleus reticularis ventralis tegmenti). Reticulothalamic fibers have recently been traced by Nauta and Kuypers. It may, therefore, be assumed, at least with some degree of assurance, that impulses from the inner ear reach the so-called *nonspecific or diffuse thalamic projection system.* Furthermore, Muskens and, more recently, Hassler have pointed out that fibers ascending in the medial longitudinal fasciculus end around cells of the nucleus interstitialis of Cajal and the nucleus Darkschewitsch. In these nuclei, tertiary neurons could originate which, according to Muskens, are supposed to end in the *pallidum.*

Efferent pallidofugal fibers end, as is known from the studies of Ranson and others, in cells of the nucleus ventralis lateralis and ventralis anterior thalami; from the first projections to the motor and premotor areas have been traced; the latter is part of the diffuse thalamic projection system.

In dogs in which the author produced circumscribed lesions of the vestibular nuclei, Whitaker and Alexander described Marchi degeneration in the medial longitudinal fasciculus (MLF), not only to the oculomotor nuclei but also to the *nucleus of the posterior commissure and the nucleus interstitialis* of Cajal, to the *nucleus ruber,* and to the *nuclei of the medial thalamus* (nucl. medialis C, nucl. proprius of Meynert's tract, nucl. filiformis, and nucl. paraependymalis). From the ruber a projection to the nucleus ventralis lateralis thalami is well known and, as mentioned, from here fibers ascend to the motor and premotor area. From the medial nuclei the frontal association areas may receive impulses.

Winkler, and later Gerebetzoff, assumed that vestibular impulses enter the *lateral lemniscus.* Ferraro et al. observed degeneration in fibers entering the lateral fillet after injury to the medial vestibular nucleus; they commented, however, that these degenerations might be due to injury of acoustic fibers. While some authors observed changes in the electrical activity of the inferior colliculus on

Aided by Grant NB-04418, from the National Institute of Neurological Diseases and Blindness, National Institutes of Health, USPHS, Bethesda, Md.

vestibular stimulation (Gerebetzoff with macroelectrodes, Gernandt with microelectrodes also in the medial geniculate body), Mickle and Ades had negative results.

Finally, Hassler's hypothesis should be mentioned that the fasciculus tegmenti dorsolateralis on the dorsolateral border of the pontine reticular formation receives impulses from the vestibular nuclei (homolateral nucleus Deiters and Bechterew, contralateral nucleus tractus spinalis vestibularis) and is continued in *Forel's tegmental fasciculi.* These fasciculi lie lateral to the MLF; at the level of the superior colliculi they ascend at the border of the central grey matter as far as the level of the posterior commissure and are supposed to end in the so-called nucleus ventro-intermedius externus of the thalamus. Other authors, however, trace the origin of Forel's fasciculi into the principal trigeminal nucleus (Carpenter) or into cell groups of the reticular formation (Lewandowsky, Russell).

In our experience not only elimination of the *cerebellum* combined with transection of the medial longitudinal fasciculi (Price and Spiegel), but also a lesion interrupting these fasciculi as well as Forel's tegmental fasciculi and the decussation of the superior cerebellar peduncles (Spiegel, Szekely, and Gildenberg) did not prevent the conduction of vestibular impulses to the cerebral cortex.

This brief sketch may suffice to show the scarcity of our knowledge regarding anatomical connections of the labyrinth to the cerebral cortex, and one has to agree with the statement of Brodal, Pompeiano, and Walberg that the existence of vestibulo-thalamic pathways has so far scarcely been proved.

PHYSIOLOGICAL STUDIES

In view of the lack of a well-defined anatomical system that would serve the conduction of corticopetal labyrinthine impulses, in contrast to the well-established cochlear projection to the cortex, a physiological and a clinical approach have been attempted by the author. It is known that *local strychninization* of a sensory projection area hypersensitizes this area to the afferent impulses originating in the respective peripheral receptors, as shown by Amantea in the somatic sensory cortex and by Clemente in the optic, acoustic, and olfactory centers. Following such a local strychninization of a sensory cortical area, the impulses reaching this area on stimulation of the respective receptors may spread to the motor cortex and elicit epileptiform convulsions. This effect of local cortical strychninization was used by the author in 1932 in order to study the question of a cortical projection of the labyrinth. In dogs and cats, various cortical areas outside the motor zone were exposed (under morphine-ether anaesthesia in dogs, under ether anaesthesia in cats), and after the effect of the anaesthetic had subsided, small pieces of filter paper moistened with a 1 per cent—2 per cent solution of strychnine nitrate solution were applied. The solution was stained with Toluidin blue so that the place of hypersensitization could be localized, and an undesirable spread of the solution could be recognized.

After the dorsal parts of the gyri ecto- and suprasylvii posteriores were hypersensitized in this way, in all 5 dogs and in 50 per cent of 18 cats treated by rotation on a Bárány chair (usually 10 rotations in 20 seconds) epileptiform clonic convulsions were induced. As a rule the cloni started in the lid and ear muscles contralateral to the strychninized cortex; in some cases they spread to the bilateral face muscles and eventually became generalized, in that first the opposite foreleg, then the hind leg and then the whole body was involved. The strychninization of middle or anterior parts of these gyri or of the frontal lobe did not have such an influence. Extirpation of the frontal lobe in front of the motor area did not prevent the appearance of these epileptiform convulsions but undercutting of the gyri- ecto and suprasylvii posteriores prevented the seizures. Following strychninization of the gyrus ectosylvius posterior, such convulsions could also be elicited by acoustic stimulation, but not by painful stimulation, by shaking the animal, by stimulation of the central stump of the cut vagal nerves, or by passive eye movements. They still appeared despite exclusion of visual impulses and despite nearly complete extirpation of the cerebellum. From these experiments, it was inferred that *labyrinthine impulses may reach the area of transition of the temporal to the parieto-occipital region by way of extracerebellar pathways.* These experiments were later confirmed and extended by Aronson who found that the medial longitudinal fasciculus is also dispensable for the cortical vestibular projection.

If one compares the strychninized areas with recent maps of the cerebral cortex of the cat, for instance that by Woolsey, one finds that the region from which these effects were obtained corresponds partly to the so-called *secondary visual area* (visual area II, Talbot), an area where an integration of visual impulses with other sensory modalities takes place, and partly to the posterior ectosylvian auditory area EP; according to Bremer et al., the inferior part of EP has the characteristics of a secondary (psychosensory) area and is in close functional association with the primary auditory area. A comparison with a cytoarchitectonic map shows that the strychninized field includes Broadman areas 18, 19, 21, and 22.

These experiments were continued by *electrocorticographical studies* (Spiegel, 1934). It was found that labyrinthine excitation by rotation increased the potential discharges led off from the dorsal part of the posterior ectosylvian and suprasylvian gyri in cats paralyzed by curare or in bulbocapnine catalepsy. Such an effect was not prevented, if the eyes were closed, the vagi cut, the spinal cord severed at the uppermost segments, or the frontal lobe with the motor zone or the parietal lobe was extirpated. This effect was rather sensitive to anaesthesia; it disappeared in deep anaesthesia. After bilateral labyrinthectomy or after an incision into the white matter severing the connection of the posterior suprasylvian and ectosylvian gyri with the subcortex, the electrogram of these gyri was not changed by rotation. A postrotatory increase of the potentials in the parietal lobe depends on the intactness of the posterior suprasylvian and ectosylvian gyri and of the frontal lobe; after combined extirpation of the frontal and the temporal lobe, rotation could not longer increase the currents led off from the parietal lobe. Postrotatory changes were noticed in the electrograms of the frontal lobe even after extirpation of the temporal lobes; but a definite effect of the rotation was no longer observed, if this extirpation was combined with high transverse section of the spinal cord. The experiments seemed to indicate that *labyrinthine impulses can enter the cortex, particularly parts of the temporal lobe near the parietal and occipital lobes.* It was considered also possible that *rubro-thalamofrontal tracts are used as a common path* by the labyrinthine as well as by other impulses. An increase of the potential discharges particularly in the posterior ecto- and suprasylvian gyri was also observed on labyrinthine stimulation by rotation by Gerebetzoff (1938, 1940), Bohm and Gernandt (1951), and by Infantellina, Sanseverino and Urbano (1963). On caloric stimulation, Kornmueller found a modification of the potentials in areas 6a and 19.

In recent years, *microelectrode studies* were carried out by Grüsser and his associates in Jung's laboratory on cats in whom an encéphale isolé preparation was produced by high transection of the spinal cord. The authors found that nearly all neurons in the "visual cortex" (apparently striate, peri- and parastriate cortex) were activated when the labyrinth was polarized by the positive or negative pole of a weak D.C. Most frequent was activation at onset and on cessation of the polarization; rarely it was found at onset or at cessation only. In most neurons of the visual cortex the critical flicker frequency was significantly raised by labyrinthine polarization. In all light-responsive neurons, the bursts of their discharges induced by brief light flashes were increased. Thus, labyrinthine and retinal impulses seemed to converge and to be integrated at neurons of the visual cortex. Grüsser et al. found that the neurons of the optic cortex reacted to vestibular stimulation after rather variable, often long latent periods (25-200 msec.); they considered, therefore, the possibility that the activation of the optic cortex by labyrinthine impulses is transmitted by a multisynaptic system such as the pontomesencephalic reticular formation and "nonspecific" thalamic relay nuclei.

Continuing these experiments, Kornhuber and Fonseka arrived at the conclusion that the neuronal convergence of opto-vestibular afferents is chiefly a convergence of specific visual and nonspecific vestibular impulses in the striate cortex and its vicinity. They found this nonspecific activation not only in the visual but also in the paravisual areas, including the cranial part of the gyrus ectosylvius posterior and within the primary somatic cortex. A closer study of their data reveals that they found a nonspecific activation on vestibular stimulation in the gyrus ectosylvius and suprasylvius anterior (that they call "vestibular area") in only 13 per cent of the investigated neurons, in the gyrus suprasylvius medius in 20 per cent, in the gyrus postcruciatus (primary somatic area) in 54 per cent, and in the gyrus lateralis anterior in 12 per cent, in the auditory area (gyrus ectosylvian medius) in 38 per cent; but much higher values in the gyrus ectosylvius posterior (73 per cent), in the posterior part of the gyrus suprasylvius medius (79 per cent, and in area 17 and 18 (74 per cent). These differences in the percentages of the neurons activated by the labyrinthine stimulation in various areas show that chiefly the visual cortex and its vicinity is stimulated by these so-called nonspecific vestibular impulses. In other words, there is a greater density of "nonspecific" vestibular projections to the visual cortex and its vicinity than to other cortical areas. If this response is elicited by the so-called diffuse or nonspecific thalamic projection system, one would have to conclude that those parts of the diffuse projection system are particularly reached by the vestibular impulses that project to the visual cortex and its vicinity. For the reticular activating system, Moruzzi already pointed out that sensory stimuli of low intensity might activate only some parts of this system, while on strong and abrupt stimulation a mass discharge of reticular neurons is likely to occur.

The electrographic studies reported so far were performed in awake or unanaesthetized encéphale isolé preparations; in most of these experiments, except the microelectrode studies, the labyrinth was stimulated by an adequate stimulus—i.e., by production of an endolymph movement by rotation. In contrast, a number of authors ascertained in anaesthetized animals the cortical areas from which evoked potentials could be recorded on electric stimulation of nerve fibers originating in the labyrinth (Walzl and Mountcastle; Mickle and Ades; Kempinski); in these studies stimulation of the nervus intermedius could not be excluded with certainty. This is the more important, since the afferent fibers of the nervus intermedius seem to project to the same cortical area (second sensory area, Patton) as found for the nervus vestibularis on electric stimulation. Stimulation of other afferent fibers could be excluded with more assurance in the experiments reported by Andersson and Gernandt, in which single branches of the vestibular nerve were stimulated or in those of Massopust and Daigle, in which the vestibular nuclei were the site of the stimulating electrodes.

These studies have shown that labyrinthine impulses elicit short latency responses in the gyrus ectosylvius anterior and adjacent parts of the gyrus suprasylvius anterior. This projection is part of the so-called *second sensory area* (Adrian, Woolsey) that receives also impulses from other receptors (touch, deep sensation, cochlea, pain; recently Berman; Carreras and Andersson) so that vestibular impulses can here interact with other modalities. It seems, therefore, hardly justified to describe this area as the "vestibular cortex" as some authors (e.g., Kornhuber) do. One could describe it just as well as auditory or somatic sensory cortex, since a considerable number of cells of this area receive also short latency responses from these receptors, and afferent impulses from several receptors may converge on single cells of this area. It would seem, therefore, that the designations "composite sensory projection area" (Mickle and Ades) or "multisensory" or "*polysensory area*" best reflect these findings.

The integration of the various impulses that may reach the second sensory area apparently takes place, at least partly, at subcortical levels, since the second sensory area receives impulses from the so-called *posterior group of thalamic nuclei* (Knighton; Rose and Woolsey; Locke), particularly from the *pars magnocellularis of the medial geniculate body*, where not only pain afferents (Whitlock and Pearl) but also acoustic impulses (Moore and Goldberg) and vestibular impulses (Spiegel, Szekely, and Gildenberg) enter. In experiments of Spiegel, Szekely, and Gildenberg, it could be shown by using a computer of average transients that evoked potentials could be elicited in the pars magnocellularis on stimulation of the vestibular nuclei, and that destruction of the magnocellular portion, including parts of the suprageniculate nucleus and other cells of the posterior thalamic groups prevents the response of the gyrus ectosylvius anterior to stimulation of the vestibular nuclei.

In the macaque brain the second sensory area lies in the upper bank of the sylvian fissure (Woolsey). In man the corresponding cortical area probably lies in a similar location but is not clearly defined as yet. Locke, Angevine, and Marin found that the magnocellular medial geniculate nucleus projects to a parietotemporal field. The smallest lesion inducing degeneration of this nucleus involved the supramarginal gyrus, parietal operculum, and posterior insula.

The location of the second sensory area at the upper bank of the Sylvian fissure may explain why in Gildenberg's experiments on stimulation of the vestibular nuclei evoked potentials were recorded chiefly dorsal from, but close to, the Sylvian fissure. It may also explain why Spiegel and Alexander in an analysis of vertigo in brain tumors found that particularly tumors in the vicinity of the Sylvian fissure (dorsal part of the temporal lobe or ventral part of the central gyri) were associated with the appearance of vertigo (see later).

From Brodmann's area 19, Gildenberg was only occasionally able to record potentials on stimulation of the vestibular nuclei. This difficulty he experienced in obtaining evoked responses may be due to the use of excessively deep anaesthesia, and further exploration of this region in the macaque brain is being undertaken.

CLINICAL STUDIES

In clinical studies Spiegel and Alexander (1936) examined the problem of whether *vertigo in brain tumors* is simply due to a general increase of intracranial pressure or whether it may appear, at least in some instances, as a local symptom of certain cortical areas. From the First Surgical Clinic of the University of Vienna, 192 cases were selected in which the location of the tumor could be established by operation or postmortem examination and a single, more or less circumscribed process was found. There were in this series 41 tumors of the frontal lobe, 52 of the central gyri, 28 of the parietal lobe, 46 of the temporal lobe, 11 of the occipital lobe, and 14 of the basal ganglia and corpus callosum.

In analyzing this material one has first to decide which types of vertigo complaints should be considered as related to the disturbances of labyrinthine function. One has to bear in mind that the labyrinth is a receptor not only for sensations elicited by rotation but also for those caused by linear ("progression") movements and by various positions of the head in space. Thus, patients with diseases of the labyrinth or its rhombencephalic nuclei and pathways complain not only about sensations of turning of their surroundings or of their body but also about sensations of rectilinear movements in a horizontal or vertical direction. The patient may experience, for instance, the sensation of plunging into an abyss or of being lifted or of being pushed or pulled to the left or right side. Or one may find delusions regarding the position of the head; the patient may feel as though the head were in an oblique position. The sensation may also be confused and lack any direction (Abels; Alpers; Brunner; Fischer and Kornmueller; Stein). Thus, one has to consider as vertigo positive not only cases that have a turning sensation but also those with the types of vertigo just described.

According to these criteria, the frequency of vertigo in tumors of each region (frontal lobe, central gyri, etc.) was determined. The complaint of vertigo was most frequent in tumors of the temporal lobe (70.0 per cent); next in frequency are tumors of the basal ganglia (64.2 per cent) and then those of the occipital lobe (42.8 per cent), while rather low values were obtained in tumors of the parietal lobe (27.1 per cent), central gyri (21.7 per cent), and frontal lobe (16.6 per cent). These figures, however, do not give as yet a correct conception of the role of the cortical localization of the tumors in the genesis of vertigo, because many of these cases were complicated by pressure upon the labyrinth.

It seemed, therefore, necessary to devote special consideration to those cases in which the labyrinthine function was tested and to exclude cases in which the appearance of vertigo was explained by abnormal excitability of the labyrinth (mostly overexcitability, in some cases differences in excitability between both sides). Sometimes such an examination may fail to detect slight differences in the state of excitation of the left and right labyrinths, but such differences may induce vertigo and become manifested by the appearance of spontaneous nystagmus. Such cases as well as cases with diplopia must, of course, also be excluded. One has also to bear in mind that patients with cerebral tumor often complain of vertigo, if there exists a disturbance of equilibrium or a tendency to fall; this may be due to a disorder of cerebellar function caused by pressure upon the cerebellum or upon its brachia or by injury to the long descending cerebral pathways. Thus, all cases were also excluded in which spontaneous nystagmus, diplopia or disturbances in equilibrium indicating a cerebellar involvement might have been responsible for the appearance of vertigo. Also, if the material was restricted in this way, the result was that tumors of the temporal lobe were most frequently (26.4 per cent) associated with vertigo (frontal and parietal lobe 10.2 per cent each, central gyri 17.6 per cent, occipital lobe 17.8 per cent, basal ganglia 11.1 per cent).

It was further tried to ascertain whether, within the various lobes, some localizations were more conducive to the appearance of vertigo than others. In this respect only this can be said: In tumors of the central region, vertigo occurred more frequently in those of the ventral parts than in those of the dorsal parts. In eleven tumors close to the dorsal margin, vertigo was only twice noticed, while it appeared four times in twelve tumors of the ventral parts of the central region. The reverse seems to be valid in temporal lobe tumors, in so far as the smallness of the material permits such conclusions. In 20 cases a dorsal and ventral localization respectively could be distinguished. The group of 13 dorsal tumors showed vertigo ten times (77 per cent); the group of 7 ventral tumors showed this symptom four times (57 per cent of the respective subgroup). In agreement with this experience is the fact that temporal lobe abscesses usually are not accompanied by vertigo (Leidler) since they start at the base of the temporal lobe (Brunner).

It is only with the greatest caution and reserve that one may draw conclusions from these observations in respect to the cortical localization of labyrinthine projections. Such a caution is dictated by the relative smallness of the material and by the uncertainty to which a localization is subject that is based upon diseases complicated by increased intracranial pressure. At any rate, one cannot neglect the fact that there exists a different frequency of vertigo in tumors of the various areas of the cerebral cortex. If this symptom were simply due to a distant effect (pressure) upon basal nerves, the labyrinth, or the cerebellum, one should expect that more ventrally located tumors would be more frequently associated with vertigo than tumors close to the vertex. This was found in tumors of the central region, but just the opposite in tumors of the temporal lobe. The striking frequency of vertigo in tumors of this region, found even after cases with vestibular overexcitability, nystagmus, diplopia, or cerebellar symptoms were excluded, seems to indicate that the temporal lobe or closely adjacent areas receive labyrinthine impulses.

In agreement with this concept are other clinical observations that followed Spiegel's initial experiments. Barré, Vincent, and Helle reported a case of temporal lobe tumor with typical turning sensation. Penfield and Gage described tumors of this region that induced *epileptiform convulsions* with attacks of dizziness. Such attacks could also be produced by electrical stimulation of the affected region of the cerebral cortex. The study of certain cases of so-called genuine epilepsy may also shed some light upon our problem. Stauder, for instance, observed such cases. In one patient the aura was characterized by a quick succession of acoustic and olfactory hallucinations; somewhat later a severe "vestibular syndrome" developed (everything turned around the patient). Finally, the optic perceptions were also affected; simultaneously amnesic-aphasic and paraphasic disturbances respectively appeared. In a second patient there was, during the aura, a succession of olfactory, vestibular, and paraphasic disturbances. The author interpreted his observations as confirming the assumption of a cortical representation of the vestibular system in the temporal lobe.

In relatively rare instances labyrinthine stimulation may evoke epileptiform seizures (Marie and Pierre; recently Behrman and Wyke; Molnár et al.). The last-named authors found that caloric stimulation was able to activate particularly epileptogenic foci in the temporal lobe, but in some cases also foci outside this lobe. The appearance of the convulsions may be associated with generalized seizure discharges in the EEG. In some of Molnár's epileptics, the labyrinthine stimulus suppressed the paroxysmal waves of the EEG. Behrman and Wyke, as well as Molnár et al., suggested that the labyrinthine effects upon the cortex were transmitted by way of the reticular formation.

For the problem of a cortical projection of the labyrinth, *EEG observations during vertiginous auras* are of more interest. They showed focal EEG disturbances in the temporal and parietal regions. (Hécaen, Gastaut et al.) In some patients with vertiginous attacks, Spiegel (unpublished observations) could also observe seizure discharges in the temporal leads in the intervals between the attacks.

On *electric stimulation of the cortex* of the temporal lobe in the vicinity of the Sylvian fissure, Penfield was able to elicit vertiginous sensations in awake epileptics. In single instances, Foerster observed tumors in the region of the interparietal fissure associated with rotatory vertigo and was able to induce such sensations by faradic stimulation of this region. This effect may have been due to a spread to the somatic sensory area II at the dorsal bank of the Sylvian fissure or to the peristriate area (visual area II); a definite answer to this problem does not seem possible at present.

In contrast to the appearance of labyrinthine symptoms in irritative pathologic processes in the temporo-parietal region or on electric stimulation of this area, is the *lack of definite labyrinthine deficiency symptoms after elimination* of the posterior ecto- and suprasylvian gyri (Bohm and Gernandt), as well as after ablation of the second sensory somatic area including the labyrinthine projection (Lehman in the author's laboratory). After uni- or bilateral destruction of this field in cats, Lehman found only that the animals hesitated to descend on an oblique ladder. In view of the fact that the second sensory somatic area contains also projections from cutaneous and proprioceptive receptors, this symptom can hardly be attributed only to the elimination of cortical endings of labyrinthine afferents. Similarly, Escabedo (in the author's laboratory) failed to find specific labyrinthine deficiency symptoms after ablation of the parietal lobe.

Recently we have attempted to develop a method that would permit one to record *potentials evoked in the EEG of awake persons by vestibular stimulation.*

For a study of central responses to stimulation of the labyrinth, production of an endolymph flow seems to be the adequate stimulus. Using the methods usually employed in the clinic (10 rotations on a Bárány chair in 20 seconds; calorization), EEG studies (Lovell, Garski, and Lyman; Baudouin and Caussée) demonstrated that the excitation tends to affect the whole cortex, apparently because the stimulation is too intense, so that the vestibular impulses induce a mass discharge of the reticular formation and activate the diffuse thalamic system in toto.

Such an overexcitation may be avoided, if one performs only single rotations with relatively low speed and records the reactions elicited by cessation of each rotation; these responses are summed up by means of a computer of average transients (author's experiments with Szekely, Moffet, and Robbins).

The experiments were performed on 37 cats and 43 awake human subjects. The cats were maintained in bulbocapnine catalepsy. In some instances, the effect of additional pentobarbital anaesthesia was ascertained. In cats the electrodes (stainless steel balls, diameter 1.2-1.3 mm., soldered to teflon-coated silver wire) were placed epidurally through a small drill hole in the skull and kept in place by fixing the connecting wire in the drill hole by a plastic plug. In men the usual Grass scalp electrodes were applied.

During these experiments, the eyes of the experimental animals or human subjects were kept closed in order to prevent optokinetic responses. The wires connecting the cerebral or scalp electrodes with the recording system were conducted in the axis of the rotating chair over the head of the tested subject. The average duration of each rotation was 3 seconds. Following each rotation—e.g., in clockwise direction—the chair was slowly returned to the starting position in order to avoid excessive twisting of the connecting wires. After a pause of one minute, the rotation was repeated and the responses from 10 to 30 or more rotations were averaged by the computer. After each series of ten rotations, the averaged response was displayed on an X-Y plotter, so that not only the effect of the summation but also possible changes in the excitability of the labyrinth and/or of its centers—e.g., habituation effects—could be observed. The reaction to rotation in the opposite direction, e.g. counterclockwise, were studied at a later period at the same day, sometimes on another day.

These experiments showed that, following rotation in cats (Fig. 1), electric responses can be elicited not only from the region of the gyrus ectosylvius anterior but also from the posterior parts of the hemisphere, from the posterior and middle ecto- and suprasylvian gyri. While in many instances the reactions recorded from various cortical areas showed a rather uniform shape, cases could be observed in which the responses from the posterior part were more pronounced, lasting a longer time. The peak latencies were rather long, varying from 0.3-0.6 seconds. These reactions were rather sensitive to anaesthesia; pentothal anaesthesia diminished or abolished them.

In order to ascertain whether the responses in the posterior part of the hemisphere were due to a propagation or spread from the region of the gyrus ectosylvius anterior, which some regard as the 'vestibular cortex," this area was extirpated uni- or bilaterally. These ablations did not prevent the appearance of the responses in the posterior part of the hemisphere (Fig. 1).

For an analysis of the origin of these responses, transverse sections of the cord at the first cervical segment were performed. Neither such transverse sections, interrupting the ascending impulses from the spinal segments, nor immobilization by Flaxedil prevented these reactions. They could no longer be elicited after bilateral elimination of the labyrinth by injection of 70 per cent alcohol or 4 per cent formalin into the round window. The results did not differ whether the noise from an adjacent room was excluded or not, so that acoustic stimuli of low intensity did not seem to change the results.

Apparently one deals here with a so-called secondary evoked response. The long-peak latency and sensitivity to anaesthesia suggest a polysynaptic afferent pathway, possibly using the diffuse thalamic projection system. There exist, however, certain local differences in the reaction, particularly in man, in that these reactions were more prolonged in the posterior part of the hemisphere, in the vicinity of the visual cortex, than in anterior parts. It would seem that those parts of the diffuse thalamic projection system are particularly activated by the vestibular impulses that project to the vicinity of the visual cortex.

In man, either diffuse responses or responses limited to, or prevalent in, preoccipital areas were noted (Figs. 2 and 3). These reactions also showed long latencies and were sometimes multiphasic in character. In parts of these studies, electronystagmo-

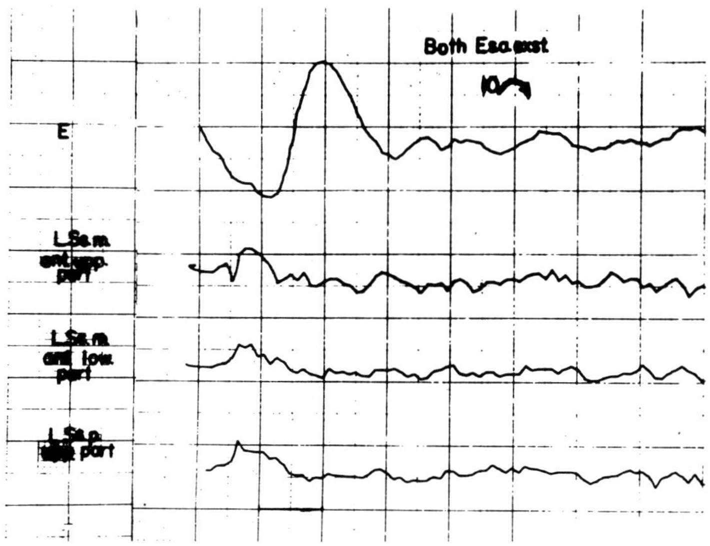

FIG. 1. Cat: Both gyri ectosylv. ant. (ESA) ablated. Averaged reactions to 10 single rotations ⤺ (computer record). E, eye movements (corneo-retinal potentials). Electrograms of the left gyr. suprasylv. medius (L Ssm) and suprasylvius posterior (L Ssp). Time calibration 0.4 sec. (in this and the following records).

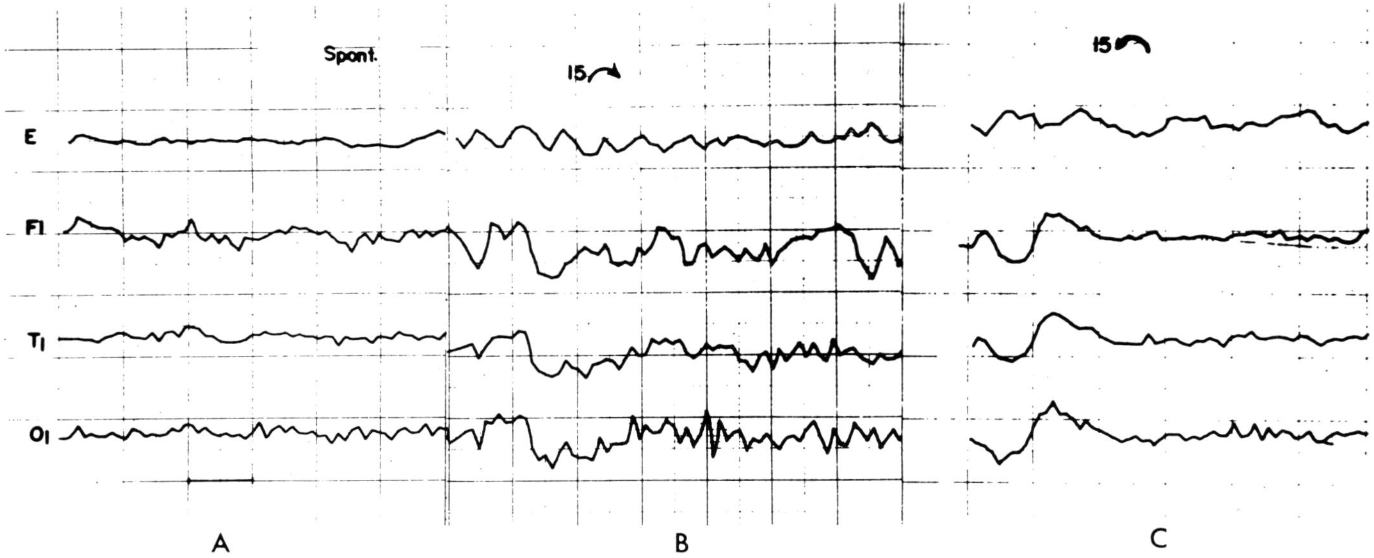

Fig. 2. Normal human subject. Eye movements (E) and monopolar scalp EEG from the frontal (F), temporal (T), and occipital (O) regions. (A) Spontaneous activity (15 sweeps averaged). (B) Averaged reactions to 15 → rotations. (C) Averaged reaction to 15 ← rotations.

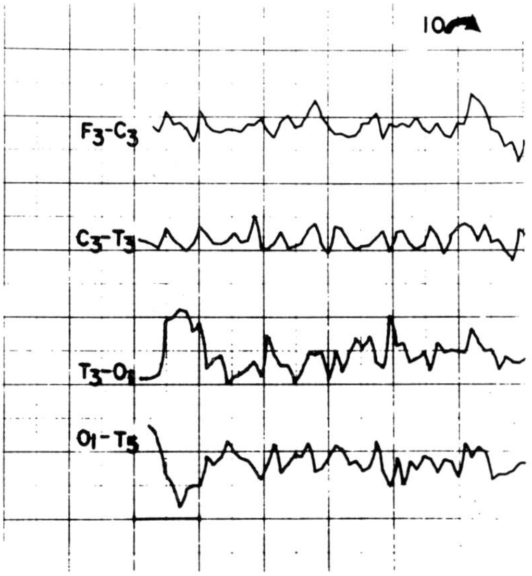

Fig. 3. Normal human subject. Bipolar scalp EEG. Averaged reactions to 10 ↷ rotations. F, frontal; C, central; T, temporal; and O, occipital leads.

grams, in other electromyograms of the neck muscles were simultaneously recorded. An interference of corneo-retinal or neck muscle potentials occurred only rarely, and such cases were not considered useful for valid conclusions. In the great majority of the records this factor played no role, and a cerebral origin of the potential discharges must be assumed. The preoccipital response may be part of the reaction of the diffuse thalamic projection system, particularly of a system synapsing in the pulvinar, or due to responses propagated from the second somatic sensory area that is supposed to lie in the human in or around the upper bank of the sylvian fissure (Locke). These problems are under study.

SUMMARY

A cortical area in which the labyrinth would be represented alone, without other receptors, could not be found as yet. Evoked reactions to vestibular stimulation could be obtained in animal experiments chiefly from the second somatic and the second visual area. In man, diffuse reactions were recorded and responses chiefly from the preoccipital area that is probably homologous to the second visual area. These studies seem to indicate that the labyrinth has multiple cortical projections, as is known for other sensory modalities. The vicinity of the preoccipital area to the posterior part of the temporal lobe makes it understandable that pathologic processes inducing a stimulation of the temporal lobe may be associated with subjective labyrinthine symptoms. Definite specific deficiency symptoms could not be found from any of these areas, while their stimulation by electric currents or by pathologic processes may induce spatial disorientation, i.e., the subjective symptoms of vertigo. The fact that a cortical area to which the labyrinth would project alone, independently of other receptors, could not be found as yet may become understandable if one bears in mind that the labyrinth is phylogenetically a rather old receptor and, therefore, similar to pain receptors has a direct representation only in the subcortex. In the subcortex, integrations with other modalities may take place, and the impulses resulting from these subcortical integrations may be projected to the cortex.

REFERENCES

1. Abels, H.: Ueber Nachempfindungen. Z. Psychol. 43:269-374, 1906.
2. Adrian, E. D.: Afferent discharges to the cerebral cortex from peripheral sense organs. J. Physiol. 100:159-191, 1941.
3. Alexander, A., and Spiegel, E. A.: Zur Frage der kortikalen Labyrinthzentren. Oest. Otol. Ges. Monatschr. Ohrenheilk. 70:363, 1936.
4. Alpers, B. A.: Vertigo and Dizziness. New York, Grune & Stratton, 1958.
5. Amantea, G.: Ueber experimentelle beim Versuchstier infolge afferenter Reize erzeugte Epilepsie. Pflüger Arch. Ges. Physiol. 188: 287-297, 1921.
6. Andersson, S., and Gernandt, B. E.: Cortical projection of vestibular nerve in cat. Acta Otolaryng. (Stockholm) Suppl. 116:10-18, 1954.
7. Aronson, L.: Conduction of labyrinthine impulses to the cortex. J. Nerv. Ment. Dis. 78:250-259, 1933.
8. Barré, F. H., Vincent, C., and Helle, Mlle.: Tumeur temporale. Rev. Neurol. 40:377, 1933.
9. Baudouin, A., and Caussée, R.: Influence des

stimulations vestibulaires sur les ondes de l'encéphalogramme chez l'homme. C. R. Soc. Biol. 137:195-196, 1943.

10. Behrman, S.: Vestibular Epilepsy. Brain 78: 471-486, 1955.

11. Behrman, S., and Wyke, B. D.: Vestibulogenic seizures: A consideration of vertiginous seizures, with particular reference to convulsions produced by stimulation of labyrinthine receptors. Brain 81:529-541, 1958.

11a. Berman, A. L.: Overlap of somatic and auditory cortical response fields in ant. ectosylv. gyn. of cat. J. Neurophysiol. 24:594-607, 1961.

12. Bohm, E., and Gernandt, B. E.: Locomotion after removal of inferior colliculi or cortical vestibular projection area. Acta Physiol. Scand. 23:320-332, 1951.

13. Bremer, F.: Nouvelles récherches sur le mécanisme du sommeil. C. R. Soc. Biol. 122:460-464, 1936.

14. Bremer, F., Bonnet, V., and Terzuolo, C.: Étude électrophysiologique des aires auditives corticales du chat. Arch. Int. Physiol. 62:390-428, 1954.

15. Brodal, A., Pompeiano, O., and Walberg, F.: The Vestibular Nuclei and Their Connections, Anatomy and Functional Correlations, Edinburgh & London, Oliver & Boyd, 1962.

16. Brunner, H.: Symptomatol. der Erkrankungen d. Nerv. Vestibul. Handb. d. Neur. d. Ohr. (Alexander-Marburg), Vienna, Urban & Schwarzenberg, 1924.

17. Brunner, H.: Discussion of Alexander and Spiegel. Monatsschr. f. Ohrenhk. 70:368, 1936.

18. Carpenter, M. B.: The dorsal trigeminal tract in the Rhesus Monkey. J. Anat. 91:82-90, 1957.

19. Carreras, M., and Andersson, S. A.: Functional properties of neurons of the anterior ectosylvian gyrus of the cat. J. Neurophysiol. 26:100-126, 1963.

20. Clementi, A.: Stricninizzazione della sfere corticale visiza and epilessia sperimentale da stimoli luminosi. Arch. Fisiol. 27:356-387, 1929.

20a. Escabedo. In print Confin. Neurol.

21. Ferraro, A., Pacella, B. L., and Barrera, S. E.: Effects of lesions of the medial vestibular nucleus. J. Comp. Neurol. 73:7-36, 1940.

22. Fischer, M. H., and Kornmueller, A. E.: Der Schwindel in Handb. Norm. Path. Physiol. 15 (I):422, 1930, Berlin, Springer.

23. Foerster, O.: Sensible corticale Felder. *In* Handb. Neurologie. Vol. 6. O. Bumke and O. Foerster, Eds. 1936, Berlin, Springer, pp. 358-448.

24. Gerebetzoff, M. A.: Des effets de la stimulation labyrinthique sur l'activité électrique de l'écorce cérébrale. C. R. Soc. Biol. 131:807-813, 1939.

25. Gerebetzoff, M. A.: Recherches sur la projection corticale du labyrinthe. I. Des effects de la stimulation labyrinthique sur l'activité électrique de l'écorce cérébrale. Arch. Int. Physiol. 50:59-99, 1940.

26. Gerebetzoff, M. A.: Recherches sur la projection corticale du labyrinthe. II. Etude anatomo-expérimentale de la voie vestibulo-cérébrale. J. Belge Neurol. Psychiat. 8:417-432, 1940.

26a. Gildenberg, P.: Personal communication.

27. Godlowski, W.: Les centres sous-corticaux du regard et des mouvements associés des globes oculaires. Trav. Clin. Mal. Nerv. de'L'Univ. Cracovie, 1936, p. 1.

28. Grüsser, O. J., and Cornehls, U.: Mikroelektrodenuntersuchungen zur Konvergenz vestibulärer und retinaler Afferenzen an einzelnen Neuronen des optischen Cortex der Katze. Pflüger Arch. Ges. Physiol. 270:227-238, 1960.

29. Grüsser, O. J., Grüsser-Cornehls, U., and Saur, G.: Reaktionen einzelner Neurone im optischen Cortex der Katze nach elektrischer Polarization des Labyrinths. Pflüger Arch. Ges. Physiol. 269:593-612, 1959.

30. Hassler, R.: Forels Haubenfaszikel als vestibuläre Empfindungsbahn. Arch. Psychiat. 118:23-53, 1948.

31. Hassler, R.: Die Anatomic des Thalamus. Arch. Psychiat. Z. Neur. 184:249-251, 1950.

32. Hécaen, H., Gastaut, H., Bancaud, J., and Rebufat-Deschamps, M.: Clinical and EEG aspects of the problem of cortical localization. *In* Cerebral Localization and Organization. G. Schaltenbrand and C. N. Woolsey, Eds. Madison, Univ. of Wisconsin Press, 1964, pp. 67-88.

33. Held, H.: Die anatomische Grundlage der Vestibularisfunktionen. Beitr. Anat. Physiol. Path. Ther. Ohres, Nase, Halses 19:305-312, 1923.

34. Infantellina, F., Riva Sanseverino, E., and Urbano, A.: Electroencephalographic changes as a result of labyrinthine stimulation after strychninization of the paraflocculus in the dog. Arch. Ital. Biol. 101:430-443, 1963.

35. Kempinsky, W. H.: Cortical projection of vestibular and facial nerves in cat. J. Neurophysiol. 14:203-210, 1951.

36. Knighton, R. S.: Thalamic relay nucleus for

the second somatic sensory receiving area in the cerebral cortex of the cat. J. Comp. Neurol. 92:183-191, 1950.
37. Kornhuber, H. H., and da Fonseca, J. S.: Optovestibular integration in the cat's cortex. *In* The Oculomotor System. M. B. Bender, Ed. New York, Hoeber Med. Div., Harper and Row, 1964, pp. 239-277.
38. Kornmueller, A. E.: Biologische Erscheinungen der Hirnrindenfelder, Leipzig, Thieme, 1937.
39. Leidler, R.: Discussion of Alexander and Spiegel. Monatsschr. f. Ohrenheilk. 70:365. 1936.
39a. Lehman. *In* print. Conf. Neurol.
40. Lewandowsky, M.: Untersuchungen über die Leitungsbahnen des Truncus Cerebri. *In* Neurobiologische Arbeiten. O. Vogt, Ed. Jena. G. Fischer, ser. 2 Vol. 1, Part II, 1904, pp. 63-150.
41. Locke, S., Angevine, J. B. Jr., and Marin, O. S. M.: Projection of the magnocellular medial geniculate nucleus in man. Brain 85:319-330, 1962.
42. Locke, S.: The projection of the magnocellular medial geniculate body. J. Comp. Neur. 116:179-194, 1961.
43. Lovell, H. W., Garski, T. J., and Lyman, R. S.: Effect of vestibular stimulation on brain waves. Chinese J. Physiol. 14:389, 1939.
44. Massopust, L. C., Jr., and Daigle, H. J.: Cortical projection of the medial and spinal vestibular nuclei in the cat. Exp. Neurol. 2:179-185, 1960.
45. Mickle, V. A., and Ades, H. W.: A composite sensory projection area in the cerebral cortex of the cat. Amer. J. Physiol. 170: 682-689, 1952.
46. Mickle, W. A., and Ades, H. W.: Rostral projection pathway of the vestibular system. Amer. J. Physiol. 176:243-246, 1954.
47. Molnár, L.: Die Bedeutung der Labyrinthimpulse in der Spontan-und-Krampftätigkeit der Grosshirnrinde, Arch. Psychiat. Z. Neurol. 198:554-573, 1959.
48. Molnár, L. Kekesi, F., and Gosztonyi, G.: Die Wirkung der Labyrinthreizung auf das normale und pathologische Elektrencephalogramm beim Menschen, Arch. Psychiat. Z. Neurol. 199:152-171, 1959.
49. Moore, R. Y., and Goldberg, J. M.: Ascending projection of the inferior colliculus in the cat. J. Comp. Neurol. 121:109-119, 1963.
50. Moruzzi, G.: The physiological properties of the brain stem reticular system. *In* Brain Mechanisms and Consciousness, J. F. Delafresnaye, Ed. Oxford, Blackwell, 1954, pp. 21-53.
51. Muskens, J. J.: Das Supravestibuläre System bei Tieren u. beim Menschen, N. V. Nord. Holl. Uitgev. Amsterdam, Maatschappij, 1935.
52. Obersteiner, H.: Anleitung beim Studium des Baues der nervösen Zentralorgane, 5th Edition, Wien, Deuticke, 1912.
53. Patton, H. D., and Amassian, V. E.: Cortical projection zone of chorda tympani nerve in cat. J. Neurophysiol. 15:245-250, 1952.
54. Penfield, W., and Gage, L.: Cerebral localization of epileptic manifestations. Res. Ass. Nerv. Ment. Dis. 13:593, 1934.
55. Penfield, W.: Vestibular sensation and the cerebral cortex. Ann. Otol. 66:691-698, 1957.
56. Poljak, S.: The main afferent fiber systems of the cerebral cortex in primates. Univ. Calif. Pub. Anat. 2:1-370, 1932.
57. Price, J. B., and Spiegel, E. A.: Vestibulo-cerebral pathways. A contribution to the central mechanism of vertigo. Arch. Otolaryng. 26:658-667, 1937.
58. Ranson, S. W., and Ranson, S. W., Jr.: Efferent fibers of the corpus striatum. Res. Pub. Ass. Nerv. Ment. Dis. 21:69, 1941.
59. Rose, J. E., and Woolsey, C. N.: Cortical connections and functional organization of the thalamic auditory system of the cat. *In* Biological and Biochemical Bases of Behavior. H. F. Harlow and C. N. Woolsey, Eds. Madison, Univ. Wis. Press, 1958.
60. Spiegel, E. A.: Cortical centers of the labyrinth. J. Nerv. Ment. Dis. 75:504-512, 1932.
61. Spiegel, E. A.: Rindenerregung (Auslösung epileptiformer Anfälle) durch Labyrinthreizung. Versuch einer Lokalisation der corticalen Labyrinthzentren., Z. Ges. Neurol Psychiat. 138:178-196, 1932.
62. Spiegel, E. A.: Labyrinth and cortex. The electroencephalogram of the cortex in stimulation of the labyrinth. Arch. Neurol. Psychiat. 31:469-482, 1934.
63. Spiegel, E. A., and Alexander, A.: Vertigo in brain tumors, with special reference to the results of labyrinth examination. Ann. Otol. 45:979-987, 1936.
64. Spiegel, E. A., Szekely, E. G., and Gildenberg, P.: Vestibular projection to meso-diencephalic nuclei and basal ganglia. Fed. Proc. 23:415, 1964.
65. Spiegel, E. A., Szekely, E. G., and Gildenberg, P.: Vestibular responses in midbrain, thalamus and basal ganglia. Arch. Neurol. 12: 258-269, 1965.

66. Stauder, K. H:. Epilepsie u. Vestibular Apparat. Arch. Psychiat. 101:739, 1934.
67. Stein, S. v.: Schwindel. Leipzig., O. Leiner, 1910.
68. Talbot, S. A.: A lateral localization in the cat's visual cortex. Fed. Proc. 1:84, 1942.
69. Walzl, E. M., and Mountcastle, V.: Projection of vestibular nerve to cerebral cortex of the cat. Amer. J. Physiol. 159:595, 1949.
70. Whitaker, J. G., and Alexander, L.: Die Verbindungen der Vestibularis-kerne mit dem Mittel-und Zwischenhirn. Studien auf Grund experimenteller Verletzungen. J. Psychol. Neurol. 44:253-376, 1932.
71. Whitlock, D. G., and Perl, E. R.: Thalamic projection of spinothalamic pathways in monkey. Exp. Neurol. 3:240-255, 1961.
72. Winkler, C., and Potter, A.: An anatomical guide to experimental researches on the cat's brain—a series of 35 frontal sections. Amsterdam, W. Versluys 1914.
73. Winkler, C.: The central course of the nervus octavus and its influence on motility. Verh. Akad. Wet. Amsterdam 14:1-202, 1909.
74. Woolsey, C. N.: Organization of somatic sensory and motor areas of the cerebral cortex. *In* Biological and Biochemical Bases of Behavior. H. F. Harlow and C. N. Woolsey, Eds. Madison, Univ. Wis. Press, 1958, pp. 63-81.

CHAPTER 3

History

Clinical History

Martin Spector

DEFINITION

The term "dizziness" is used here in the broad sense of any unpleasant sensation of disturbed relationship to surrounding objects in space. It may also be defined as a sensation of instability of position in relation to space and surrounding objects. Webster's definition of vertigo is "the disturbance in which objects, though stationery, appear to move in various directions and the person affected finds it difficult to maintain an erect posture." According to Spiegel, "vertigo is the subjective experience of a disturbance in the relationship of the individual to his surroundings." The subject feels either that he is moving in space or that the outer world is moving about him. The term "vertigo" will be largely used here according to the restricted definition of Soma Weiss—i.e., an experience in which the patient has the sensation that his surroundings are whirling about him or that he himself is whirling in space. The term dizziness will be used in a broader sense where the more specific term vertigo does not apply. The terms vertigo and dizziness are often used interchangeably in the general literature for the very good reason that it is often impossible to make a differentiation in the individual patient. A sensation of movement is critical to both terms.

DESCRIPTION OF COMPLAINT

The examiner must ascertain what the patient means by vertigo or dizziness. To a patient, dizziness may signify a to-and-fro motion, an up-and-down movement, a sensation that the floor is rocking, a sinking feeling, mental confusion, blurring of vision, uncertainty, unsteadiness, apprehension, fearfulness, giddiness, reeling, swaying, swimming sensation in the head, drunk feeling, or pressure in the head. The patient may say his brain is moving inside his head. Patients undergoing the cold caloric test may describe their sensations as other than that of rotation, but there is always some sensation of motion. A feeling of lateral pulsion is not uncommon, nor is a to-and-fro movement. Sometimes unsteadiness of the environment during motion may be the complaint. If the patient disclaims any disturbance of equilibrium during the dizziness, it must be regarded with skepticism unless the vertigo is so fleeting as to cause no impairment of balance.

It may be difficult to elicit an exact description of the sensation experienced by the patient. Sometimes, even after careful questioning, one cannot ascertain whether the patient has dizziness, faintness, unsteadiness, fear, or nausea. It is well to repeat the questions at a second visit. The patient may give a more precise description after deliberation. When the patient remains uncertain in the description, the examiner must rely on other symptoms and signs for confirmation. Also it is well to compare his symptom with the vertigo elicited by a mass caloric test. If there is any doubt, it is safer to assume that there is dizziness. The direction and character of the motion are not as important as the fact that there is an unreal sensation of motion, a hallucination of movement.

Vertigo is sometimes divided into subjective vertigo, in which the patient himself rotates, or objective vertigo, in which the room rotates. However, often this is an artificial separation, since it may depend on whether the patient keeps his eyes open or closed. When the patient keeps his eyes closed, he himself may rotate; whereas when he opens his eyes, the room tends to rotate. The direction of the rotation is in the direction of the quick component of the nystagmus. In a peripheral lesion, the direction of the vertigo is toward the good side. In a central lesion, the rotation is toward the side of the lesion. However, it is often difficult for a patient to reliably identify the direction of his vertigo.

Severity of Attack

Dizziness may vary in severity, from a mild unsteadiness to a severe whirling sensation. Nausea, vomiting, pallor, sweating, tachycardia may accompany vertigo. In very severe vertigo, the patient lies immobile in bed, fearing that movement may exaggerate his symptoms. He usually lies with the affected ear up. The severity of the attack is judged by whether nausea, falling, or staggering are present. If the patient must remain recumbent, the attack is considered severe; a very mild attack will not force the patient to remain recumbent. If the patient tends to fall and cannot stand without support, it indicates a severe type of vertigo. A severe initial attack may so frighten a nervous patient that she may confine herself to bed for a prolonged period in spite of only minimal residuals. The intensity of the vertigo is often related to the rapidity of the onset; the more rapid the onset, the more intense the vertigo. The vertigo which accompanies a peripheral vestibular disturbance will be roughly proportional in intensity to the nystagmus.

Vegetative Reflex Actions of the Labyrinth

Excitation or disease of the labyrinth is usually accompanied by vegetative disturbances such as nausea, vomiting, vasomotor reactions, facial pallor, palpitation of the heart, and perspiration. The reflex nature of a great many of these manifestations is readily demonstrable in animal experiments. Both caloric and galvanic stimulation of the labyrinth lead to fall of the blood pressure. The mechanism involved here is similar to that involved in the reflex action of the depressor vagi nerves (e.g., Spiegel). An action on the digestive apparatus is indicated by the observation that an excitation of the labyrinth may be followed by vomiting. This reaction is brought about largely by reflex stimulation of both vagal nerves. This reflex action through the cranial autonomic nervous system also causes an increased secretion of saliva. Dilatation of the pupils is also observed.

The nausea and vomiting can be a very misleading feature. Because of this the digestive system is almost always blamed in the first instance for an attack of vertigo.

Head Movement in Relation to Dizziness

Practically all labyrinthine forms of vertigo will be aggravated by motion of the head. The headshaking test is used to initiate vertigo and nystagmus. Dizziness may be precipitated by changes of position, particularly positions involving the neck, such as bending the head or looking up. Relief here may be obtained by lying down. It is particularly common for dizziness to occur in the morning when first arising, and this may occur from vascular causes, from the neck, etc. This is the type that is prevalent in elderly people and is commonly ascribed to the inability of the cerebral circulation to adapt quickly enough to a change of position. In Meniere's disease, movement seems to have no distinct effect except for aggravation of the vertigo—that is, the vertigo may arise when the patient is sleeping quietly. However, during an attack, if the patient moves his head, the nausea, vomiting, and the vertigo will be aggravated.

Positional Vertigo

The term "positional vertigo and nystagmus" denotes the vertigo and nystagmus which appear only when certain positions of the head and body are assumed. Positional vertigo is a relatively common form of dizziness. The vertigo occurs particularly in the supine positions—i.e., head hanging or head to the left or right, and sometimes looking up or twisting the neck may elicit this vertigo. It is typically transient. Positional vertigo is distinctive in that it occurs in the recumbent positions. Where we use either the term positional nystagmus or positional vertigo, it is inferred that both vertigo and nystagmus are present, and nystagmus must accompany the vertigo for the vertigo to be considered the positional type. (See also Chapter 4 ["Examinations"] and the clinical section [Part II] of this volume.)

Number of Attacks

It is important to ascertain if there was only one attack or multiple attacks of dizziness. Meniere's disease is characterized by multiple attacks and the attacks tend to occur in clusters. The intervals at which attacks occur and the circumstances may help in the diagnosis. For instance, positional vertigo occurs in the supine position. Meniere's disease is intermittent with long spells of freedom from attacks. A progression in severity is found with otologic infection such as suppuration involving the labyrinth. A gradual progression without severe attacks is found with acoustic neurinoma. A single attack of vertigo is found with acute toxic labyrinthitis, the viral type, and vascular lesions. A prolonged single attack occurs in vestibular neuronitis.

Onset

It is important to determine whether the symptom appeared abruptly or was gradual in onset; whether a single episode of severe dizziness or vertigo was followed by a slow and gradual recovery; whether the recovery was complete or if there were residuals. Mawson has classified the onset into the following categories:

1. Sudden Semicircular Canal Failure

a. Complete: Acute unilateral failure provides the most extreme clinical example of vestibular disturbance. The patient is at first totally disabled, unable to rise from the ground where he had fallen, and disinclined to move at all for the accentuation of vertigo and vomiting that movement provokes. Immobility may continue for several days and is accompanied by gross nystagmus with the slow component to the affected side. Adaptation to the loss of one labyrinth is slow but usually enables the patient to regain his feet by the end of three weeks. It rarely lasts more than three weeks. Vomiting generally ceases within three days and the vertigo gradually subsides together with nystagmus, so that during the second week the patient is ready to sit up in bed and perhaps do some reading. Ultimately, the patient is little affected by the failure of his labyrinth although he may always be prone to momentary vertigo on sudden movement.

b. Incomplete: Partial or temporary loss of labyrinthine function is accompanied by less severe clinical manifestations. The disablement may not amount to more than a sharp attack of vertigo and vomiting accompanied by a desire to lie down or sit in a chair for a few hours, or a sudden transient dizziness with nausea accompanied by the necessity to pause and hold on to something. If the patient is walking he may lurch violently to one side or even fall.

2. Gradual

Patients are sometimes encountered in whom caloric testing reveals impairment of vestibular function without previous symptoms having occurred to occasion the seeking of medical advice. When one vestibular end organ or nerve is gradually involved by a pathologic process, if this involvement is sufficiently gradual adaptation my take place without the subject being conscious of any loss of vestibular function and without apparent disturbance in balance.

A sudden disturbance can be due to a vascular accident, an acute viral or toxic process, as well as an episodic attack of endolymphatic hydrops. Vertigo may awaken a patient in the middle of the night, and Meniere's disease, positional vertigo, or vascular occlusions may do this. Attacks early in the morning or on first arising may denote vertebral-basilar artery insufficiency. Vertigo with menstrual periods may be due to hypotension, retention of fluids, or endocrine disturbance. Occurrence of vertigo during a meal may indicate dental malocclusion, while the occurrence of vertigo after a meal has been related to gallbladder trouble or food allergy. A head-bent position, as in a cook or a dentist, or after anteflexion of the head on a large pillow may precipitate attacks. This type is prone to occur with the so-called "cervical" vertigo.

Falling

Lateral pulsion or falling with attacks is usually significant of a labyrinthine lesion. The falling is always toward the side of the diseased labyrinth. Sudden falling attacks have been reported due to utricular stimulation. Falling may also be due to a lesion of the rhombencephalon. In basilar artery disease the patient sometimes falls to one side and sometimes the other side as the basilar artery is a single artery which supplies both sides. True vestibular vertigo is associated with pastpointing in the plane of but in the direction opposite the direction of vertigo. There is no pastpointing in nonrotatory dizziness. Lateral pulsion when walking with the eyes closed is a sort of generalized pastpointing.

If the patient loses his balance in the dark or while swimming, it indicates a bilateral loss of vestibular function.

Duration of Individual Attacks of Dizziness

The length of each attack can be differentiated according to Alpers' classification: (1) transient attacks lasting moments; (2) paroxysmal attacks lasting hours to a few days; or (3) continuous dizziness lasting weeks.

Transient or transitory attacks may last from a few seconds to minutes. Transient attacks are encountered in practice much more commonly than more lengthy attacks. After a transient attack of dizziness, the patient may require rest for many minutes before he is completely recovered. Transient attacks can occur with almost any form of dizziness—i.e., peripheral, central, medical, or psychogenic—and are not diagnostic in themselves. Transient attacks are often initiated by change in posture or movement. The transitory postural dizziness which occurs when the patient arises from bed in the morning or arises from a sitting position or which occurs when the head is raised is not specifically helpful in diagnosis, for it seems to arise from a wide variety of conditions. This condition is often ascribed to vascular abnormality without definite proof. The postural vertigo which occurs when the patient assumes a supine or lateral position is more significant. This postural vertigo is discussed in more detail under that heading. Postural hypotension is ruled out if symptoms occur when the patient is recumbent.

Paroxysmal attacks are exemplified by endolymphatic hydrops. This condition is characterized by recurring paroxysms of vertigo, although transient attacks may also occur. Direct trauma, vascular occlusions, middle ear infections, or mastoiditis involving the labyrinth can also produce paroxysms of vertigo. Lesions in the brainstem involving the vestibular nuclei, such as tumors, multiple sclerosis, or thrombosis of the posterior-inferior cerebellar artery can induce paroxysms of vertigo. Other central causes of paroxysmal vertigo include syphilitic meningitis involving the vestibular nerve (a rare cause) and lesions in the vicinity of the vestibular nuclei causing Bruns' syndrome. The most common diagnosis with a single paroxysm of vertigo is the condition popularly called acute toxic labyrinthitis.

The complaint of continuous dizziness usually indicates one of three things:

1. Most commonly the patient means that he has ataxia or staggering.
2. Continuous dizziness may be psychogenic in derivation. The psychogenic constitute the most numerous subgroup among our continuous cases.
3. A continuous dizziness is found in some intracranial conditions.

If a single attack continues for more than two weeks, we should rule out a central or psychogenic origin.

After a severe crisis of vertigo subsides, or after a labyrinthectomy, sudden movement of the head may elicit dizziness for months. Chronic dizziness, in its slightest degree, may be present only on movement.

SITE OF ORIGIN AND MANIFESTATIONS OF DIZZINESS

Dizziness has been ascribed to disturbances in proprioception, central portions of the nervous system, statokinetic system, circulation, systemic medical conditions, foci of infection, and the psyche. Some cases are ascribed to the endocrine system, allergy, dental malocclusion, cervical pathology, or ocular pathology.

Severe vertigo usually limits the investigation to the statokinetic system—usually the labyrinth but also the vestibular nerve or vestibular nuclei and their tracts in the brain stem may be implicated. From a numerical viewpoint, severe vertigo with nausea and vomiting is in most cases due to the end organ. The closer the lesion is to the peripheral labyrinth, the more active tends to be the vertigo, and it is said that stimulation of the end organ produces a more marked reaction than irritation of the vestibular nuclei in most instances. Vertigo may be due to hyper- or hypofunction, destruction or stimulation of the labyrinth. Mechanisms of production include inflammation, hydrops, tumors, disturbances of circulation, and injury. Several factors may cooperate to initiate the vertigo. In some people, there is a predisposition to vertigo so that relatively minor lesions may incite dizziness.

William House reported that 83 per cent of the cases in his series of acoustic neuroma at some time during their history had prodromal symptoms related to the vestibular system. The symptoms included a sensation of unsteadiness, especially with turning the head suddenly or with turning in bed from one position to another or with bending over or getting up suddenly. This unsteadiness seemed to persist over a long period of time and, even though it fluctuated somewhat, was more or less constantly present once it started. However, in some of these patients, the symptoms would appear for a time and then disappear, only to reappear again. A few patients had episodic vertigo, not unlike that seen with Meniere's disease. Vestibular symptoms of any type were absent throughout the history in some patients. Severe vertigo, associated with nausea and vomiting, is rarely found with an acoustic neuroma, and the vestibular symptoms of acoustic neuroma cause far less distress on the whole than those in Meniere's disease.

Elliott feels that all patients with true vertigo have an organic disorder rather than a functional disorder although Sloan reports otherwise.

Fainting

Various distinctly different sensations are described by patients as dizziness; notable among these are blackouts, lightheadedness, or faintness. The term lightheadedness should be reserved for faintness, weakness, or blackout without sensation of motion. Faintness may be occasionally associated with severe attacks of vertigo but syncope, rarely if ever, occurs in labyrinthine disease. On the other hand, faintness or blackout is highly indicative of a medical, neurologic, or psychogenic ailment rather than labyrinthine disease. Faintness may be described by the patient as dizziness, but is easily differentiated on detailed questioning. The sensations of giddiness or lightheadedness where there is no sensation of motion indicate nonlabyrinthine disease. Engel points out that the most important differential point between fainting and vertigo is the increase in symptoms which occurs on movement of the head in vertigo. Also, nystagmus is not associated with fainting.

Episodes of Unconsciousness

When there is clouding of consciousness, convulsive disorders such as psychomotor seizures, petit mal, and grand mal should be considered. A period of sleepiness follows a typical epileptic attack. Loss of consciousness with an attack is rarely, if ever, found in labyrinthine vertigo. An unconscious episode may also signify an intracranial space taking or vascular lesion, and Bruns syndrome is one example.

Ataxia

Many patients complain of dizziness when they mean staggering. When a patient states he is dizzy continuously, he often means that he staggers whenever he walks. This has a distinctly different connotation than dizziness, for staggering, as the sole complaint, often indicates a neurologic condition. Some impairment of balance accompanies an attack of dizziness and is an integral part of the picture but ceases when the dizziness ceases. Ataxia, loss of balance, or staggering between attacks of vertigo or dizziness arouses the suspicion of a lesion outside the labyrinth. This unsteadiness is accentuated by arising or turning. Such unsteadiness or ataxia may be present in brain stem lesions, diseases of the cerebellum, diseases of the proprioceptive system, psychogenic ailments, or complete destruction of both statokinetic labyrinths. Unsteadiness is also ascribed to cardiovascular diseases such as arteriosclerosis, hypertension, and chronic hypotension. Although sensations of dysequilibrium may be caused by aberrations of the proprioceptive and ocular mechanisms, these symptoms are not commonly confused with the vertigo and dizziness which occurs with the disturbances in function of the vestibular apparatus. The patient is unsteady on walking, but the complaint is not present in the sitting or recumbent posture. The vestibular symptoms caused by an acoustic neuroma usually consist of gradually increasing unsteadiness or episodes of unsteadiness.

Fullness in the Ear

Fullness, stuffiness, or pressure in the ear is a typical complaint of patients with Meniere's disease. Alfaro reports that fullness in the ear is a very frequent complaint, and furthermore it is one of the earliest complaints with Meniere's disease. Fullness of the ear is reported with other conditions. Also, William House reported its presence in 10 per cent of his cases of acoustic neuroma.

Hearing Loss

Hearing loss (and tinnitus) may indicate a labyrinthine or eighth nerve etiology for the dizziness. However, the hearing loss may be due to an unrelated condition so hearing tests are mandatory (See Chapter 4, "Examinations").

Tinnitus and Vertigo

Duncan Hatton

Tinnitus is a sensation of noise in the ears or in the head which originates autogenously.[1] When the vertiginous patient complains of tinnitus, it is not unreasonable to suppose that the cause of the syndrome lies somewhere in the stato-acoustical organ or the eighth cranial nerve and/or its central connections. Conversely, vertigo resulting from diseases of the brain or brain stem is rarely, if ever, accompanied by tinnitus.

Tinnitus may be divided into two groups according to the mode of origin. The extrinsic or vibratory tinnitus is that which is produced by actual vibrations of the structures in and about the ears, head, and neck. These vibrations are transmitted to the cochlea and are received in the auditory cortex as sound. These vibrations may be produced by the flow of blood through the vessels, the contractions of muscles, the movements of the joints, and the opening and closing of the eustachian tubes. The second type of tinnitus is the intrinsic or nonvibratory which is thought to be due to irritations or destruction of the auditory neural elements (cochlea, auditory nerve and its central connections). The exact mechanism of this nonvibratory tinnitus is not thoroughly understood, but it seems likely that the irritations or the destruction of the neural elements produces a 'firing" of some of the cochlear hair cells or of some of the neurones of the auditory nerve which produces a sensation of sound in the auditory cortex. This "phantom" sensation is somewhat analogous to that which is often experienced by the recent amputee who complains of pain or dysesthesia in a member which is no longer a part of his body.

LOCATION

Tinnitus may be reported as being heard in one ear or both (tinnitus aurium) or in the head (tinnitus capitum). Some patients will state that the noise is in both ears and head. A definite location by the patient of the tinnitus to one ear, especially if a hearing loss can be demonstrated on that side, would indicate that the vertigo is caused by a lesion of the ipsalateral stato-acoustical organ or nerve. If the tinnitus, on the other hand, cannot be localized to one or both ears but is heard, indefinitely, in the head, the diagnostic value is reduced.

DURATION

Tinnitus may be constant or intermittent. Even the so-called constant tinnitus may become inaudible at times, but these remissions do not last very long. Constant tinnitus is more often than not associated with vertigo of inner ear and/or auditory nerve origin. The intermittent tinnitus, on the other hand, is more likely to be of external or middle ear origin thus, the tinnitus, and vertigo, from impacted cerumen lasts only until the offending foreign matter is removed. Rhythmic tinnitus usually results from the pulsations of the blood in the vessels and may be constant as long as the disturbance that is causing it remains.

SOUND FREQUENCY CONTENT

Most patients attempt to describe their tinnitus by comparing it to a sound that is common to both themselves and the examiner. Thus, it may be likened to the sound of crickets, the wind in the trees, the sigh of a seashell, a motor hum, a bell, the escape of steam, and many other common things. It may be said, as a general rule, that tinnitus with predominant high-frequency characteristics is of inner ear or eighth nerve origin while that with low-frequency tones is from a middle ear or external ear dysfunction. Thus, the tinnitus that accompanies such conductive problems as otosclerosis, acute and chronic inflammation of the middle ear, impacted cerumen, to name a few, will usually be low pitched; the tinnitus of presbyacusis, head trauma with injury to the auditory neural elements, drug intoxication, noise trauma and other sensorineural lesions will be of a predominantly high pitch. Some recent investigations in which the pitch of the tinnitus of many patients with various disorders of the hearing apparatus was matched against tones of known frequency content support this view.[2-3] The tinnitus that accompanied conductive hearing losses was found to have a median frequency of 490 cps with a range of 90 to 1450 cps. The tinnitus of the sensorineural group had a median frequency of 3900 cps and a range of 545 to 7500 cps. An exception to this finding was the frequency characteristics of the tinnitus that accompanied Meniere's disease. While this syndrome is classified as a sensorineural disease, the frequency content of the tinnitus was found to be confined to the same low frequency range as that associated with conductive hearing losses. The Meniere's group showed a median frequency of 320 cps and a range of 90 to 900 cps.[3]

Meniere's Syndrome, while not a common condition in the accepted sense of the word, is seen, at one time or another, by almost every physician. The tinnitus may precede any other sign of the disorder by many years or may appear only with the first attack of the vertigo. It is usually continuous, but its loudness may swell and diminish. It may or may not increase during the attack.[5]

Tinnitus that precedes or accompanies a slowly progressing unilateral deafness should alert one to the possibility of an acoustic nerve tumor. These may be the only symptoms for months or years although vertigo, dizziness, and giddiness can be an early complaint.[5] In Scott's series of 35 cases of acoustic nerve tumors, he found one patient who had unilateral deafness and tinnitus for 25 years and four others whose symptoms had preceded operation by 11 - 15 years.[5] Tinnitus, however, is not as frequent a symptom as is impaired hearing. A review of 140 cases of acoustic neurinomas by Erickson et al. disclosed that 35 had no tinnitus but only 4 were without some hearing impairment.[4]

Tinnitus that accompanies vertigo should be considered carefully, and while it must be emphasized that the character of the noise will not in every case provide sufficient data for a precise diagnosis, it will, in many instances, be a useful adjunct to the information secured from the other procedures detailed in this volume.

REFERENCES

1. Erickson, L. S., Sorenson, G. D., and McGavran, M. H.: Laryngoscope 75:601, 1965.
2. Graham, J. T., and Newby, H. A.: Arch. Otolaryng. 75:162, 1962.
3. Nodar, R. H., and Graham, J. T.: Arch. Otolaryng. 82:28, 1965.
4. Scott, M.: Arch. Otolaryng. 79:139, 1964.
5. Williams, H. L.: Meniere's Disease. Springfield, Ill., Charles C Thomas 1952.
6. Winston, J.: Med. Clin. N. Amer.: 40:1781, 1956.

Neurological History and Past Medical History

Martin Spector and J. U. Toglia

NEUROLOGICAL HISTORY

Certain features help to distinguish vertigo of peripheral origin from that of central origin. The vertigo associated with lesions of the central nervous system is usually not paroxysmal but rather continuous and of longer duration than the vertigo of peripheral origin. It is more a subjective sensation than a rotatory hallucination of movement, and it is not influenced by positions of the head. Patients afflicted by central vertigo have no hearing difficulties, unless the acoustic nerves are involved. Very rarely does brain stem involvement alone cause deafness. Autonomic disturbances are mild or absent, but the patients frequently have some of the following symptoms: headaches, disturbances of consciousness, visual disturbances, diplopia, dysarthria, dysphagia, paresthesia, especially numbness of the face or around the mouth, ataxia, tremor, weakness of the extremities, and hoarseness.

Headaches

Many patients with dizziness also complain of headaches, and the complaint of headache arouses the fear of intracranial disease. In our series, occipital headaches were particularly common among the cases of intracranial disease. The term vertiginous migraine has been applied to a combination of migraine and vertigo; it seems to be an uncommon syndrome. Hypertension is a common cause for throbbing headaches, but dull throbbing headaches have also been found with hypoglycemia. In the obese with headaches and dizziness, hyperostosis frontalis interna may occasionally be found. Frequent or almost constant dull headaches may accompany hypothyroidism. Head injury and cerebral arteriosclerosis are other conditions characterized by a combination of headache plus dizziness. In Meniere's disease, patients may describe an ache in the mastoid region, but a sense of pressure in the ear is much more common.

PAST MEDICAL HISTORY

Inquiry should be always made for history of head trauma, infections of the central nervous system, chronic and acute intoxications, lues, migraine, epilepsy, cerebrovascular diseases, endocrine and metabolic diseases, and familial degenerative diseases. Any coincidental condition at the onset of the dizziness should be noted.

It is pertinent to inquire about the use of tobacco, past or present ear infections, mental ailments, allergy, problems in dental bite, and problems in the neck.

The following list of questions is suggested:

Does the room turn?

Are there fainting spells or periods of unconsciousness?

Do you stagger when you walk?

Date of onset (with description of the initial attack and number and frequency of attacks)?

Does any other complaint precede the dizziness?

Do nausea and vomiting accompany the attack?

Under what circumstances do attacks occur?

Do they occur after a meal?

Time of day of the vertigo?

Does the vertigo follow menstrual periods?

Does the occupation have any relationship to the vertigo? Has there been exposure to heat, fumes, paint, poisons, tobacco, or alcohol?

Past history of head trauma?

Does diet play a part? Does the patient consume excessive salt?

What medications has he taken?

Does the disorder seem to affect the ears? Is there a sense of pressure?

Does the dizziness occur on lying down?

Does the dizziness occur on first arising in the morning?

Does the dizziness occur in certain positions?

Is tinnitus or deafness present?

To the patient, dizziness is serious and a careful history and examination is imperative. Nothing is more annoying to such a patient than to have the complaint treated lightly.

REFERENCES

1. Alpers, B. J.: Vertigo and Dizziness. New York, Grune & Stratton, 1958.
2. Cogan, D. G.: Neurology of the Ocular Muscles. 2nd edit. Springfield, Ill., Charles C Thomas, 1956.
3. DeWeese, D.D.: Dizziness, An Evaluation and Classification. Springfield, Ill., Charles C Thomas, 1954.
4. Engel, G. L.: Fainting—Physiological and Psychological Considerations. Springfield, Ill., Charles C Thomas, 1950.
5. House, W. F.: Transtemporal bone microsurgical removal of acoustic neuromas (monograph). Arch. Otolaryn. 80: 1964.
6. Kane, C. A., and Strong, M. S.: Dizziness and vertigo, diagnosis and treatment. Med. Clin. N. Amer. 1229-1244, 1957.
7. Mawson, S.: Diseases of the Ear. Baltimore, Md., Williams and Wilkins Co., 1963.
8. Portmann, G.: Diseases of the Ears, Nose, and Throat, Baltimore, Md., Williams and Wilkins Co., 1951.
9. Rachlis, B.: Meniere's syndrome, a proposed classification. Arch. Otolaryng. 52:373-379, 1950.
10. Spiegel, E. A., and Sommer, B.: Neurology of the eye, ear, nose, and throat. New York, Grune & Stratton, 1944.
11. Weiss, S.: The treatment of vertigo and syncope. J.A.M.A. 118:529-535 (Feb.) 1942.
12. Williams, H. L.: Meniere's disease. Springfield, Ill., Charles C Thomas, 1952.

CHAPTER 4

Examinations

Spontaneous Nystagmus

G. O. Proud

A search for the presence or absence of spontaneous nystagmus is an integral part of the otoneurological examination. Spontaneous nystagmus may be of the pendular type in which both components have the same speed, or the presence of a slow and fast component may place it in the category of jerk nystagmus. The former usually stems from faulty central vision and is actually a searching effort to keep all areas of the visual field in view. Pendular nystagmus of a fine and rapid type is seen in some individuals who work in poorly lighted mines. It also may be of congenital origin, and a few persons can produce it voluntarily. Spasmus nutans is another example of the pendular type and is associated with oscillations of the head in the same plane in which the nystagmus occurs.

Jerk nystagmus originates from peripheral (labyrinth), intermediate (VIII nerve trunk), or central nervous system disease as a rule; but it may be of congenital origin. Ocular muscle weakness may be responsible for it as well. If, for example, a weakness of the left lateral rectus muscle exists and the eyes are intentionally brought into left lateral gaze, they will wander slowly to the primary position due to the superior strength of the medial rectus muscle. The subject realizes, after a time, that his gaze has shifted, and the eyes are forcibly and quickly brought back into lateral gaze. This type of jerk nystagmus is referred to as muscle paretic nystagmus.

Nystagmus is classified according to its severity into grades I, II, and III. When it can be provoked only by conjugate gaze in the direction of the quick component the term "nystagmus of the first degree" applies. The designation "second degree" implies that nystagmus is present during forward gaze as well as during gaze toward the direction of the quick component. When nystagmus is apparent while conjugate gaze is directed toward the side of the quick component, straight ahead, and toward the side of the slow component, it is called nystagmus of the third degree.

Nystagmus is also categorized as vertical, oblique, horizontal, or rotatory according to the plane in which the eye movements occur. "Frequency" is a term used to indicate the number of eyeball oscillations per unit time, and the term "amplitude" applies to the distance of each excursion of the eyes. Accordingly, a given nystagmus may be said to be coarse or fine. The length of time which nystagmus persists is called the duration, and the terms unidirectional and multidirectional indicate that the oscillations appear in one or several directions of gaze.

Proper evaluation calls for observation of the eyes while the patient looks to the right, left, upward, downward, and in the primary position. The last is important, for pendular nystagmus may exhibit a jerk pattern when the subject's eyes leave the primary position. Pendular nystagmus in the primary position may be invisible unless the eyes are examined with an ophthalmoscope which affords 13 power magnification. The examiner must instruct the patient to follow his finger with his eyes, and the finger is moved to the new positions slowly in order to avoid saccadic movements. A few flicks of nystagmus frequently are seen in many individuals in pronounced lateral gaze. This is the normal phenomenon of accommodation and suggests no disease or localization. It is sometimes referred to as end-point nystagmus. The physician should note whether the nystagmus is unidirectional or multidirectional. The direction of nystagmus is named by the direction of the quick component, for it is most easily seen. However, it is the slow component which is initiated by the labyrinth, whereas the fast phase is probably of central origin.

UNIDIRECTIONAL SPONTANEOUS NYSTAGMUS

Unidirectional nystagmus is usually of peripheral origin, occurs in the horizontal plane, and the quick component is toward the uninvolved side. It is usually accompanied by hypoactivity or absence of a caloric response. For example, a subject with Meniere's Disease involving the right ear will show a left nystagmus. The same may be said of the recipient of right-sided inner ear surgery or injury. Usually the nystagmus is enhanced when the gaze is directed toward the side of the quick component. Indeed, it may show itself only in this direction of gaze. Such unidirectional nystagmus is transient and disappears when healing occurs or the end-organ dies. Since unidirectional nystagmus ordinarily is of peripheral origin, any lesion which injures or destroys the labyrinth may be responsible for its genesis. Along with the causes previously listed one must include head trauma, nonspecific virus infections of the inner ear, and purulent labyrinthitis. The nystagmus following unilateral labyrinthectomy disappears after about six days, and the subject again responds normally to body rotation. If the second labyrinth is destroyed nystagmus reappears. This is called the compensatory nystagmus of Bechterew,[1] and it may be explained by the assumption that the vestibular nuclei assume the resting discharge of the destroyed labyrinth.

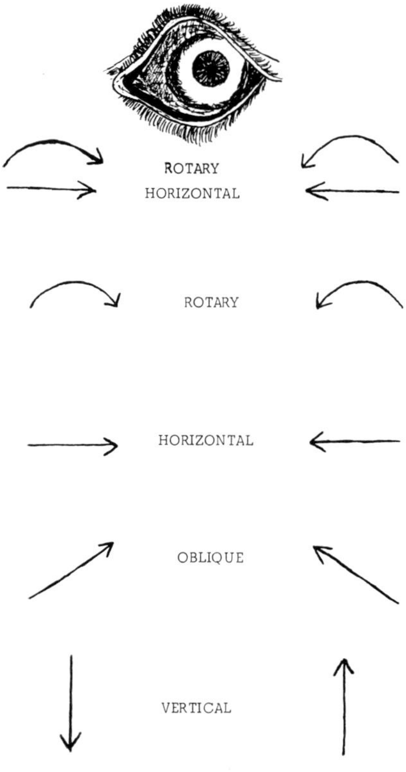

FIG. 1. Forms of nystagmus.

When the caloric test is normal, a unidirectional nystagmus may be of central origin.

MULTIDIRECTIONAL SPONTANEOUS NYSTAGMUS

When nystagmus is present in multiple directions of gaze, central involvement should be suspected. Such a nystagmus may be accounted for by a lesion anywhere in the brain. It even may be supratentorial in location, for the entire vestibulocerebellar complex is regulated by the corticopontine cerebellar system. As a rule, however, multidirectional nystagmus speaks for localization to the posterior fossa wherein is contained the bulk of the vestibulocerebellar units such as the vestibular nuclei and the vestibulocerebellar interrelation.

The quick component of nystagmus of central origin is usually toward the side of the lesion, and a normal postcaloric response is the rule. Unlike nystagmus of peripheral origin, central nystagmus is permanent and is less apt to be accompanied by true vertigo, although ataxia may be evident.

Retractile Nystagmus

An in-and-out nystagmus is a rare one, and it is usually associated with paralysis of upward gaze. Midbrain lesions are the usual cause.[2]

Oculomotor Asthenia

Since the cerebellar hemisphere adds the stamp of smoothness to muscular activity initiated elsewhere, a hemisphere lesion may cause oculomotor asthenia. No quick component is seen nor is the eye movement rhythmical. A nonsensical searching motion of the eyes is observed in most directions of gaze.

POSTROTATIONAL NYSTAGMUS

The testing of the labyrinth by rotation of the subject is of limited value since any rotation which affects one canal system will inevitably stimulate the other as well. Fluorens[3] showed that the eyes move in the plane of the canal stimulated, and slow component is in the direction of endolymphatic fluid motion. If, therefore, a patient is placed in a rotating chair with the horizontal canal in a position whereby it is maximally stimulated, rotated to the right 10 revolutions in 20 seconds and stopped abruptly, the endolymph will continue to move to the right. The eyes will move to the right (slow component), and the nystagmus (quick component) will beat toward the left. The nystagmus persists for as long as it takes the cupula to return to the summit of the crista ampullaris, and the average time is 30 seconds after the cessation of rotation. Equipment for the test is bulky, and the information gained by the practitioner from the test is restricted since unilateral canal testing is impossible.

REFERENCES

1. von Bechterew, W.: Durchschneidung des nervus acusticus. Arch. Ges. Physiol. 30:312, 1883.
2. Koerber, H.: Trois observations de mouvements de retraction de bulbe (Nystagmus retractorius). Clinique Ophth., p. 147. Abs. Jahresb. Ophth. 34:683, 1903.
3. Flourens, J. P.: Recherches Experimentales sur les Proprietes et les Functions du Systeme Nerveux, dans les Animaux Vertebres, Edit. 2, Paris, J. B. Balliere, 1844.

Positional Nystagmus and Ear, Nose, and Throat Examination

Martin Spector

POSITIONAL NYSTAGMUS AND VERTIGO

The examination for positional nystagmus is conducted as shown in Figure 1. To simplify examination, positional nystagmus is sought with the patient's eyes in the second degree position—i.e., with the eyes looking straight ahead. The patient is placed in a sitting position on a table or couch and is instructed to gaze directly forward. Spontaneous nystagmus is first sought. The patient is told that he will be placed in various positions and that it is imperative to keep the eyes open at all times and announce the presence of any vertigo. The patient's head is held by the examiner who stands behind the patient. The patient is placed in a supine position with the head hanging over the edge of the table. He is laid down quickly within three seconds. If nystagmus does not occur within 60 seconds, the patient is raised to the sitting position. Then he is placed with his

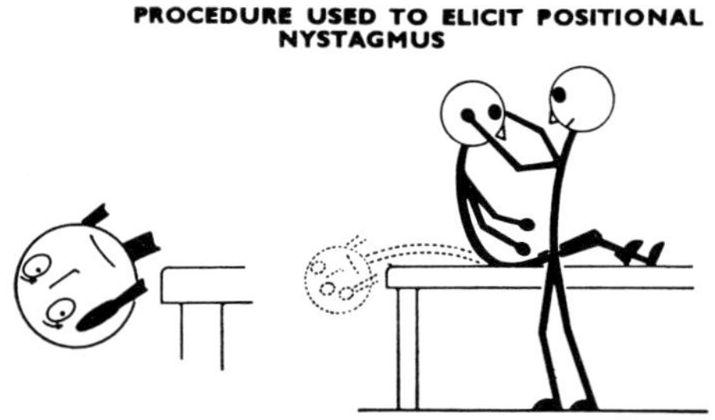

FIG. 1. Procedure used to elicit positional nystagmus. (From Cawthorne, Dix, Hallpike, and Hood: The investigation of vestibular function. Brit. Med. Bull. 12:141, 1956. By courtesy of the British Council, Publisher.)

head hanging over the edge of the table and face directed to the left (Fig. 2). If nystagmus is not observed within 60 seconds, he is returned to the sitting position. Then he is placed in the supine position with the head hanging over the edge of the table and the face directed to the right. In a positive response, there is often a period of latency lasting from 2 to 10 seconds before vertigo and nystagmus appear. If nystagmus is noted with the patient in any position, that position is held until the nystagmus subsides. However, if the nystagmus continues for more than 60 seconds, it is considered as persistent. The transitory type is that which lasts less than 60 seconds. In the vast majority of cases, vertigo accompanies the nystagmus. In some cases, positional nystagmus may fail to appear if a change of position is made slowly, but if made rapidly, nystagmus will appear. If a slow change of position fails to elicit a response (in the presence of a positive history), the position can be changed more rapidly. If there is a positive history and one examination is negative, the test is repeated after a delay. Positional nystagmus may not recur at every test. It may be necessary to test on different days. If nystagmus appears, the patient is returned to the upright position, rested, and placed again in the same position that provoked the nystagmus to determine whether it will recur or is fatigable. The three positions described seem the most informative. Other positions, such as looking up or stooping, are only used when the patient states that they cause vertigo. The straight supine position, with head hanging over the edge of the table, is the position which most commonly elicits positive findings (Fig. 3).

When spontaneous nystagmus is present, the nystagmus may be intensified by brisk

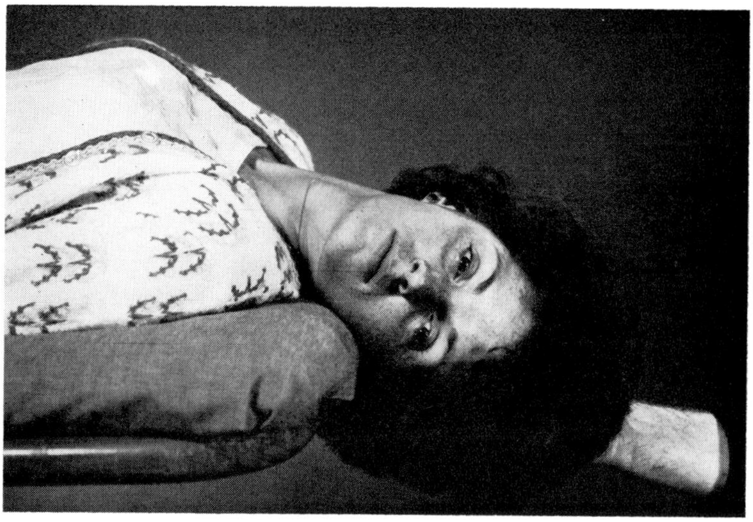

FIG. 2. Test for positional nystagmus and vertigo in head to the left position. Head supported by examiner's hand.

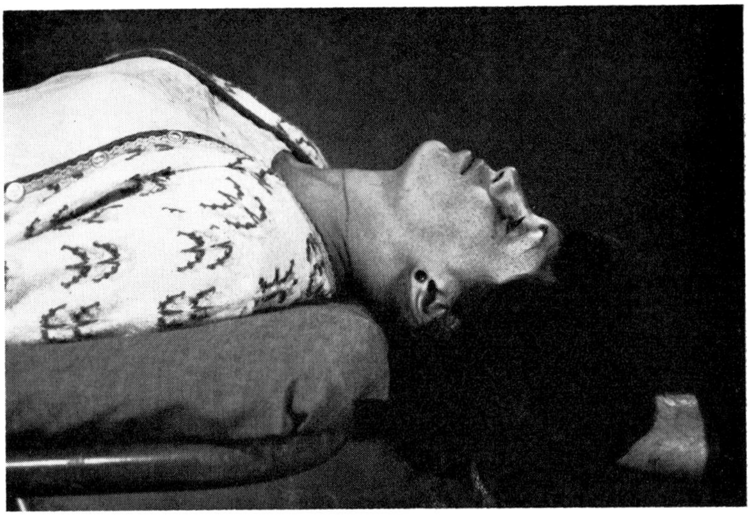

Fig. 3. Test for positional nystagmus in the supine head hanging position. Head supported by examiner's hand.

movement of the head, as by head shaking or posture testing. Rapid head shaking may also bring out a latent spontaneous nystagmus. A spontaneous nystagmus may in some cases be altered or reversed in direction depending upon the position of the head. Most observers include as positional nystagmus spontaneous nystagmus which changes its form or intensity in certain positions of the head. A broad definition for positional nystagmus is one which is in some way clearly altered by the assumption of another position of the head (Lindsay and Perlman). In contrast, spontaneous nystagmus is present whatever the position of the head; i.e., it continues to be present in similar intensity regardless of alteration in position of the head.

Frenzel glasses magnify, aid observation of the eyes, and prevent inhibition by fixation. (Frenzel glasses are spectacles with plus 20 diopter lenses. See Fig. 4.) They are helpful but not essential.

Positional nystagmus may be in any direction, i.e., horizontal, rotatory, vertical, or may be so tumultuous that the observer cannot judge. The nystagmus has been reported to change direction. Often when a patient is brought from the supine to the sitting position there is a recurrence of vertigo. There may be nystagmus in the opposite direction, the same direction, or no nystagmus after rising to the sitting position. With persistent forms of positional nystagmus, the position of the head seems the determining factor. For transitory positional nystagmus, movement of the head to a new position also plays an important part—often a dominating one. Rarely nystagmus may appear only after the position is maintained for more than one minute.

Jan Stahle, by electronystagmography, reports that there may be a secondary reversal of nystagmus. That is, if the patient's head is held in the critical position after the paroxysm has disappeared, new nystagmus beats in the opposite direction may sometimes ap-

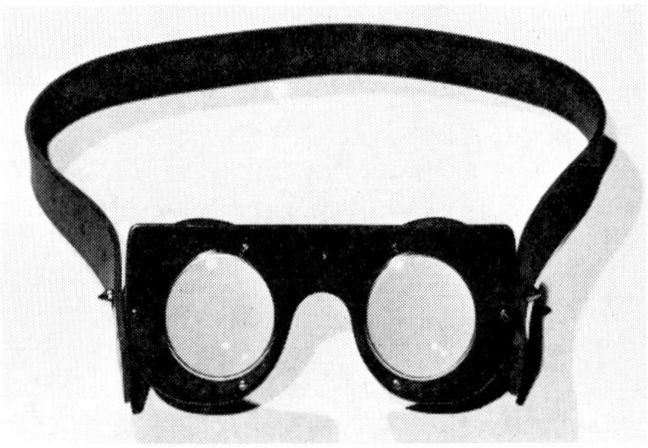

Fig. 4. Frenzel glasses.

pear. Among 55 cases, a secondary reversal was recorded in 15 cases. Between the paroxysm and the secondary period, there is a brief quiescent interval of 5 to 10 seconds. The nystagmus during the second period is usually much weaker in intensity than the primary paroxysm but is of considerably greater duration and may be persistent. In the secondary nystagmus, the patient does not experience vertigo.

Value

Since the examination is short and simple and can be performed in the office, positional nystagmus and vertigo should be sought in every patient with vertigo. It is especially important because so frequently the remainder of the examination is negative. Nylen states that positional nystagmus must be considered to be one of the surest, most objective, and most easily demonstrated signs of disturbance in the human vestibular system. Hugh Barber found positional nystagmus in 18.8 per cent of all his dizzy patients.

Classification

A. Nylen

Nylen's nomenclature represented an early classification. He classified positional nystagmus into three types:

Type I—The direction of the nystagmus changes with different positions of the head.

Type II—The direction of the nystagmus remains constant in different positions. If it is observed in different head positions, it is stronger in a particular position.

Type III—The nystagmus is irregular, characterized by variations in its behavior. It is thus sometimes direction changing, sometimes direction fixed, and sometimes changes its direction in the same head position. This type includes all forms of positional nystagmus which cannot be classified in Type I or Type II.

B. Aschan

Aschan's classification: This takes note of the duration of nystagmus:

Type I—The nystagmus is persistent, direction changing.

Type II—The nystagmus is persistent, direction fixed.

Type III—All varieties of transitory positional nystagmus.

C. British Classification

This has been described by the English authors Dix, Hallpike, and Cawthorne, and it will be the classification primarily used in our discussion. It divides positional vertigo into two groups:

I. Peripheral Type—manifested by:

a. Latency: There is an interval of 2 to 10 seconds between the time the new head position is assumed and the nystagmus jerks begin.

b. Limited duration: The nystagmus and vertigo stop spontaneously in a short time, i.e., within 30 seconds and often within 10 seconds without change of position.

c. Fatigability: The reaction is less apparent on successive repetitions of the test, and the nystagmus fails to appear by the third or fourth time the critical position is assumed. A rest period is necessary before the positional nystagmus may be demonstrated again.

d. Incidence: This group constitutes almost 90 per cent of the total.

e. Fixed Nystagmus: The nystagmus appears only in one head position, i.e., the left lateral position or possibly also the supine head hanging position. The direction of the nystagmus is only to one side, i.e., to the left side. The direction of the nystagmus is usually in the direction of the undermost ear.

II. Central Type

a. There is no latent period; the nystagmus begins immediately on assuming the critical position.

b. Persistence: The nystagmus continues for more than one minute and may continue as long as the critical position is maintained.

c. No fatigability: The nystagmus reappears each time the critical position is assumed.

d. The incidence is about 10 to 15 per cent of the total of cases of positional nystagmus.

e. Direction changing: The nystagmus changes direction with changes of position in the head.

f. Occasionally vertigo may be present.

g. This type should lead one to be highly suspicious of a central lesion.

D. Site of Origin

A further classification may be attempted on the basis of site of origin.

1. Peripheral labyrinth.
2. Neck.
3. Intracranial.

SIGNIFICANCE

According to Nylen, positional nystagmus may sometimes appear in normals as weakly pronounced, inconsistent vertical nystagmus, directed down toward the chin, when the patient's head is in the hanging position. A vertical nystagmus which is transient and fatigable is not likely to be significant or central in origin. However, a very marked vertical nystagmus is found with supratentorial tumors. Normals may show coarse nystagmic beats during movement with eyes open—a form of optokinetic nystagmus. With these exceptions, positional nystagmus has been generally accepted as pathological and taken to indicate a disturbance in the vestibular system. Positional nystagmus established an organic disturbance as opposed to a psychogenic disturbance.

Fernandez and Lindsay state that "there is no variety of positional nystagmus which per se may be evaluated with absolute certainty as a sign of localization." Changes in the peripheral labyrinth may cause positional nystagmus not only of the direction-fixed but also of the direction-changing type. In the absence of obvious end-organ disease, persistent and nonfatigable positional nystagmus, especially if the accompanying vertigo is slight or absent, is considered good evidence of a central etiology. Positional nystagmus of the so-called benign paroxysmal type, showing latency, fatigability, and evanescence, is usually ascribed to a peripheral lesion. Even so, Riesco MacClure found this specific type of positional nystagmus in a case of surgically proven astrocytoma of the inferior vermis of the cerebellum. Dizziness on head movement without nystagmus has been ascribed to trauma, foci of infection, fatigue, neck lesions, or hypometabolism. It also occurs for some days or weeks at the termination of an attack of positional nystagmus. Most commonly circulatory deficiency is incriminated. The postural dizziness which accompanies emotional stress, cardiovascular problems, and carotid sinus syndrome is not accompanied by nystagmus. This dizziness occurs particularly when the patient arises from bed in the morning. On the other hand, positional nystagmus without vertigo is intracranial in origin.

TABLE 1. Differences Between Peripheral and Central Positional Nystagmus

	Peripheral	*Central*
Latency:	2 to 20 seconds	None
Persistence:	Disappears within 50 seconds	Lasts longer than one minute
Fatigability:	Disappears on repetition	Repeatable
Positions:	Present in one position	Present in multiple positions
Vertigo:	Always present	Occasionally absent, and only nystagmus present
Direction of Nystagmus:	One direction	Changing directions in different positions.
Incidence:	85 per cent of all cases	10 to 15 per cent of all cases

Positional nystagmus is uncommon in endolymphatic hydrops or vestibular neuronitis. A word of explanation is in order here. Positional nystagmus is reported to occur as an aggravation of spontaneous nystagmus in certain positions during an active attack of Meniere's disease. This is particularly found with electronystagmography. However, positional tests with Frenzel glasses in the free periods between active vertigo attacks have never discerned positional nystagmus in endolymphatic hydrops in the author's experience. Thus, as a general rule, the presence of positional nystagmus would help rule out a diagnosis of endolymphatic hydrops or vestibular neuronitis.

Positional nystagmus may appear only when the head is in a certain relation to the rest of the trunk regardless of the position of the head in space. Interference with the neck must be considered in this type. The condition may be differentiated on examination by using a plaster of Paris collar or neck brace to hold the neck and shoulders steady while doing the positional tests. This should elicit no reaction with the cervical syndrome. On the other hand, if the head is extended and forcibly rotated to each side when the patient is erect and positional nystagmus is found, pathology in the neck rather than the peripheral labyrinth may be inferred. These positions compress the vertebral vessels. The examiner may perform the positional tests by side bending the patient into the left and right positions while holding the head so there is little or no twist or relative movement of the neck. The patient lies on his left, while testing the left lateral position and on his right side for the right lateral position. This will avoid and help differentiate the cervical syndrome.

Bosko Milojevic has put forth the interesting idea that latent nystagmus elicited by head shaking, direction-fixed positional nystagmus, directional preponderance, and secondary phase nystagmus are all different aspects of spontaneous nystagmus.

EAR, NOSE, AND THROAT EXAMINATION

Ear Examination

About 30 per cent of all dizziness is considered to be of aural origin. Most of these cases will reveal no pathologic features on inspection of the ear. However, the ears should be routinely examined since the origin of some of the cases will be detected by this examination. Although cerumen rarely causes serious dizziness, it must be removed to obtain an unimpaired view of the tympanic membranes. The tympanic membranes are usually examined by the magnifying otoscope, but examination with the binocular microscope, in special situations, will detect features unseen by a regular examination. The examiner looks for perforation, exudate, granulomas, crusts, or retraction pockets particularly in the posterior superior part of the tympanic membrane, for this is the region close to the vestibular apparatus. In particular, a perforation in Shrapnell's membrane is sought, and white flakes of keratinized squamous epithelium emanating through a perforation will reveal a cholesteatoma more certainly than radiology. A cholesteatoma is often associated with a fetid discharge, although not always. If a cholesteatoma is present, this should be considered the cause of any dizziness, until proven otherwise. If an occlusion of the Eustachian tube bears relationship to dizziness, usually exudate in the middle ear or deformities of the drum will also be present.

Nose and Throat Examination

Oral and nasal infection are reported as the most common focal infections associated with acute toxic labyrinthitis and vestibular neuronitis. Also, a stuffy nose may cause a sensation of giddiness in some patients. This sensation is not described as a rotary vertigo but as a persistent giddiness or dizziness or pressure in the head. The nasal passages are studied in cases in which nasal complaints such as stuffy nose, nasal discharge, or nasal discomfort are present. Transillumination of the anterior paranasal sinuses, politzerization or Eustachian catheterization, antral puncture and lavage, inspection of the nasopharynx with mirror, and the nasopharyngoscope may be utilized. Henry L. Williams reported two cases of vertigo associated with Thornwaldt's abscess in the nasopharynx. The pharynx is inspected for tonsillar infection, which may serve as a focus of infection. If a neurologic lesion is suspected, the larynx is examined by mirror for vocal cord paralysis. The teeth are inspected for dental decay, gingivitis, and abnormal bite, and a dentist is consulted when necessary. The neck is palpated for adenopathy. The cervical vertebrae and adjacent muscles are palpated for tenderness and inspected for restricted motion. Williams stated that unilateral otitis interna or a tumor of the acoustic nerve may lead to rotation of the head toward the affected side while lesions of the pons or midbrain may lead to the rotation of the head toward the normal side.

Caloric Tests of Semicircular Canal Function and Signs of Intracranial Involvement on the Caloric Test

CALORIC TESTS OF SEMICIRCULAR CANAL FUNCTION

Martin Spector

The outstanding advantage of caloric tests is that they make it possible to study each ear separately. If the external auditory canal is irrigated with cold water, the air in the middle ear and the surrounding bone will also be cooled. Such cooling will result in convection currents in the endolymph of the membranous labyrinth with a downward flow of the colder endolymph. This disturbance will induce nystagmus with the slow component in the direction of the endolymph motion. If hot water is used, the convection flow and, in turn, the nystagmus will be reversed. Provided the cold stimulus is colder than body temperature and the hot, hotter than body temperature, some stimulation will take place. It has been shown in caloric tests that the temperature of the horizontal semicircular canal after about 20 seconds is altered; a 20° C. difference in external temperature results in a 1° C. change in the semicircular canal.

The duration of the nystagmus seems to be the easiest measurement of the gross caloric test. The latent period does not seem to be an important measurement since differences in the auditory meatus, tympanic membrane, and cellularity of the temporal bone play too great a part. The latency (and the number of beats) vary too much from one subject to another as well as in the same individual and are not considered significant by most observers. Sellers, however, felt that the latency should be about one to four with respect to duration. A shorter ratio indicated hypoactivity; a higher ratio indicated hyperactivity to him. Torok assessed the caloric response by the number of beats at the maximum frequency for a five second period. He called this the culmination phenomenon. The frequency rises to a maximum and then decreases. This culmination phenomenon, he felt, was an expression of the vestibular sensitivity. Other measurements will be discussed under electronystagmography. The endpoint of nystagmus is often difficult to estimate, and the opinions of several observers may vary. Five to six minute intervals between tests of each ear are advised so that all effects from the previous stimulation have disappeared.

Caloric tests reveal whether the semicircular canal function is normal, hyperactive, hypoactive, or nonreactive. Many factors may alter the response and interfere with quantitative estimation. Light interferes with the response, for vision and fixation diminish the nystagmus; closing the eyes increases the response. Attention of the patient alters the response; alerting the mental activity increases the response, while inattention and dozing dull the response. Habituation also decreases the response. Other factors affecting the nystagmus response include cellularity of the mastoid and palsy of the ocular muscles. Spontaneous nystagmus of first degree will not mask out the provoked nystagmus. Between the end of the provoked nystagmus and the reappearance of the spontaneous nystagmus, a period of eye standstill will take place.

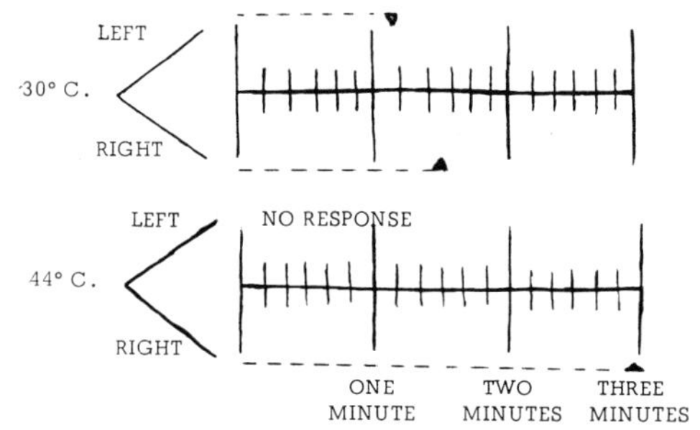

Fig. 1. Caloric responses with early involvement of left labyrinth and spontaneous nystagmus to right.

McNally and Stuart reported the sensations of patients following caloric stimulation. In many there was no sensation of turning. Faintness, unsteadiness, rocking, staggering, weakness, and swimming were experienced by different patients. If the sensation elicited is the same as the sensation of which the patient complains then one can be sure that the complaint is true vertigo.

It has been indicated that warm water may serve as a better caloric test than cold water (Bernstein; Hart). Due to involvement of one ear there may be a latent or spontaneous nystagmus of first degree to the opposite side. The response to cold water in an involved ear, although poor, will be aided by the latent nystagmus to the opposite side. On the other hand, in the good ear, the caloric re-

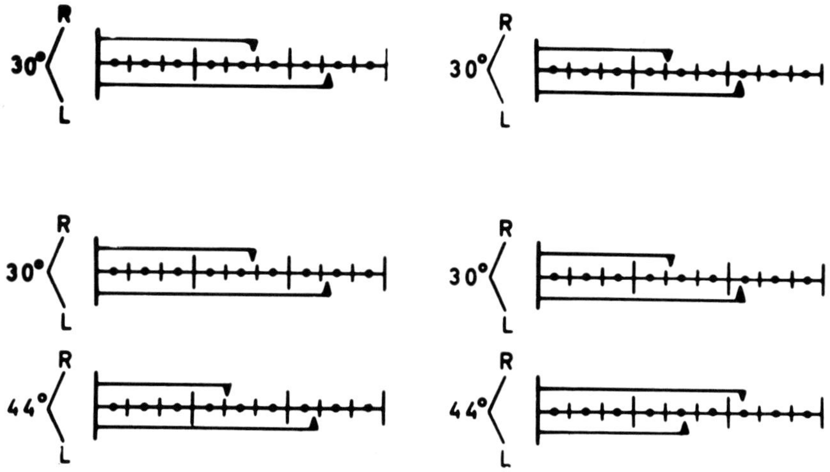

Fig. 2. Above, two cold syringing calorigrams apparently identical and with an asymmetry (two different patients). Below, the complete calorigrams for the two patients showing quite different pictures. To the left, a right-sided canal paresis (right-sided Meniere's disease); to the right, a directional preponderance to the right (central vascular lesion). This demonstrates the necessity of using both cold and hot stimuli to obtain a correct diagnosis. (From Aschan, G.: *In* Neurological Aspects of Auditory and Vestibular Disorders listed. Edited by Fields and Alford. Springfield, Ill., Charles C Thomas, 1964. Reproduced with permission of Charles C Thomas, Publisher, Springfield, Ill.)

sponse to cold water will be hindered by the latent nystagmus. The sum effect is that the responses to cold water on the two sides will be equal although smaller than usual. However, with warm water the caloric response of the involved ear will be nil or almost nil. Between the hypoactivity of the involved labyrinth and the latent nystagmus to the opposite side there will be little to no response in the involved ear to warm water. The sound ear will give an exaggerated response due to the boost of the latent nystagmus. These effects make for a distinct, unmistakable response to hot water but a blurred indefinite test with cold water in certain cases.

It is preferable that both hot and cold water should routinely be used in caloric tests. In addition to the advantages outlined in the previous paragraph, the additional finding of directional preponderance can be elucidated with the use of both hot and cold water.

Indications for the Caloric Test:

1. Every case of vertigo should undergo a caloric test as part of routine testing.
2. Every case of unilateral perceptive deafness should have a caloric test, especially to help rule out the presence of a cerebello-pontine angle tumor.
3. It may sometimes be of advantage to do a caloric test on bilateral cases of perceptive hearing loss and cases of tinnitus, even in the absence of vertigo.

There are many methods for doing a caloric examination, and several will be detailed with their specific advantages and disadvantages.

DIRECTIONAL PREPONDERANCE, BITHERMAL, OR FITZGERALD HALLPIKE TEST

The directional preponderance test is the

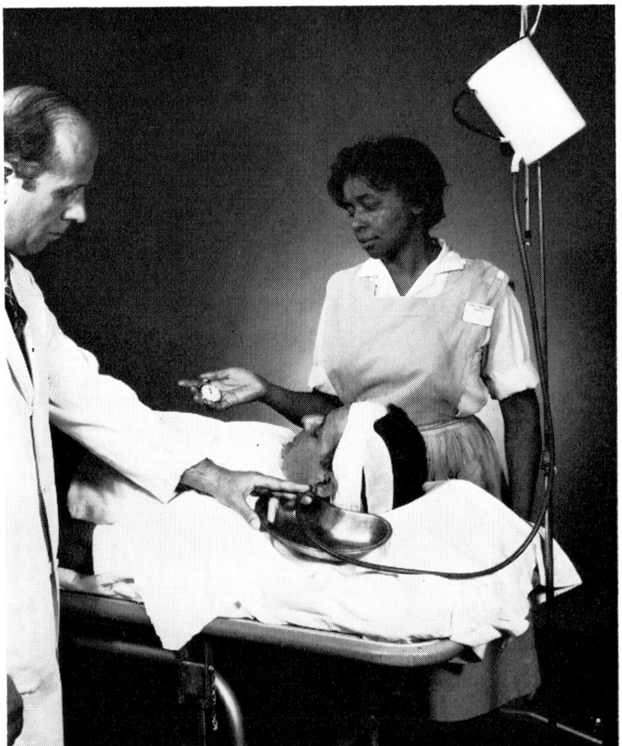

FIG. 3. Bithermal caloric test in office.

most standardized test, and it has gained wide acceptance. It is not too disturbing to the patient. Its great disadvantage is the lengthy time for the performance of the test—about 30 minutes per patient. Its great advantage is that it reveals both canal paresis and directional preponderance.

Technique

The lateral semicircular canal is relatively superficial compared with the posterior and superior canals and is separated from the tympanic membrane by only a few millimeters. If the patient is made to lie supine and the head is flexed through 30 degrees, the lateral semicircular canal will then be in the vertical plane with the ampulla uppermost. Water from a 2 pint douche can fixed about two feet above the ear is allowed to flow for 40 seconds into the ear. The diameter of the outflow nozzle (4 ml.) is such that not less than 8 ounces flows through during the 40 seconds, the average amount being from 12 to 14 fluid ounces. Each ear is douched in turn with water at exactly 30° C. (86° F.), and then with water at exactly 44° C. (112° F.), the temperature being measured in the douche can immediately before the flow is started. The water lying in the tubing should be discarded to assure that the irrigation is the proper temperature. Jongkees stated that at 30° C. and 44° C. vestibular reactions are nearly maximal. At least 5 minutes pause is allowed between each syringing. During each test the patient is instructed to fix his gaze upon some relatively distant object straight ahead of and slightly above him, so that the eyes are voluntarily held in the midway position; no true endpoint is observed but rather the time at which the nystagmus ceases to be visible to the unaided eye at a distance of ten inches with good illumination. The duration of nystagmus is noted in minutes and seconds from the onset of the stimulus to the endpoint of the nystagmus. It is found that the response to cold water averages 2 minutes and the response to hot water averages 1 minute and 40 seconds.

KOBRAK TEST

In the Kobrak test, ice water is used in varying amounts from 0.2 cc. up to 5 cc. instilled against the drum. There is a latency period from 20 to 40 seconds, and the duration of the nystagmus averages from 60 to 120 seconds. The response is considered hypoactive when the nystagmus is less than 30 seconds. The patient is seated for the test. Linthicum used a modification wherein only 0.2 cc. of water was used. The ice water was instilled into the ear canal and allowed to remain there 20 seconds. The head was then tilted to the opposite side so that the water drained out of the ear canal. The patient was then instructed to look at a spot on the ceiling with the head tipped back 60 degrees. A small scleral blood vessel was observed for nystagmus. If the vertigo brought on by this was bothersome to the patient, 0.2 cc. of warm water was instilled into the canal to neutralize the cold effect. If there was no response to 2 cc. of ice water, the labyrinth was considered nonreactive by Linthicum. The advantage of this test is its speed and simplicity. The chief disadvantage is that, without using hot water in a test, one cannot test for directional preponderance or overcome the effects of spontaneous nystagmus, either latent or manifest. The parameters of

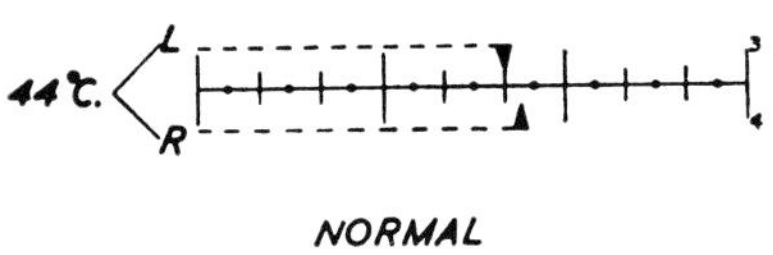

FIG. 4. Caloric test results obtained in an average normal subject. Continuous lines: time (3 min. divided into intervals of 10 sec.) Dotted lines: response durations. (From Cawthorne, Dix, Hallpike, and Hood: The investigation of vestibular function. Brit. Med. Bull. 12: 133, 1956. Reproduced with permission of the British Council, Publisher.)

this test are not as standardized as the bithermal test. There is also discomfort from the ice water.

VEIT'S MINIMAL CALORIC TEST

Frenzel glasses are applied to the patient's eyes. These spectacles have 20 plus diopter lenses which magnify the eyes so any movement can be readily observed. The patient is in a sitting position. Five cc. of water at 80° F. is instilled against the posterior superior quadrant of the tympanic membrane through an ear speculum using a syringe and a metal cannula. The water is instilled over a period of three to four seconds. The duration is counted from the insertion of the water until the nystagmus ceases. The patient looks straight ahead with his head bent downward 30 degrees to the horizontal. If no nystagmus appears in 35 seconds then the patient's head is turned so he faces up toward the ceiling. The duration of the nystagmus is counted (mean—90 seconds, average—75 to 120 seconds). The amplitude of the nystagmus is roughly estimated as coarse, medium, or small. The frequency of jerks is usually 6 to 18 per 10 seconds. The range of nystagmus jerks is 68 to 115 with a mean value of 94. With this test, it is hypoactive when there is no response in the face front position and the duration in the face up position is less than 50 seconds. The chief advantage of the minimal caloric test is the lack of disturbance to the patient. The test rarely produces any vertigo. The test is rapid. This is particularly advantageous when testing in the presence of recent vertigo as a stronger caloric test may often precipitate bouts of vertigo. The disadvantages include the fact that if the test elicits no response, a stronger caloric test must be used. Also, in doubtful cases of vertigo, the patient has no sensation to compare to his complaint.

BARANY MASS CALORIC TEST

This test is performed by irrigating water at 62° F. into the ear while the patient is in a sitting position. The irrigation is administered from a douche can about two feet above the head through a rubber tube and nozzle into the ear. The irrigation is continued until nystagmus begins. If no nystagmus ensues in

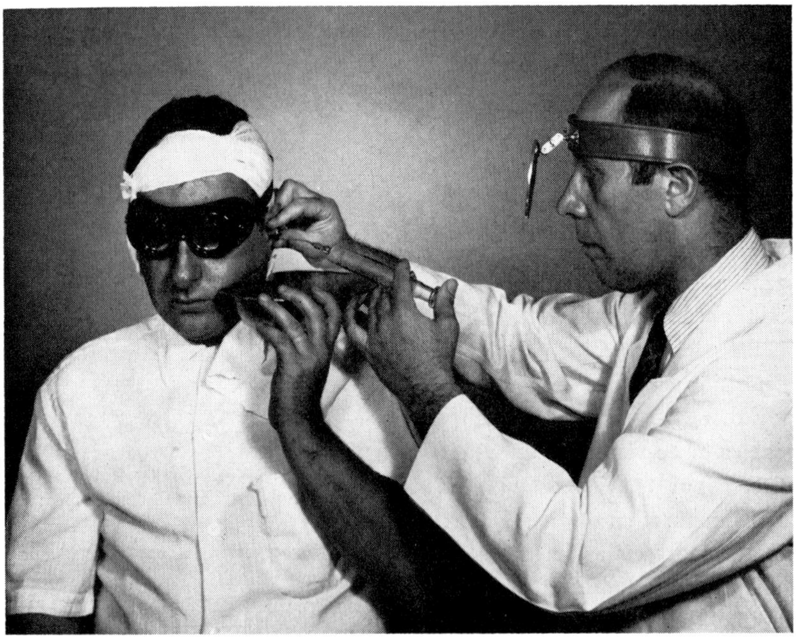

Fig. 5. Minimal caloric test (modified after Veit).

about four minutes, the labyrinth is considered dead. Otherwise the irrigation is stopped as soon as nystagmus begins. The patient is observed for the duration of nystagmus for falling and pastpointing. The nystagmus duration is measured in the face front position for the vertical canals and in the face up position after the nystagmus in the face front position has ceased. An interval of 5 minutes is allowed and then the other ear is tested. No hot water is used in this test.

The disadvantage of this test is the severe vertigo which is induced. The test is rather uncomfortable and has not been as popular of late years as it was formerly. Also, the fact that hot water is not used does not allow measurement of directional preponderance. Its proponents claim that this test is most valuable for central nervous system diseases.

DUNDAS GRANT COLD AIR TEST

In infected ears or ears with perforated drums, one may wish to avoid use of water since it may cause a flareup of middle ear infection. To avoid this, a Dundas Grant tube is used where the air is cooled by a spray of ethyl chloride. Cold air is blown against the tympanic membrane for 30 seconds (some use 15 seconds). The temperature can be reduced to 55 to 60° F. The duration of the nystagmus which ensues is 2 to 2½ minutes. Shuster employed a little ice water to determine the viability of the vestibular apparatus. He stated no ill effects were encountered if the ear was immediately dried. Laff suggested instillation of alcohol as a test.

ABNORMAL RESPONSES

Hypoactive Response or Canal Paresis

In canal paresis the labyrinth gives a weaker response both to cold and hot water than is normal—or as compared to the other ear if the other ear is normal. The usual way to judge whether a canal paresis is present is to compare the values of syringing one ear to those obtained from the other. Differences up to 40 seconds are accepted as normal variations for the bithermal test.

Labyrinth

The coordinate reduction of all the charac-

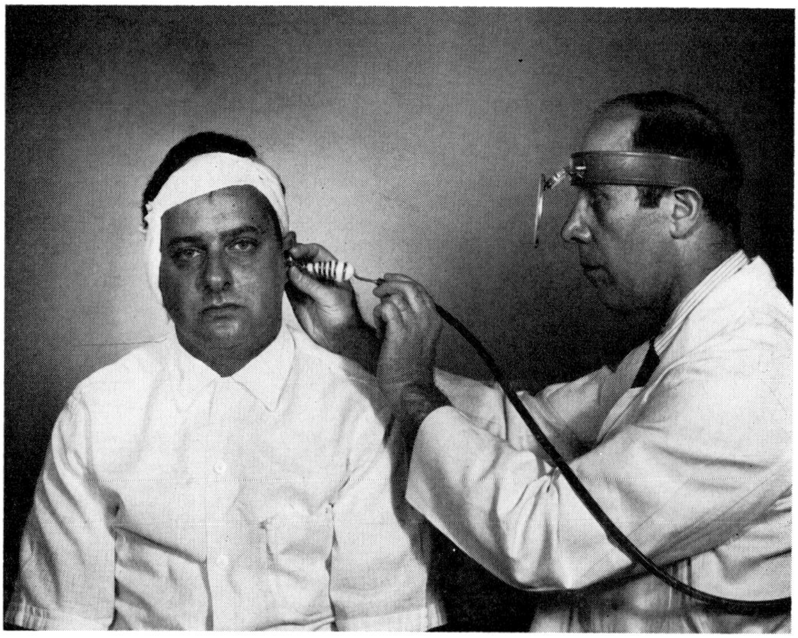

Fig. 6. Caloric test with cold air.

ters of the provoked nystagmus seems to be typical when a lesion is localized in the labyrinth. Hypoexcitability of the vestibular apparatus may be caused by degeneration of the inner ear after chronic inflammation or diffuse labyrinthitis. About 70 per cent of cases of endolymphatic hydrops present hypoactivity. Many cases of endolymphatic hydrops have a normal caloric response, however. The caloric test in hydrops bears no consistent relationship to either the audiogram or severity of the disease. A Meniere's patient with a depressed response on caloric testing does have less vertigo after a labyrinthectomy than patients with normal responses. Arnwig found the great majority of children with congenital deafness gave a normal caloric response. In congenitally deaf children he found that abolished vestibular function often was accompanied by retinitis pigmentosa. Vestibular function is abolished in most postmeningitis cases. With severe sensorineural deafness the caloric response may be hypoactive in adults. Streptomycin toxicity diminishes the intensity even more than the duration according to one study. Harbert reported that with occlusion of the anterior vestibular artery there is no response of the horizontal semicircular canals to caloric stimulation.

Fractures and Head Injury. After a transverse fracture of the petrous bone there results a markedly paretic or inactive caloric response. In longitudinal fractures of the petrous bone normal or mildly paretic caloric responses are obtained. Hugh Barber reported that with fracture 43 per cent had normal caloric response but without a fracture 85 per cent had a normal caloric response among those head injured patients with vertigo. Cawthorne reported that among 58 patients with head injury, 56 showed deviations from the normal in their response to caloric stimulation and of these 56 only 24 had damage to the cochlea.

Eighth Nerve

When a vestibular root is damaged, severe hypoflexia or areflexia results. Trauma, neuritis, or tumor may affect the eighth nerve. In vestibular neuronitis the incidence rate of abnormal responses comes close to 100 per cent, and here hypoactivity is the outstanding diagnostic sign. Diminished or absent response to caloric stimulation is an outstanding and early sign of a cerebello-

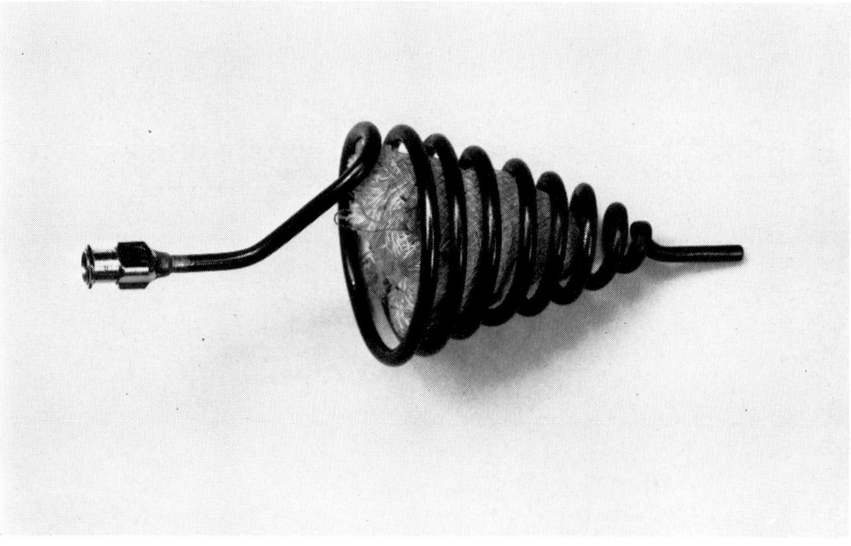

FIG. 7. Dundas Grant coiled copper tube with gauze saturated with ethyl chloride.

pontine angle tumor. Cystic arachnoiditis is another central cause for a unilateral hypoactive response with auditory symptoms.

Brainstem or Other Central Lesions

Hypoactivity may be a sign of a lesion of the vestibular nuclei or the fibers to the medial longitudinal fasciculus. Some mental disturbances particularly schizophrenia, have been reported to induce a hypoactive vestibular response.

Complete Absence of Response

A rather benign cause is vestibular neuronitis. Complete absence of vestibular response may result from destructive labyrinthine disease, such as suppurative labyrinthitis; from toxins, such as streptomycin, kanamycin, and neomycin; labyrinthectomy; meningitis; and transverse fracture of the petrous bone. Cerebellopontine angle tumor is outstanding as a central cause. Unilateral total vestibular paralysis to caloric stimulation in the presence of a spontaneous nystagmus to the same side is found with cerebellar abscess of otic origin.

Absence of response even to ice water, doesn't always signify a dead labyrinth. Hugh Barber reported a case in which 90 seconds of irrigation with ice water elicited no response but a labyrinthectomy on that side induced spontaneous nystagmus indicating that there must have been some vestibular activity. This point must be remembered in judgment of a labyrinthectomy which has failed to give symptomatic relief.

Bilateral Canal Paresis

Meningitis; severe toxins such as streptomycin, kanamycin, and neomycin; vestibular neuronitis; bilateral acoustic neurinoma (von Recklinghausen's disease); and brain

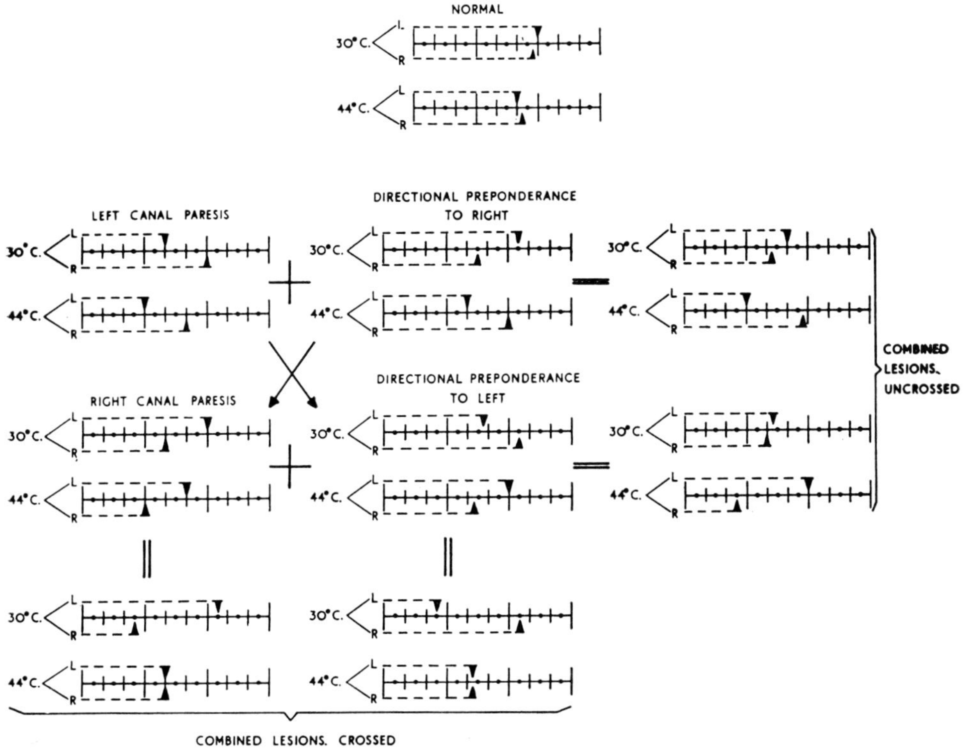

FIG. 8. Full range of abnormalities of caloric test results. (From Cawthorne, Dix, Hallpike, and Hood: The investigation of vestibular function. Brit. Med. Bull. 12:133, 1956. Reproduced with permission of the British Council, Publisher.)

stem lesions involving the vestibular nuclei may cause bilateral hypoactive responses.

Directional Preponderance

Directional Preponderance signifies a preponderance of the nystagmus in one direction, as obtained by cold water in one ear and hot water in the other, as opposed to the nystagmus in the opposite direction. A directional preponderance is detected by adding the cold syringing value from the one ear to the hot syringing value from the other ear to give one sum, and the two remaining values to give another sum, and then one sum is subtracted from the other.

Jongkees and Philipzoon described a quantitative method for estimating canal paresis and directional preponderance. We quote:

> We gave the numbers 1, 2, 3, and 4 according to the traditional standards to the irrigations, i.e., 1 = left cold (30 degrees Centigrade), 2 = right cold (30 degrees Centigrade), 3 = left hot (44 degrees Centigrade), and 4 = right hot (44 degrees Centigrade). The difference in excitability between the left and right was expressed in the percentage of the total excitability as follows:
>
> $$\frac{(1 + 3) - (2 + 4)}{(1 + 2 + 3 + 4)} \times 100 \text{ per cent.}$$
>
> When the right labyrinth is less than the left one, we get a positive value and a negative value in the reverse case. The directional preponderance was also expressed as a percentage, as already proposed by Jongkees in 1948. The difference between the right and the left beating nystagmus was expressed in the percentage of the total excitability:
>
> $$\frac{(1 + 4) - (2 + 3)}{(1 + 2 + 3 + 4)} \times 100 \text{ per cent.}$$
>
> Consequently, we find in case of a directional preponderance to the right a positive value and a negative value in case of a directional preponderance to the left. On the strength of these findings we called a difference in excitability or a directional preponderance abnormal in our patients when the values differed more than the double standard deviation from the mean. We called a difference between left and right pathological as regards duration when it exceeded the values minus 14 per cent or plus 14 per cent. We called a directional preponderance pathological as regards the duration when we found its value exceeding minus 30 per cent or plus 30 per cent.

Directional preponderance has been reported with partial unilateral lesions of the labyrinth. It has been reported in 26 per cent of one series of cases with endolyphatic hydrops (Hallpike). It has been thought to indicate a utricular lesion on the opposite side in some cases (Hallpike). Directional preponderance has been reported with tumors of the eighth nerve and also with head injuries. Carmichael, Dix, and Hallpike studied the caloric responses in unilateral vascular lesions of the vestibular centers within the brain stem. In the majority of their cases, directional preponderance to the opposite side

Table 1. Caloric Test Responses

Hyperactive	*Hypoactive*	*Absent*	*Normal*
Perforated tympanic membrane	Toxins, i.e., streptomycin	Suppurative labyrinthitis	Some cases of Meniere's disease
Neurosis	Vestibular neuronitis	Vestibular neuronitis	Most intracranial diseases
Intracranial, especially supratentorial	Posterior fossa diseases	Labyrinthectomy	Positional vertigo
Head injury (occasional cases)	Acoustic neurinoma	Transverse fracture of petrous bone	Basilar insufficiency
	Head trauma (peripheral)	Acoustic neurinoma	
	Meniere's disease	Toxins, i.e., kanamycin	
	Some forms of perceptive deafness	After meningitis	

was found. With infarction of the brain stem below or caudal to the level of entry of the eighth nerve the chief abnormality was directional preponderance to the opposite side without deafness. Canal paresis was less common and occurred if the lesion extended above the entry level of the eighth nerve. Thus with occlusion of the posterior inferior cerebellar artery directional preponderance was found. In the elderly with basilar insufficiency who display short attacks of vertigo, the caloric test is normal. Directional preponderance may be due to a tumor of the posterior part of the temporal lobe. The lesion here is homolateral with the direction of the preponderance.

Directional preponderance has been found in a certain percentage of normals, and this has detracted from its importance as a significant finding. Directional preponderance is found consistently in the presence of spontaneous nystagmus. Directional preponderance may well be a manifestation of latent spontaneous nystagmus, and we may derive the same significance from directional preponderance that we derive from spontaneous nystagmus.

Hyperactive Responses

Hyperexcitability of the vestibular apparatus occurs rarely in peripheral diseases, but more frequently in diseases causing irritation of the central vestibular nuclei or their pathways, or release of these from inhibitory centers. Where the tympanic membrane is ruptured, a hyperactive reaction is to be expected. Hyperactive caloric responses are encountered in psychogenic patients. If there is a hyperactivity of the subjective responses without a coincident hyperactivity of the nystagmus, a neurosis should be suspected. Exaggerated responses of the vegetative nervous system on testing occur in neurotics, after head injury as well as in supratentorial lesions. Excessive autonomic sensitivity is manifested by marked pallor, perspiration, nausea, and vomiting. This may help differentiate a malingerer from a person with a

Table 2. Presence of Canal Paresis and Directional Preponderance in Various Conditions

Disease	*Canal Paresis*	*Directional Preponderance*
Endolymphatic Hydrops	Present in 70% of cases	Present in 25%
Positional Vertigo	Absent	Absent
Vestibular Neuronitis	Present	Absent
Cerebellopontine Angle Tumor	Present almost 100%	Sometimes present
Destructive Labyrinthine Disease	Present	Absent
Psychogenic	Absent	Absent
Systemic Medical Conditions	Absent	Absent
Thrombosis Postinferior Cerebellar Artery	Absent	Present
Basilar Insufficiency	Absent	Occasionally present
Disseminated Sclerosis	Absent	Present with spontaneous nystagmus
Epilepsy	Absent	Absent
Temporal Lobe Tumor	Absent	Present
Head Injuries	Absent	Occasionally in central injuries
Fractures of Temporal Bone	Present	Absent
Normals	Absent	Present in 17%

real head injury or a neurotic, since the malingerer would not present hyperactive responses.

Hyperactive caloric responses are a significant finding in some intracranial lesions. A third degree nystagmus resulting from a caloric test is considered abnormal, and one should be suspicious of a possible intracranial lesion. Wodak wrote that a prolonged nystagmus lasting more than three minutes indicated a destruction of the central checking mechanisms.

REFERENCES

1. Arnvig, J.: Vestibular function in deafness and severe hardness of hearing. Acta Otolaryng. 45:283, 1955.
2. Arslan, M.: On the renewing of the methodology for the stimulation of the vestibular apparatus. Acta Otolaryng. (Suppl.) 122, 1955.
3. Bernstein, L.: Directional preponderance Test. Arch. Otolaryng. 76:57, 1962.
4. Carmichael, E. A., Dix, M. R., and Hallpike, C. S.: Pathology, symptomatology and diagnosis of organic affections of the eighth nerve system. Brit. Med. Bull. 12:146, 1956.
5. Gulick, R., and Pfaltz, C. R.: Diagnostic values of caloric tests in otoneurology. Ann. Otol. 73:893, 1964.
6. Hart, C.: The value of the hot caloric test. Laryngoscope 75:302-315, 1965.
7. Jongkees, L. B. W.: Which is the preferable method of performing the caloric test? Arch. Otolaryng. 49:594, 1949.
8. Jongkees, L. B. W., and Philipszoon, A. J.: Electronystagmography. Acta Otolaryng. (Suppl.) 189.
9. Mahoney, J. L., Harlan, W. L., and Bickford, R. G.: Visual and Other Factors Influencing Caloric Nystagmus in Normal Subjects, A. M. A. Arch. Otolaryng. (Chicago) 66: 46, 1957.
10. Nathanson, M., and Bergman, P.: Newer methods of evaluation of patients with alerted states of consciousness. Med. Clin. N. Amer., 1958.
11. Shuster, B. H.: Vertigo: clinical considerations. Arch. Otolaryng. (Chicago) 30:536, 1939.
12. Spector, M.: The routine use of the minimal caloric test as an office procedure. Arch. Otolaryng. 69:303-306, 1959.
13. Stoner, L.: Use and interpretation of vestibular testing. Trans. Amer. Acad. Ophthal. Otolaryng. 59:721, 1955.
14. Torok, N.: Significance of frequency in caloric nystagmus. Acta Otolaryng. 36:38, 1948.
15. Torok, N.: Assessment of vestibular sensitivity. J. Int. Coll. Surg. 36:649, 1961.

SIGNS OF INTRACRANIAL INVOLVEMENT ON THE CALORIC TEST

Martin Spector and J. U. Toglia

In diseases of the central nervous system, vestibular tests are often normal. Shuster stated that signs of intracranial involvement were best elicited with a mass caloric test such as the old Barany test with water at 68° F. The deviation reaction of the arms or pastpointing should be studied. It is normal to have a deviation reaction after vestibular testing. The arms deviate from four to eight inches after a mass caloric test. However, today the directional preponderance test is more commonly performed.

Diminished or absent response to caloric testing is an outstanding and early sign of a cerebellopontine angle tumor, such as acoustic neurinoma. House in a recent series of 53 cases found only two who had normal caloric responses. This gives an incidence of 96 per cent and is the general experience of many investigators. Normal response to a caloric test is a strong but not absolute indication that an acoustic neurinoma is not present. Shuster reported the results of the Barany caloric tests with cold water in various intracranial diseases: postencephalitis with Parkinson's syndrome, multiple sclerosis, tabes dorsalis, dementia, cerebrospinal lues, prolonged use of barbiturates, but there were no characteristic findings. In induced sleep, such as with barbiturates, and in various stages of coma or anesthesia, syringing the ears with ice water produces the following ocular responses: (1) in lighter or intermediary stages of unconsciousness, tonic conjugate deviation of the eyes to the side of stimulation; (2) in deeper states of consciousness, no ocular response.

The following abnormal responses strongly indicate a central lesion:

1. Inverted nystagmus, i.e., directed to the left when a right beating nystagmus is expected. The observer must be watchful for the influence of spontaneous nystagmus.
2. Perverted nystagmus, i.e., vertical or oblique instead of horizontal.
3. Monocular nystagmus or dissociated eye movements. If both eyes do not work in unison following the test—i.e., one eye goes up to the right and the other down to the left, or some similar dissociation—a central lesion should be suspected. One must be watchful that weakness or paralysis of an eye muscle does not cause an apparent dissociation. The lesion will usually be found in the brain stem as long as extraocular motion is normal.
4. Conjugate deviation of the eyes to one side without nystagmus, i.e., absence of a fast phase.

These abnormal findings following a caloric test suggest a central lesion:

1. Third degree nystagmus resulting from a caloric test.
2. Long-lasting changes of head posture and somnolence during the examination.
3. Absence of any autonomic reaction, i.e., absence of nausea, pallor, and vertigo occur with infratentorial lesions even with a mass caloric test.
4. Absence of horizontal nystagmus and normal vertical nystagmus or vice versa. Failure of response from the vertical canals may also result from a weak caloric stimulus.
5. Very large amplitude or small, rapid eye movements.
6. Absence of the rotatory component of caloric nystagmus.

Electronystagmography

J. U. Toglia

Electronystagmography (ENG) is the latest and most used technique for recording nystagmus and other ocular movements. It is based on the existence of a corneoretinal potential, first discovered by Dubois-Reymond in 1849. The cornea is electropositive with respect to the retina: When the ocular globe moves, its anterior pole conveys positive electrical charge to the nearest electrodes, which is then amplified and recorded by the writing system. In 1936 Mower and associates first recognized that the potentials utilized in electronystagmography originated in the metabolism of the retina and not of the muscles. The basic bioelectrical potential between the anterior and the posterior poles of the ocular globe is about 600 microvolts when the eye is at rest in darkness. This potential, however, may increase upon illumination of the eye, as first demonstrated by Holmgreen in 1865; the effects of light and darkness on the corneoretinal potential have been further studied by several investigators. Large fluctuations are present from day to day in each individual. The cause of this remains obscure, but no demonstrable correlation exists between metabolic changes in the human body and variation of the corneoretinal potentials. Among other factors influencing the corneoretinal potentials are acapnia, anoxia, ischemia of the retina, and administration to the patient of adrenaline and other drugs. A great amount of literature on this subject and on the technique of ENG is available in the monographs of Aschan et al., Megighian, Jongkees et al., Aboulker et al.

In our medical center, we are routinely performing ENG studies on all patients who complain of vertigo, dizziness, difficulty with balance and ataxic gait. Our patients receive, prior to the ENG studies, complete audiological, otological, and neurological examinations. The neurological examination has been described in a separate section of this book.

Periorbital biopotential skin electrodes are used as demonstrated in Figure 1. The electrodes are applied in place after the skin has been cleansed with alcohol. Calibration is performed by recording eye movements of 10° visual angle as 10 mm. of pen deflections. Calibration tests are performed at the beginning and at the end of each test, since corneoretinal potentials easily fluctuate between tests. The examining room has controlled temperature in order to eliminate sweating which affects the basic amount of electrical potential utilized in ENG. The room is kept dark during the caloric tests. The recording apparatus is a multichannel Offner Dynograph, which has available DC and AC amplifiers with a time constant varying from 3 to 10 seconds. Multiple paper speeds are available from 1 mm./sec. to 100 mm./sec.

Our routine ENG studies include the following examinations:

1. Search for spontaneous nystagmus in the direct forward gaze.

2. Search for gaze nystagmus in both vertical and horizontal planes.

3. Search for positional nystagmus with eyes closed or open in the dark, the patient supine with his head straight then rotated to either side and finally with his head hanging, straight and rotated to each side.

4. Recording of optokinetic nystagmus in both horizontal and vertical planes using a rotating Kestenbaum drum.

5. Recording of caloric nystagmus using the well-known Fitzgerald-Hallpike technique. The latter tests include irrigation of each ear for 40 seconds first with water at temperature of 30° centigrade, then at 44°. The patient is lying down, the head flexed 30° and kept in the midline by a headholder. The patient is kept alert by conversing with the examiner. The water used for caloric stimulation is controlled by a thermistor and kept in constant circulation, reaching the ejecting pistol through a plastic tube. Intervals

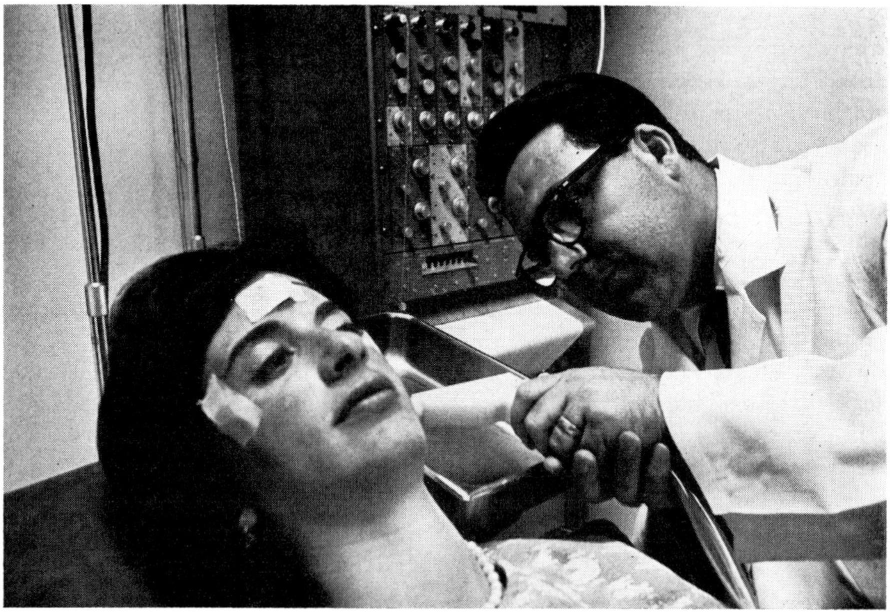

FIG. 1. The caloric tests are recorded through a multichannel Offner Dynograph.

of 5 minutes are recommended between tests. The paper speed is 2.5 mm./ sec.

The first channel of the recording apparatus (bottom line) measures latency period, frequency, amplitude, and duration of the caloric nystagmus; the second and third channels (second and third lines from below) record the speed of the fast and of the slow phases. Additional channels are used for recording, simultaneously, displacement of the eyes in the vertical plane and when it is desirable to record movements of each eye separately.

We are here particularly interested in demonstrating the value of ENG in association with caloric testing.

ELECTRONYSTAGMOGRAPHIC EVALUATION OF CALORIC NYSTAGMUS

The opinion as to which of the various parameters of the caloric nystagmus parallel vestibular sensitivity varies from author to author. The majority agree that duration and total number of nystagmic beats is the least reliable characteristic of the caloric response, since this can be easily prolonged by simply clapping the hands or by any alerting stimulus. Frequency is believed more reliable, and some authors (Buys, Torok) find that maximum frequency parallels maximum speed of the slow phase. Aschan recommends that frequency be determined for periods of 10 to 30 seconds. Arslan recommends that frequency be determined for 10 seconds at the beginning, 10 seconds in the middle, and 10 seconds at the end of each caloric response. Hennebert and Jongkees feel that frequency is not reliable since it may change often in the same patient. In our experience, frequency does not change in the same patient unless other factors are intervening, such as changes in visual fixation and alertness. The total amplitude of the nystagmus is considered by some to be very significant (Jung et al.). Most authorities agree that the speed of the slow phase directly parallels vestibular sensitivity. There is some disagreement regarding when the maximum speed of the slow phase should be averaged out. In our records the maximum speed appears at about 60 seconds from the beginning of the caloric irrigation, although it may change from patient to patient. Stahle recommends that the velocity of the slow phase be averaged from the amplitude of the spikes present in a period of 10 seconds, taken between the 60th and the 90th second, from the beginning of the stimulation. Henricksson has taught us

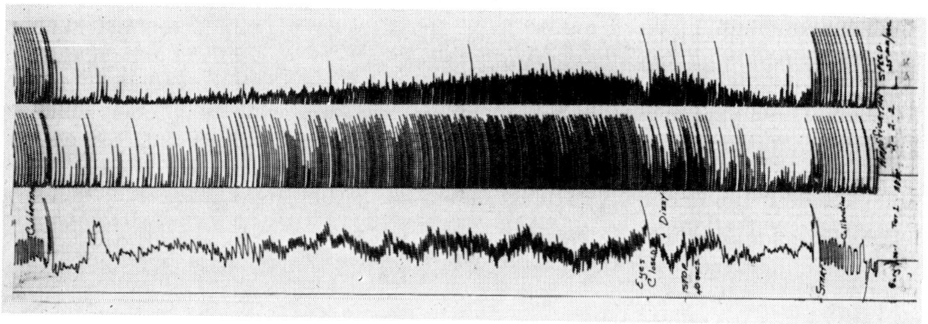

FIG. 2. Normal electronystagmogram. Latency, frequency, form, duration and amplitude of caloric nystagmus (AD30°) are recorded in the bottom line. The velocity of the fast phases is shown in the center line; the velocity of the slow phases is recorded in the upper line: the higher the spikes, the higher the velocity. Calibration deflections are observed at the beginning and at the end of the tracing. Deflections of 10 mm. in the lower line represent eye movements of 10° visual angle.

how to derive this speed directly on a separate channel, eliminating need for mathematical computations. Although velocity of the slow phase is likely the most linear measure of vestibular nystagmus, we follow Arslan's teaching that all parameters of the nystagmus should be recorded and taken in consideration for a complete evaluation of the caloric response. Evaluation of qualitative parameters (direction, form, rhythm) is of particular interest when vertiginous patients are suspected of having supratentorial syndromes.

The value of ENG, as compared to the naked eye evaluation of caloric nystagmus, is demonstrated by the following observations:

1. Caloric nystagmus may be inhibited by ocular fixation: several times when no caloric nystagmus is present with the eyes open, normal response is observed when the tests are performed in the dark or with the eyes closed. Occasionally, the caloric nystagmus is inhibited by closing the eyelids, a phenomenon which needs further evaluation.

2. Caloric nystagmus recorded in darkness or with eyes closed may show intermittent pauses, which might assume a significant clinical value.

3. Perrotatory nystagmus may only be evaluated by ENG, since it is almost impossible to observe it during rotation of the patient. This technique, of course, allows study of vestibular threshold, which is simply not possible by direct observation.

4. Only ENG permits analysis of the nystagmus of each eye, observation which is most useful in cases of vertigo due to neurological diseases.

5. When the patient has already a spontaneous nystagmus, the evaluation of caloric nystagmus is very difficult unless ENG is util-

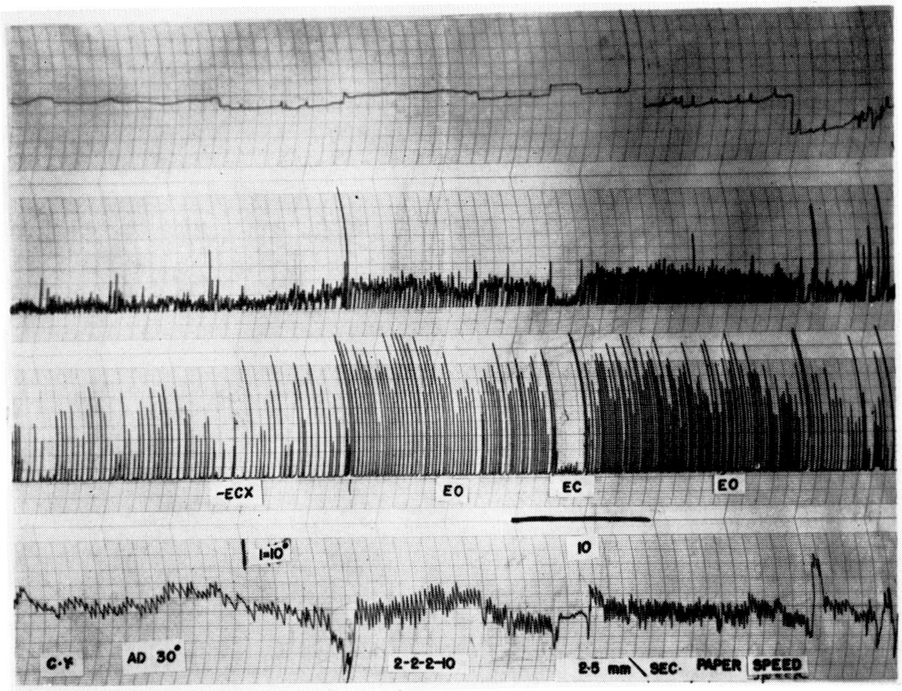

Fig. 3

Figs. 3, 4, 5, and 6. Electronystagmographs of caloric tests in a patient with Meniere's disease. Frequency of the nystagmus and velocity of the slow phases are higher in Figures 3 (AD 30°) and 6 (AS 44°) than in 4 (AS 30°) and 5 (AD 44°), indicating "directional preponderance" of the nystagmus beating toward the left side. These records also show that when the patient actively closes his eyes, their upward deviation, as demonstrated in the upper line (Bell's phenomenon) abolishes the caloric nystagmus.

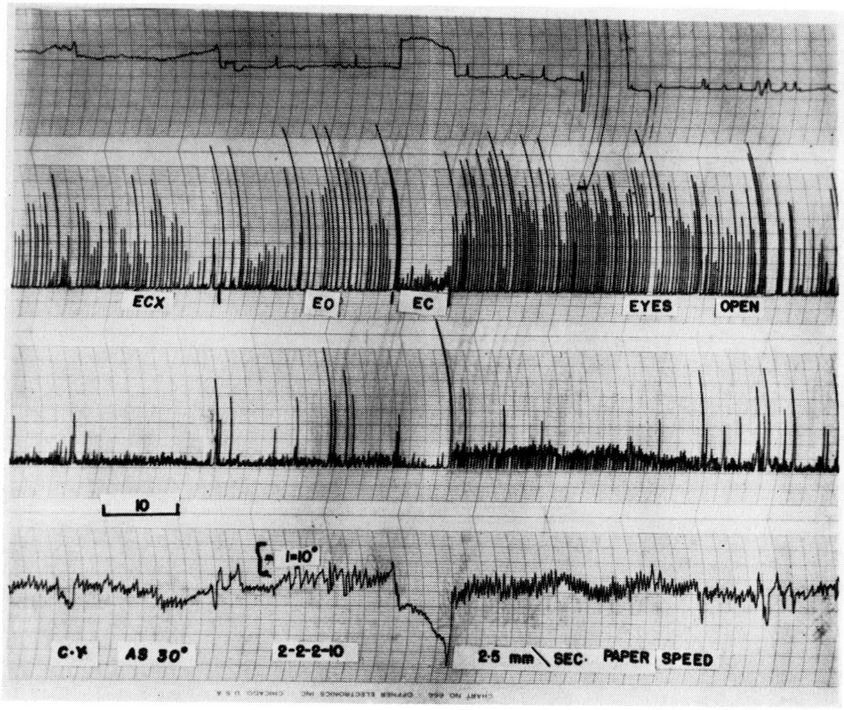
ECX
EO
EC
EYES
OPEN
10
1=10°
C·Y
AS 30°
2-2-2-10
2·5 mm\SEC· PAPER SPEED

FIG. 4.

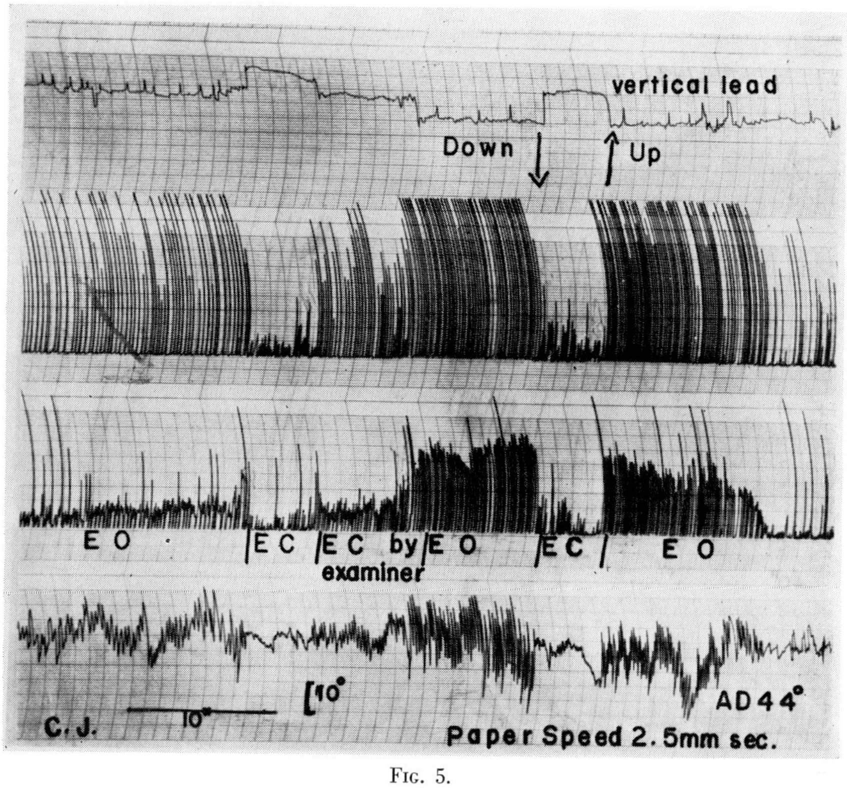
vertical lead
Down
Up
E O
E C
E C by
examiner
E O
E C
E O
10°
10°
C. J.
AD 44°
Paper Speed 2.5mm sec.

FIG. 5.

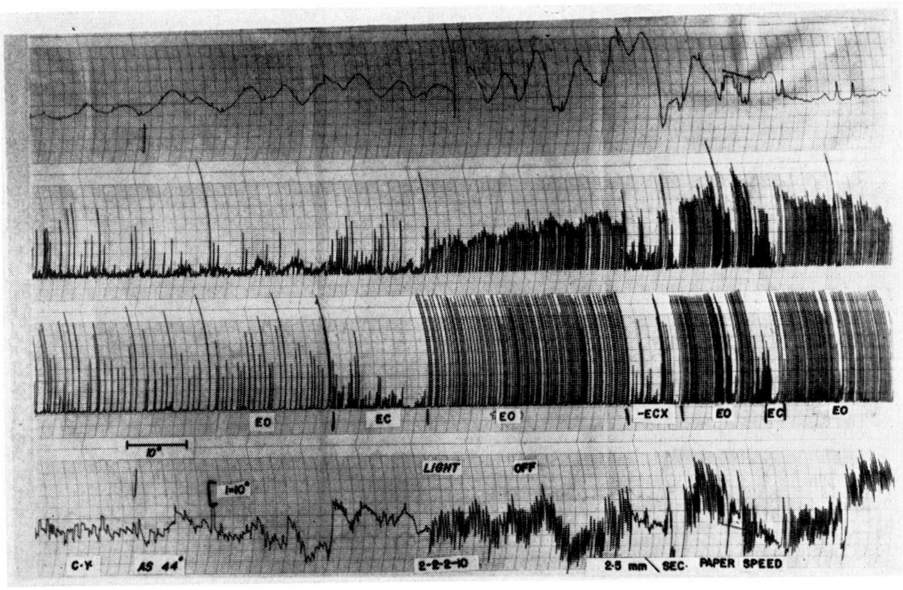

FIG. 6.

ized. Also the interference between spontaneous, gaze, optokinetic, and caloric nystagmus which is of clinical value is only possible by using ENG.

Although ENG is not a substitute for clinical diagnosis, it is very helpful in the complete evaluation of patients with vertigo and dizziness. By electronystagmographic analysis of qualitative and quantitative parameters of the nystagmus induced by caloric stimulations, the following conclusions may be suggested:

I. Caloric responses show considerable variations between individuals and in the same individual if other factors interfere such as alertness, drowsiness, intentional gaze, positions of the eyes, etc.

II. *Hypoactive Responses:*

1. Unilateral hypoactive responses determined only by the speed of the slow phase that

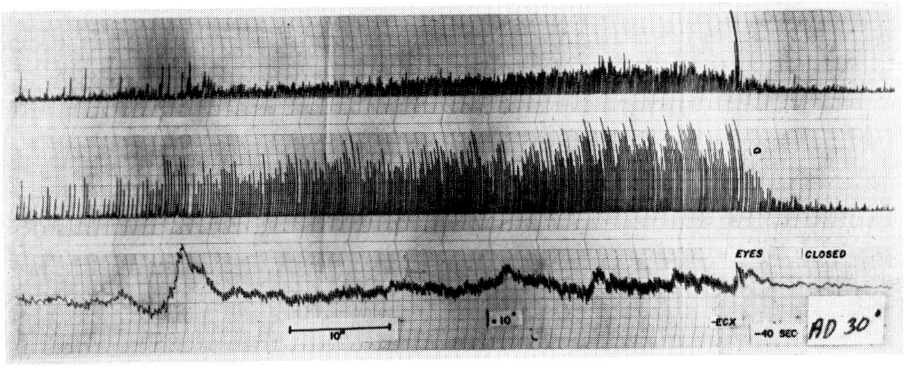

FIG. 7.

FIGS. 7, 8, 9, and 10. Electronystagmographs of caloric tests in a patient with left side acoustic neurinoma, showing "left canal paresis." Minimal response is observed in Figure 8 (AS 30°) and no response in Figure 10 (AS 44°), whereas good response is seen in Figures 7 (AD 30°) and 9 (AD 44°).

is without concomitant decrease of duration, frequency, etc., are attributed to pathology of the homolateral labyrinth. Hypoactive responses, as measured by decrease of all the parameters instead indicate pathology of the homolateral vestibular nuclei or vestibular nerve (i.e., acoustic neurinoma).

2. Bilateral hypoactive responses beyond the limits of normal variations, and not associated with gaze paresis, suggest peripheral vestibular pathology (i.e. bilateral neurinoma, streptomycin toxicity). Bilateral inexcitability of central origin is of course associated with bilateral gaze paralysis and is due to pontine pathology.

3. Bilateral hypoactive responses associated with directional preponderance suggest central compensation to older peripheral vestibular pathology. Positional nystagmus may be present.

4. If patients with vertigo show absent caloric nystagmus *only when the eyes are open*

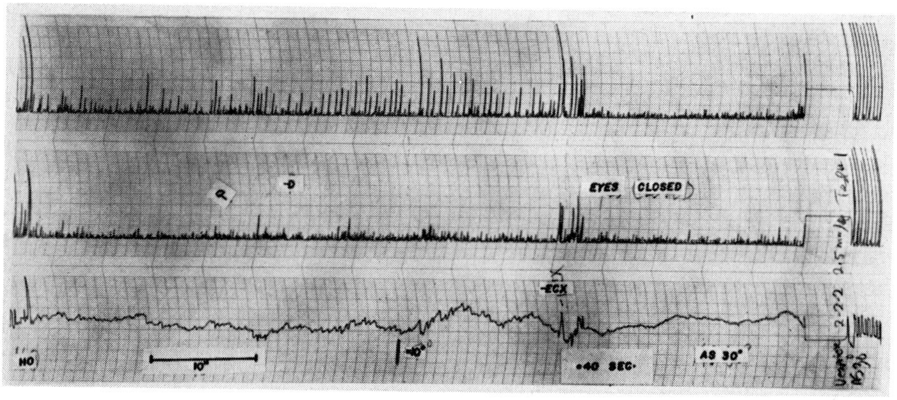

Fig. 8.

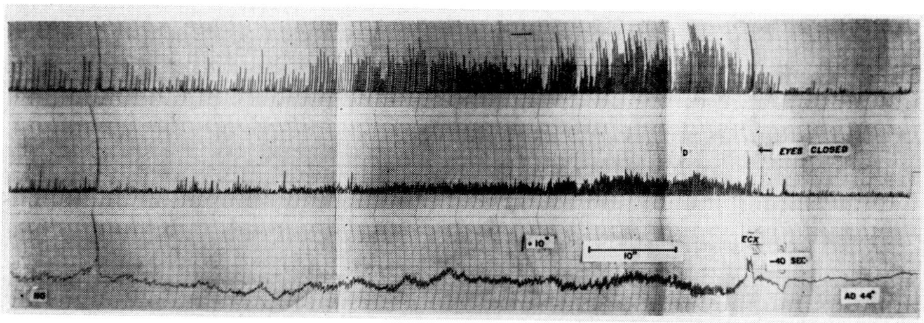

Fig. 9

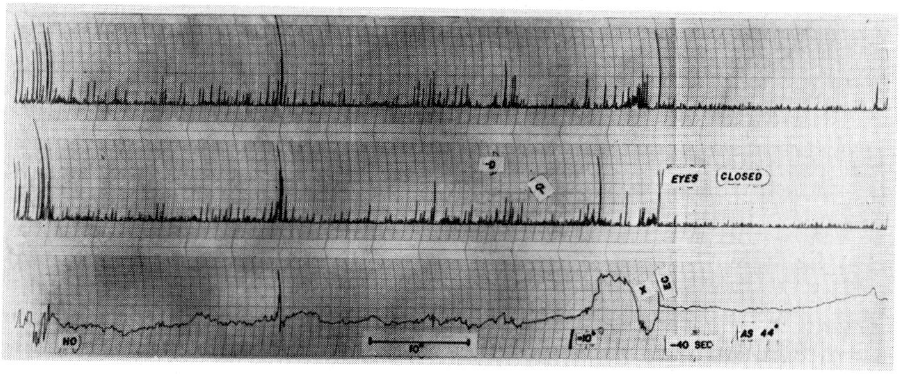

Fig. 10

and not when the eyes are closed, vertigo is most likely of psychogenic origin. Strong visual fixation may be responsible for this phenomenon.

III. *Hyperactive Responses:*

1. Bilateral hyperactive responses, determined only by duration of the nystagmus, are frequently observed in patients complaining of psychogenic vertigo.

2. Bilateral hyperactive responses relative to all parameters of the caloric nystagmus indicate central vestibular pathology.

3. Bilateral hyperactive responses with directional preponderance and without evidence of spontaneous or positional nystagmus may be caused by high brainstem lesions of the opposite side or by hemispherical lesions of the same side.

IV. Dissociation of qualitative or quantitative parameters of the caloric nystagmus between the eyes indicate brainstem pathology.

Although electronystagmography has limited value in topographic diagnosis, in our opinion this technique will be in the future as useful as electrocardiology, electroencephalography, and electromyography are today.

REFERENCES

1. Aboulker Pialoux, P., Nevew, M., Butruille, P., and Bouchet, J.: Syndromes Vestibulaires et Nystagmographie. Paris, Librairie Arnette, 1963.
2. Arslan, M., and Sala, O.: Fisiopatologia e clinica delle vie vestibolari centrali. Soc. Coop. Tipogr. Padova, 1956.
3. Aschan, G., Bergstedt, M., and Stahle, J.: Nystagmography. Recording of nystagmus in clinical neuro-otological examinations. Acta Otolaryng. (Stockholm). Suppl 129:1-103, 1956.
4. Buys, E., Dubois-Reymond, E. and Coppez, H.: Traces graphiques du nystagmus. Arch. Ophthal (Paris). 29:737-743, 1909.
5. DuBois-Reymond, E.: Untersuchungen Uber Thierische Elektrizitat. Vol. 2. Berlin, Reimer, 1849, p. 236.
6. Hennebert, P.: La nystagmographie dans les epreuves thermiques. Actaotorhinolaryng. Belg. 14:5-88, 1960.
7. Henrikson, N. G.: An electrical method for registration and analysis of the movements of the eyes in nystagmus. Acta Otolaryng. (Stockholm). 45:25-41, 1955.
8. Holmgreen, F.: Ueber die Retina-stroemer. Acta Soc. Med. Upsal. 6:419-455, 1870, 1871.
9. Jongkees, L. B. W., Maas, J. P. M., and Philipszoon, A. J.: Clinical nystagmography. Prac. Otorhinolaryng. (Basel) 24:65-93, 1962.
10. Jung, R., and Mittermaier, R.: Zur Objectiven Registrierung Und Analyse Verschiedener Nystagmusformen-Vestibularer, Optokinetischer und Spontaner Nystagmus in ihren Wechselbeziehungen. Arch. Ohr. Nas. Kehlkopfheilk. 146:410-439, 1939.
11. Megighian, D.: Electronystagmografia. Collana monagraphica. Minerva Otorinolaring. 1959.
12. Meyers, I. L.: Electronystagmographic study of action currents in nystagmus. Arch. Neurol. Psychiat. 21(1):901-918, 1929.
13. Mowrer, O. H., Ruch, T. C., and Miller, N. C.: The corneo-retinal potential difference as the basis of the galvanometric method of recording eye movements. Amer. J. Deutsch. Physiol. 114:423, 1936.
14. Schott, E.: Record of movements of eyes. Deutsch. Arch. Klin. Med. 140:3:79-90, 1922.
15. Stahle, J.: Electronystagmography in the caloric and rotatory test (a clinical study). Acta Otolaryng. Suppl. 137, 1958.
16. Torok, N., and Nykiel, F.: Frequency meter for nystagmus analysis. Acta Otolaryng. 54: 363-368, 1962.

Galvanic Test

Duncan Hatton

This test for labyrinthine function makes use of galvanic current, a direct and constant flow of electricity of low voltage and low amperage. This current, when passed through human tissue, produces various biochemical and neuromuscular effects.

The source of the galvanic current may be either a battery set or a modern galvanometer. This latter device uses house or commercial (alternating) current for its energy source.

The current is modified in the apparatus and is delivered at two terminals as direct (galvanic) current. The galvanometer should be supplied with a meter for measuring the current in milliamperes, and a convenient accessory will be a toggle switch by which the polarity of the current may be reversed. Two round or square metal discs (dia., 2½-3″) covered with felt serve as electrodes by which the patient, through flexible, insulated wire, is connected to the terminals of the galvanometer. One electrode will be the positive pole, while the other will be the negative one. The current will flow from positive to negative pole. The polarity of the electrodes can be reversed either by a convenient polarity-reversing switch or by changing the connecting electrode lead wires at the terminals of the galvanometer. Before the pads are applied to the patient, they should be well soaked in salt solution. Insufficient moisture causes poor conductivity at the skin site and thus increases the likelihood of discomfort to the patient.

ELECTRODE PLACEMENT

Bipolar. Each electrode is placed on opposite sides of the face, directly in front of the tragus (or on each mastoid prominence). Unipolar: one electrode is placed on the face, in front of the tragus, while the other is attached to the opposite wrist. The latter technique is used more than the former for, it is believed, with unipolar placement, each labyrinth can be separately tested. With this method four different electrode placements can be secured. They are (1) positive electrode (anode) on right face, negative electrode (cathode) on the left wrist; (2) cathode on the right face, anode on the left wrist;

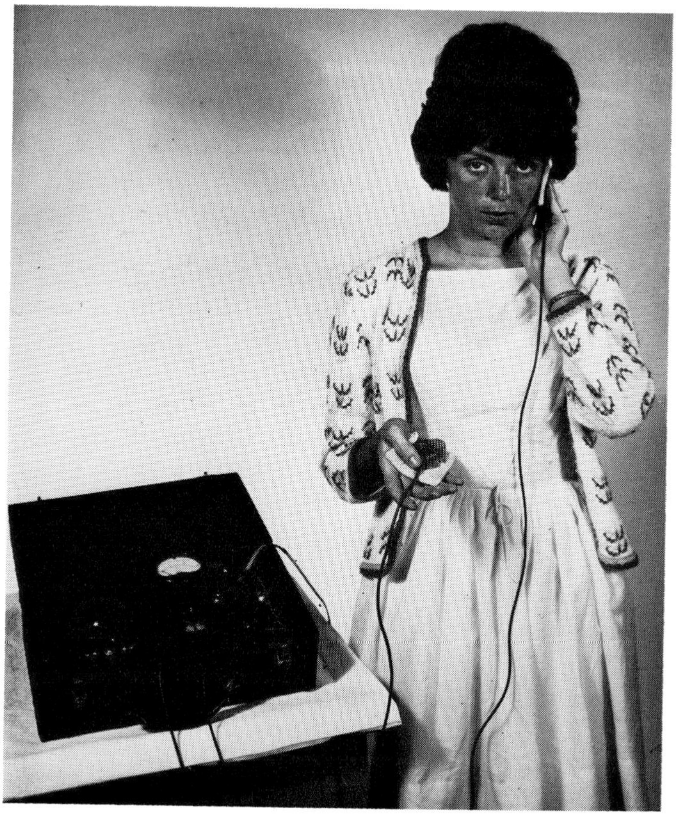

Fig. 1. Galvanic test.

(3) anode on the left face, cathode on the right wrist; (4) cathode on the left face, anode on the right wrist. Some authors maintain that it is not necessary to change the position of the wrist electrode when the face electrode is changed.

The test is done in two parts—one with the patient seated and one with the patient standing with feet and heels together. In the first part of the test, the patient is equipped wth Frenzel lenses, or other magnifying glasses, so that nystagmus may more easily be observed. With the well-soaked electrodes in position 1, above, the current is slowly advanced by an assistant while the operator observes the patient for nystagmus. If nystagmus is produced, the assistant notes the reading on the milliammeter. The current is then slowly reduced to zero. Care must be taken to advance and reduce the current slowly; too abrupt current changes cause discomfort and may unduly upset a very apprehensive patient. The same procedure is now followed in positions 2, 3, and 4. The second part of the test is done with the patient standing and the feet and heels together. When the patient is standing without sway and with the eyes closed, the examiner positions himself in back of the patient with his (examiner's) arms 4 to 5 inches lateral to the patient's shoulders. This is done to insure against a too-great fall. The assistant slowly advances the current and, if sway or fall occurs, the amount of current is noted. The current is gradually reduced and the compensatory sway or fall noted (This, of course, will usually be in the opposite direction from that provoked by the turning on of the current). The test is repeated three or four times with the electrodes in the same position so that the examiner may satisfy himself regarding the validity of the fall or sway. Then positions 2, 3, and 4 are tested in the same manner.

The passage of the galvanic current through the subject will cause a series of subjective and objective phenomena. The subjective symptoms are (1) tingling, prickling, or heat under the electrodes usually in porportion to the current strength; (2) a metallic taste in the mouth due to chorda tympani stimulation; (3) a sensation of vertigo and loss of equilibrium; (4) occasionally, tinnitus at the negative electrode or a decrease in an existing tinnitus under the positive electrode. The objective sign is rotatory nystagmus in a direction opposite to the positive electrode or to the side of the negative electrode when in place at the ear. This nystagmus is independent of the position of the head and differs in this respect from that produced by the caloric stimulation. It is not possible to produce nystagmus in every patient even at current strengths at the limit of endurance, 10-15 milliamperes. Failure to produce galvanic nystagmus should not be construed as evidence of an abnormal labyrinthine system. For this reason, many observers do not perform this part of the test.

INTERPRETATION

The interpretation of the results of galvanic testing is made difficult by the fact that there is some doubt concerning the actual site of the current's action and the degree of the spread. Some early writers believed that the induced phenomena were due to the effects of the current on the brain; others were convinced that the peripheral organ was affected (ampulae of the semicircular canals). However, most present-day investigators believe that "galvanic responses depend on the integrity of Scarpa's ganglion and the vestibular neurons central thereto and are preserved in lesions of the peripheral sense organs."[1] Further weight has been given to this opinion by the researches of Dohlman and Huizinga in 1929 and 1931, respectively. Dix and Hallpike[1] in a study of normal persons found that response to the current—swaying that could be clearly and repeatedly observed—could be produced between 0.3 and 1.9 milliamperes; the average value was 0.8 milliamperes. If swaying cannot be clearly and repeatedly demonstrated at current levels above 4 milliamperes, it may be assumed that there is a lesion of Scarpa's ganglion or the neurons central thereto. The precise location of the lesion cannot be inferred, however, for it is not known to what extent the current spreads. Thus, it may be possible to have an intact Scarpa's ganglion and its central axones with impairment of the vestibular nuclei and/or their central connections in patients who give no response to maximum stimulation. If the limitations of the galvanic test are born in mind, it can be a useful tool to differentiate between lesions of the peripheral organ and its central connections.

REFERENCE

1. Dix, M., and Hallpike, C.: Proc. Roy. Soc. Med. 45:341, 1952.

Pneumatic or Fistula Test

Martin Spector

A fistula test may be performed by pressure and suction with a Sigel otoscope or Politzer bag applied in the external auditory meatus while the eyes are observed for nystagmus. Slow alternate pressure and suction are exerted on the tympanic membrane and middle ear. In a positive test, both vertigo and nystagmus will be elicited. Under normal circumstances, the pneumatic test is negative. Shuster described instances of a positive fistula reaction in cases with an intact eardrum and this has been ascribed to lues, but a loosely fitting stapes could explain some of these reactions. A fistula reaction may occur after eustachian catheterization. The fistula test obviously can be positive only when there is retained function of the semicircular canals.

There are several pathological conditions in which the pneumatic test has diagnostic value:

1. Labyrinthine fistula.

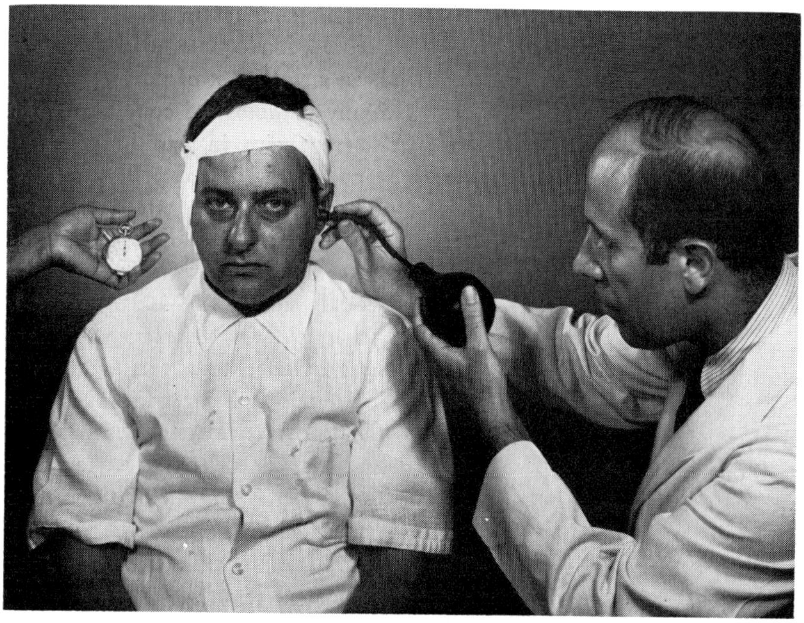

Fig. 1. Fistula test using Politzer bag.

2. Hereditary syphilis.
3. Certain cases of suppurative otitis media, especially with granuloma.
4. Temporal bone tumor.

A perforation in the tympanic membrane with a history of vertigo necessitates a fistula test. With labyrinthine fistula, the test is reported positive in as high as 93 per cent of cases, both on compression and decompression. Compression usually produces nystagmus toward the side being tested and aspiration toward the opposite side. If the reaction is immediate, it may be reproduced indefinitely. A labyrinthine fistula is usually due to cholesteatoma, and the cholesteatoma usually involves the horizontal semicircular canal in the region of the ampulla. At operation, a blue or purple area is observed at the site of the fistula. In uncomplicated suppurative otitis media with a fistula, there may result either a nystagmus or only a conjugate deviation. Here, there is a latent period of three seconds with fatigability. In late hereditary syphilis, compression usually produces nystagmus toward the side of the ear being tested; while in congenital syphilis, the fistula test may be only positive on negative pressure and may only show conjugate deviation or only result in a few bursts of nystagmus.

Audiologic Correlates of Vestibular Disorders

Philip E. Rosenberg

It was during the Devonian period of the paleozoic Era, some 300 million years ago, that the fishlike ancestor of the terrestrial vertebrates first crawled out upon dry land. The eye of that animal was an almost perfect organ. Its usefulness, however, was somewhat limited in this period of lush vegetation. The animal also brought with it a highly developed system for maintaining balance in space and for its own orientation. During the next 100 million years this complex vestibular system, or labyrinth, became modified so that the animal might react to vibratory stimulation and sensation. The ear, then, is a direct outgrowth of the phylogenetically older balance mechanism.

It seems reasonable to expect that a pathology of one portion of this system will frequently affect the other portion. It also may be expected that a generalized pathology of the entire auditory and vestibular system may occur due to a single cause. Thus, symptomatology of vestibular pathology is often accompanied by symptomatology of auditory pathology.

Any thorough examination of the vertiginous patient should include an extensive audiologic evaluation. Pure tone air and bone conduction threshold audiometry, speech reception thresholds, and auditory discrimination tests comprise a minimum battery for the determination of auditory pathology. A normal air conduction audiogram should be considered inadequate evidence upon which to base a statement of normal auditory function. Many pathological conditions exhibit various discrepancies in audition even though pure tone thresholds are well within normal limits. In addition to the minimum battery of audiologic tests mentioned above, other special tests should be used when indicated. These would include Békésy Audiometry, Psychogalvanic Skin Resistance Audiometry, loudness balance tests for loudness recruitment, difference limen tests for loudness recruitment, the Short Increment Sensitivity Index Test, and the Tone Decay Test for abnormal auditory adaptation. All of these tests should be performed in a suitable audiologic environment, with calibrated test equipment and competent examiners.

Most specific peripheral pathologies of the

labyrinth and vestibular system have concomitant auditory disorders which yield highly specific findings upon examination. Indeed, it is highly unusual for an individual to report true vertigo and to be pronounced normal by audiologic examination. A recent study at Temple University Medical Center indicated that patients who complained of "dizziness" but who had normal audiologic findings tended to have normal vestibular examinations as well. On this population the otolaryngologists and neurologists reported normal findings, while the examining psychiatrists and psychologists found significant functional disturbance. In other words, physiologic vertigo tends to be accompanied by physiologic hearing impairment. When this hearing impairment does not exist, the examiner should suspect the possibility of a nonorganic "dizziness." It is true, however, that certain forms of vestibular neuronitis cause true vertigo without causing any significant change in hearing. Furthermore, some vertigo which may be due to intercranial lesions will likewise not show a hearing deficit.

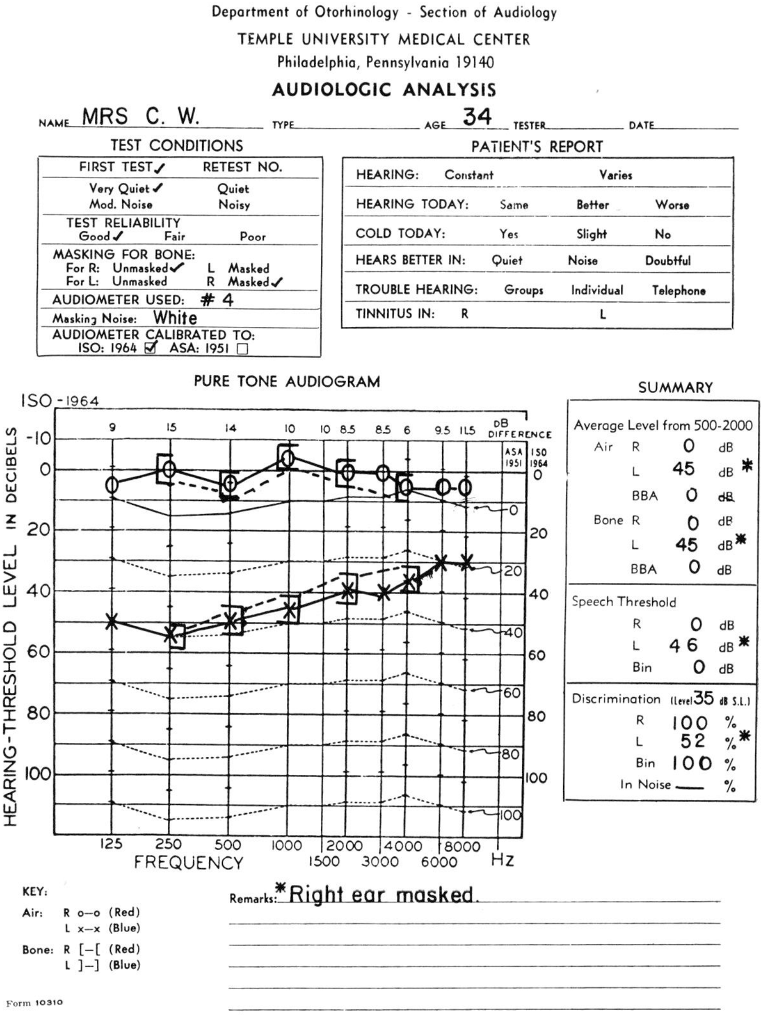

FIG. 1. Characteristic pure tone and speech audiometric findings of a patient with unilateral endolymphatic hydrops.

The most common disease entity resulting in true vertigo is endolymphatic hydrops or Meniere's disease. This causes the classic triad of symptoms—tinnitus, hearing impairment, and vertigo. Endolymphatic hydrops shows a highly typical audiologic pattern. The hearing loss is almost always unilateral. It tends to be of moderate degree, rarely exceeding 60 decibels, and is approximately equal for all frequencies. There is a slight tendency for the lower frequencies to be poorer than the higher frequencies. The loss is purely sensorineural in nature, with the air and bone conduction audiograms being identical. The unaffected ear shows normal hearing. The speech reception thresholds are the same as

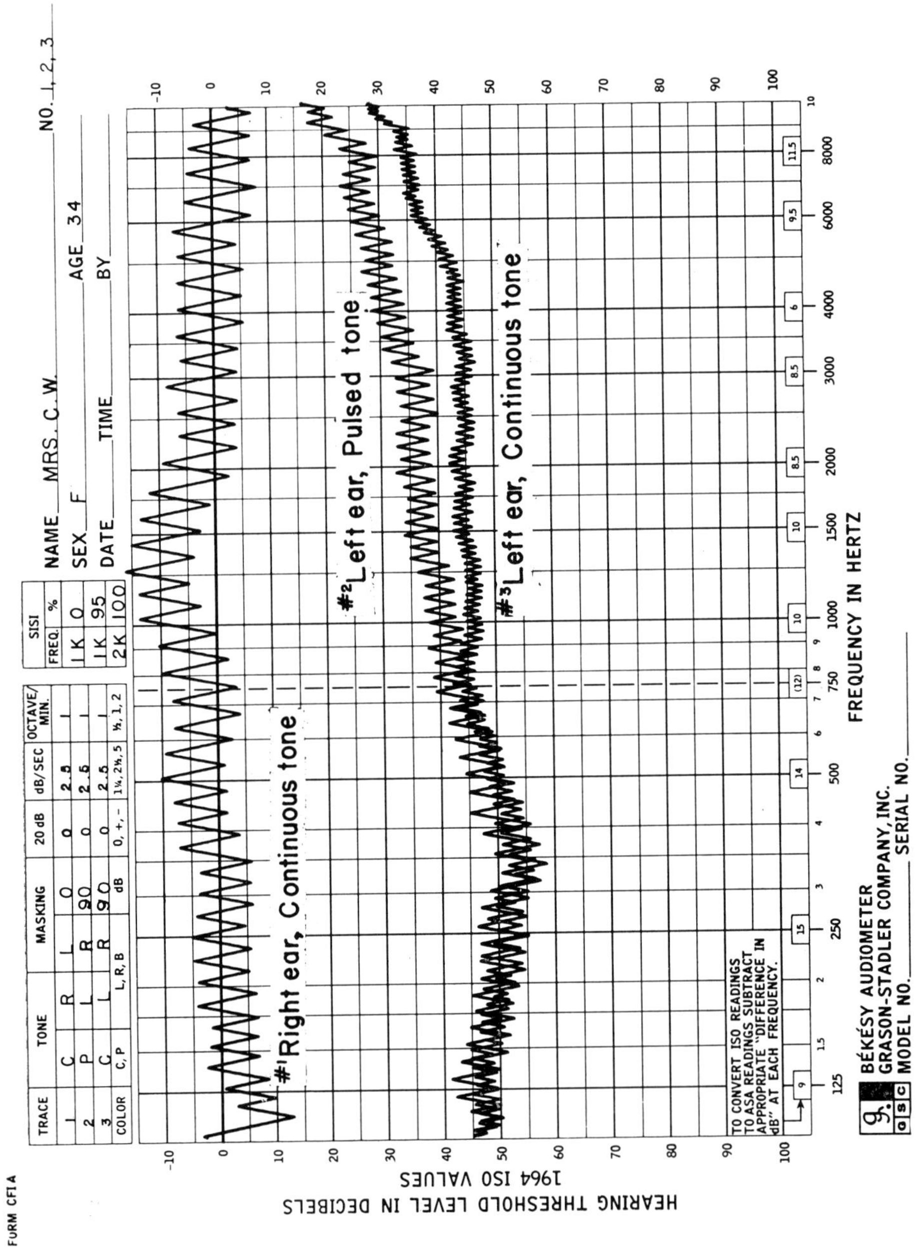

FIG. 2. Typical von Békésy test findings of a patient with endolymphatic hydrops illustrating the Type II Bekesy audiogram.

the average of the three speech frequencies: 500, 1000, 2000 cycles per second. Auditory discrimination in the affected ear tends to be considerably poorer than one would expect from the pure tone audiogram. Discrimination scores of 30 per cent to 40 per cent are quite common. The patient frequently reports that the speech signal sounds are distorted and unpleasant to him. Diplacusis is frequently observed during the pure tone examination, with the patient reporting that a similar frequency has a different pitch in each ear. He may even report that a pure tone has no tonality whatever, but sounds like noise. The typical unilateral Meniere's disease patient will show complete loudness recruitment on Fowler's Alternate Binaural Loudness Balance Test. Difference limens will be quite small at levels near threshold and the Short Increment Sensitivity Index will yield scores above 80 per cent. Both of these findings are also indicative of loudness recruitment. The Békésy audiometric test will usually show a Type II result between pulsed and continuous tone tracings. That is, the continuous tone tracing will drop slightly below the pulsed tone tracing at 1000 cycles per second and remain approximately 10 dB below for the duration of the examination. Furthermore, the continuous tone tracings will show the reduction in pen amplitude characteristic of the recruiting ear. Slight abnormal adaptation or tone decay may be found in patients with endolymphatic hydrops, but this seldom exceeds 20 dB of adaptation. It is important to note that masking must be used to temporarily eliminate the good ear for all audiologic tests upon the bad. Otherwise, deceptive test findings will be obtained that may even suggest the existence of a unilateral conductive hearing disorder. A reduced threshold of discomfort will frequently be noted during the audiologic testing of the patient with Meniere's disease. He will frequently complain that tonal and speech presentation is uncomfortably loud. His dynamic range, that is the difference between his threshold of hearing and his threshold of discomfort, is often dramatically reduced. Approximately 10 per cent of patients with endolymphatic hydrops show bilateral disease. When this occurs, the two ears tend to be quite similar and all of the tests mentioned above may be used with the exception of the alternate binaural loudness balance test. The presence of loudness recruitment may be derived from the difference limen tests and from the SISI test. While the tinnitus and vertigo may recede between attacks of endolymphatic hydrops, the hearing impairment tends to become permanent after the first few attacks. Hearing fluctuation is usually noted in the beginning of the disease but not in its later stages. The very early stages of endolymphatic hydrops show less than the complete pattern described above. A low frequency, sensorineural hearing loss will frequently be observed affecting only 125 and 250 cycles per second. At this point the patient complains of no specific hearing problem and his speech reception threshold and discrimination scores may well be within normal limits. However, the modest reduction of thresholds in the two lowest frequencies will indicate an incipient endolymphatic hydrops.

Those vestibular disorders associated with the degenerative processes of aging are almost always accompanied by a similar degeneration in the auditory system. Presbycusis tends to follow a very characteristic audiologic pattern. The pure tone audiogram shows a bilateral, high frequency, sensorineural deficit. The loss is greatest at 8000 cycles per second, and hearing is frequently normal at 125 and 250 cps. The ears are bilaterally symmetrical, and air and bone conduction audiograms intertwine. The loss may progress to any level of severity but rarely results in total deafness. The patient frequently complains that his problem is not one of hearing but rather one of understanding speech. He states that sounds are loud enough but are not clear. The speech reception thresholds agree quite well with the average of the speech frequencies. Auditory discrimination is almost always reduced. This reduction in auditory discrimination in the presbycusic patient is frequently not severe. Discrimination scores in those patients with only a moderate loss of hearing may be in the region between 60 and 80 per cent. This is due to the loss of the high frequency consonant sounds and the inability to interpret words which contain these sounds. Since the specific pathology of presbycusis may lie anywhere in the inner ear, loudness recruitment tests tend to be equivocal. If the hair cells of the organ of Corti have sustained damage, loudness recruitment will be evidenced. If the pathology is localized to the spiral ganglion or to stria vascularis, recruitment will be absent. Békésy audiometry will usually show a Type I or Type II tracing. Mild tone decay will frequently be present but will not exceed 20 to 25 decibels. Phonemic regression may accompany the presbycusic pattern. These patients understand speech much less well than other presbycusics. They are characterized by an abnormally low auditory discrimination score even in the presence of a relatively mild loss in auditory acuity. It is presumed that cerebral arteriosclerotic changes, perhaps ef-

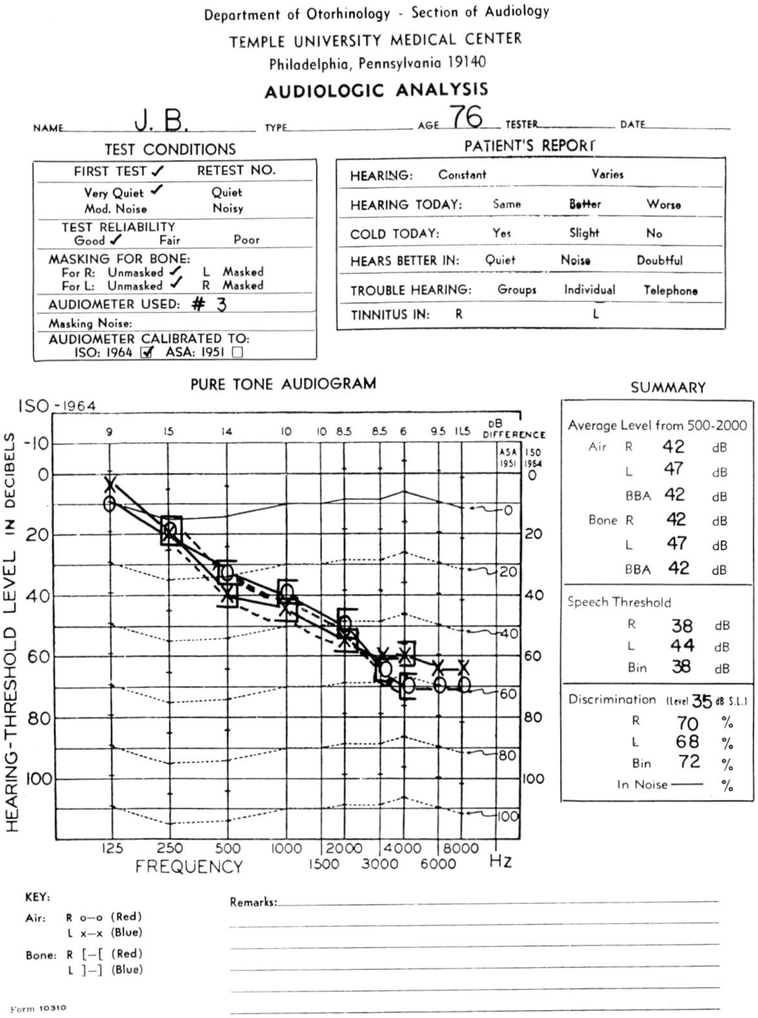

FIG. 3. Characteristic audiometric findings in presbycusis.

fecting the association areas of the cortex, have accompanied the more peripheral changes in the auditory pathways when phonemic regression occurs.

The tumor of the cerebellopontine angle, the acoustic neurinoma, also yields a characteristic pattern of audiologic examination findings. In the past, one rarely saw a patient with an acoustic tumor until the involved ear was essentially deaf. Today, however, these patients are being seen relatively early in the course of their disease, and the hearing impairment is frequently minimal. Characteristically, one ear shows normal hearing while the other shows only a mild, high frequency, sensorineural deficit. The amount of hearing acuity loss may be as little as 15 decibels in the early stages of the disease. Air and bone conduction thresholds on the affected ear will be identical, and the speech reception threshold will agree quite well with the pure tone average. Auditory discrimination is usually extraordinarily poorer. Total absence of discrimination for speech is not uncommon in patients with an acoustic neurinoma. Loudness recruitment, as determined by the alternate binaural loudness balance technique, is traditionally absent. Difference limen scores

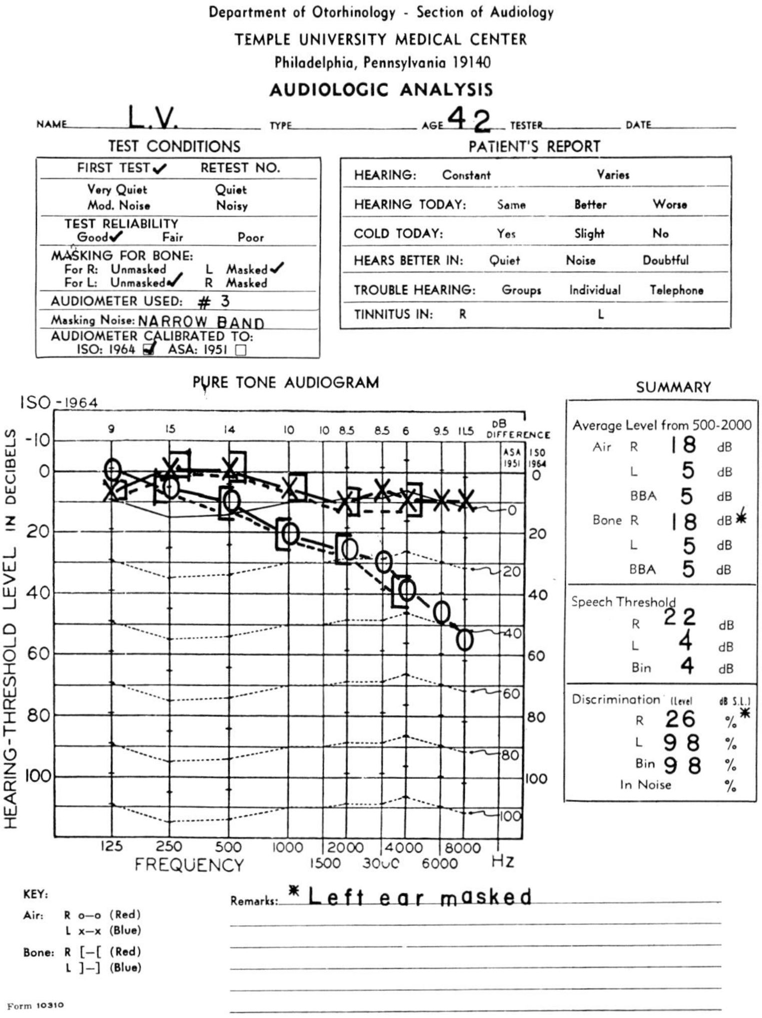

FIG. 4. Pure tone and speech audiometry in a patient with a small cerebello pontine angle tumor.

are not indicative of loudness recruitment, while the Short Increment Sensitivity Index will give a score of 0 per cent. The most remarkable audiologic finding in these patients is the large amount of abnormal adaptation or tone decay. When presented with sustained auditory stimulation, the patient with an acoustic neurinoma shows a dramatic and rapid adaptation to the tonal stimulus, frequently to the point of extinction. Within a 1 minute period, 60 or 70 decibels of tone decay is not unusual. This abnormal adaptation is also exhibited on the Békésy audiogram. A Type III Békésy is usually obtained showing a wide disparity between the threshold tracing for a pulsed tone and the trac-

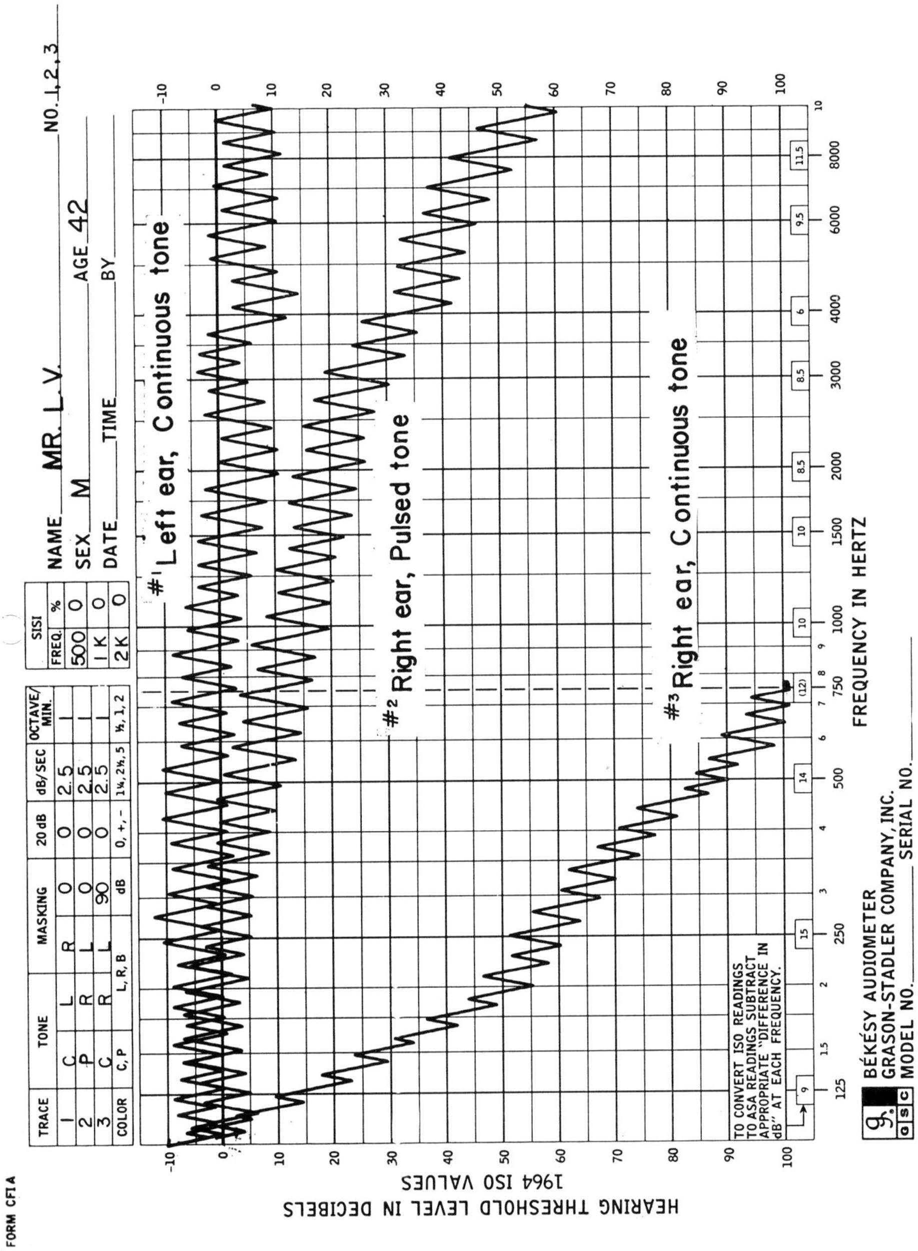

FIG. 5. Type III Békésy audiogram of a patient with an angle lesion illustrating marked abnormal adaptation for continuous tone presentation.

ing for a continuous tone. Even with a very mild loss in acuity, the continuous tone threshold will frequently decline to 100 decibels by the time the test has reached 1000 cycles per second. Momentary interruption of the test tone will permit the ear to recover its initial threshold, but prolongation of the stimulus will again result in total decay and extinction. The dramatic nature of this audiologic finding renders it unmistakable as an item of considerable diagnostic significance. A certain percentage of patients with acoustic tumors will exhibit loudness recruitment. This is frequently indicative of damage to the hair cells of the organ of Corti as a result of other pathologies such as acoustic trauma. It is, however, possible for retrograde degeneration to take place so that a lesion which begins in the internal auditory meatus as a result of pressure from the tumor may eventually cause destruction of the peripheral sensory elements themselves. In such a case, loudness recruitment will be found even though the primary pathology is retrocochlear. Certainly, any unilateral, high frequency, sensorineural hearing impairment should make the examiner suspect the possibility of a tumor of the cerebellopontine angle. Further audiologic studies as well as otologic, neurologic, electronystagmographic, and plesiosectional tomographic studies should be done.

It is not uncommon for a chronic middle ear infection to erode its way into the vestibule and the labyrinth. The resultant labyrinthitis and attacks of paroxysmal vertigo have been described elsewhere. The audiologic findings in such a case would be characteristic of the typical conductive hearing impairment. Bone conduction scores may well be normal, while air conduction thresholds would be significantly depressed. Auditory discrimination should be quite good. Loudness recruitment would be absent, SISI scores would be low, and no indication of tone decay would be apparent. A pure conductive lesion would not cause a hearing impairment of greater than 60 dB. If the infectious invasion of the labyrinth is particularly severe, a sensorineural hearing impairment may be superimposed upon the already existing conductive deficit. This sensorineural loss may be of any severity up to total deafness.

Ototoxic drugs which may effect the vestibular system, the auditory system, or both, cause a high frequency, sensorineural hearing impairment. Among these drugs are dihydrostreptomycin, streptomycin, quinine, kanamycin, neomycin, and others. The pure tone audiogram is quite similar to that obtained in presbycusis, with the highest frequencies showing the poorest thresholds. The loss tends to be bilaterally symmetrical and is gradually progressive. In some drug intoxications, the progression of the impairment ceases when the drug is withdrawn. With other drugs this is not the case, and, even after the drug has been stopped, deafness progresses to totality. Most toxic hearing impairments exhibit loudness recruitment and high SISI scores. Type II Békésy audiograms are usually obtained, and there is only minimal tone decay.

Other pathological conditions, while less common than those previously discussed, nevertheless may affect hearing. Basilar artery insufficiency, thrombosis of the posterior inferior cerebellar artery, and spasm of the internal auditory artery may well result in a relatively severe, unilateral, high frequency sensorineural hearing loss. The onset of this type of deafness is frequently quite rapid and very dramatic to the patient. Head trauma, with or without fracture, may also result in a high frequency nerve loss which is usually unilateral. A concussive injury will cause a hearing impairment of only moderate degree, while a fracture through the temporal bone will result in profound deafness. Multiple Sclerosis and Cogan's syndrome also frequently are accompanied by mild to moderate amounts of hearing impairment. The loss is of the sensorineural type and is usually progressive in nature.

In summary, true vertigo is frequently

accompanied by an auditory defect. Vestibular pathology without auditory pathology is fairly uncommon. Specific disease or pathologic entities tend to have characteristic audiologic patterns associated with them. These patterns are frequently unmistakable and are not easily confused one with the other. A thorough and complete audiological evaluation is necessary in order to achieve a definitive diagnosis of the vertiginous patient.

Testing Vestibular Spinal Reflexes

David A. Dolowitz

PHYSIOLOGY

Balance and spatial orientation are maintained by streams of afferent impulses which are generated by the ocular system, the vestibular system, and the propriocepters (muscles, joints, viscera, and skin). These impulses are acted upon and interact at conscious and subconscious levels. The proprioceptive impulses of the muscles and tendons and especially of the joints of the neck[1,2] have an extreme influence on the interaction. Regulatory systems in the brain and spinal nervous structures act like computers, taking the constant stream of impulses from the eye, ear, and proprioceptive senses, regulating them to constantly alert the body to maintain balance in its normal terrestrial position. Thus these sense organs provide a running commentary on both the external and internal environment of the individual from which the central nervous system collects an integrated pattern which maintains both equilibrium and spatial orientation and hence the ability of locomotion.

PAST POINTING WITH CALORIC TESTS

Clinical testing of the activities of the vestibular spinal tracts has long been used to determine the differential diagnosis of balance disorders. Barany demonstrated that irrigating the external ear and tympanic membrane with fluids of different temperature would produce stimulation of both the cristo-ocular and cristo-spinal mechanisms. This would produce vertigo, nystagmus, and past pointing in the calorically treated patient. He further amplified this work[10] by developing methods of recording objective measurements of these activities. In his testing of past pointing, he would have a sitting person, with eyes closed, raise one hand with the index finger pointing straight forward, then let the stretched out arm sink on his knee. While a normal individual could always touch the same spot, if the right ear was irrigated with cold water, the index finger would drift to the right in a matter of one to six inches, depending upon the activity of the labyrinth. Hot water would produce movement in the opposite direction. Irrigating the opposite ear would also produce motion in the direction of the slow component of nystagmus. Urbantschitsch varied the method to have the patients point simultaneously with both arms. To try and obtain objective measurements, Barany suggested the use of a ruler or similar rod to estimate how far the patient would past point on stimulation of the cristo-spinal reflexes. There has been interpretation of this motion by different investigators. Fischer and Wodak[11,12] considered it a form of space localization in which a vestibular stimulation produced a disturbed impression of one's position in space and caused the pseudomovements. According to their theories, space orientation is necessary in any pointing so that the patient's impression is an egocentric localization. In another paper, Wodak and Fischer[13] exposed their patients to labyrinthine stimulation and described the turning, twisting, and tilting movements of the body. They felt that the body moved in the direction of the slow component of a simultaneously provoked nystagmus. Attempting to record this test, they had a patient hold a pencil in each hand which was kept against a downward moving paper. Unfortunately this did not give adequate recording. Nyman[14] and later Behrman confirmed that past pointing almost always occurred in the predicted direction. The latter felt that the few exceptions were accidental or due to labyrinthine pathology.

STEPPING TESTS

Using another variation of this basic mechanism of the labyrinth, Guttich[15] and Wodak and Fischer,[13] and then Unterberger,[16] developed stepping tests in which they found that persons seemed to rotate on their own axis while walking in one spot (marking time). Unterberger made the comment that most right-handed people rotate slightly to the left and move a little forward even when asked to step in one spot. The problem with all of these tests has been that the authors did not report the degree of rotation or the number of patients tested. Fukuda[17] further refined these tests to see if he could not correlate this reading with diagnosis. In 1959 he had a normal series comprising 500 patients who stepped while blindfolded. That is, they walked in the same spot by alternately lifting their legs, as if in ordinary walking, but their feet remained on the same spot. They had previously been placed in the center of two concentric circles, one half and one meter in diameter, which had been divided so that the angles of 30° could be observed. Thus the rotation of the subject on his own axis and the angle of displacement were very easily seen. He measured the displacement between the initial and ultimate position. Fukuda feels that most normal people remain in the original position after as many as 50 to 100 steps. Some, however, may rotate 30 to 45 degrees and may move forward as much as one meter. He further emphasized that spontaneous changes are most important.

Peitersen and Zilstoff-Pedersen[18] in 1963 did a very careful study on 40 normal subjects, who did the stepping test blindfolded for one minute. Each subject ran through the test on eight different days. Measurements were made of the subject's rotation on their axis or any movements in any direction. In 257 of the 320 normal tests, the subjects moved forward; in 175 to the right and in 116 to the left; 166 of the subjects rotated to the right and 107 to the left. The rotations were between 30 and 60 degrees. The forward movements from 50 to 100 centimeters, while the side movements were less than 25 centimeters. They concluded that it was difficult to set up normal standards, that the values found in a single test cannot be claimed to have major diagnostic value. However, after further testing[19] they came to the conclusion that the cristo-spinal reflex, when used correctly, can produce a diagnosis of central nervous system effect through their alteration of the labyrinthine reflexes. Peitersen[20] repeatedly examined 72 patients with known inner ear pathology and 40 normal volunteers. His otoneurologic examination included the previously described stepping test. He concluded that the stepping test was of value in diagnosing peripheral labyrinthine lesions, especially in unsteady patients. Ninety-three per cent of these tested stepped in only one direction—74 per cent toward and 19 per cent away from the affected ear. Normal volunteers moved in a random fashion 85 per cent of the time. The remaining 15 per cent rotated in only one direction, but their angle of motion was less than half that of patients with peripheral labyrinthine lesions. Thus the diagnosis of both peripheral labyrinthine and central nervous lesions, could be made by their effects in altering the vestibular-spinal reflexes as measured by the stepping tests.

WRITING TEST

Further improvements were then sought by the use of Fukuda's vertical writing test.[21,22]

In this test a patient writes a vertical column of words (in Japanese) or letters (in English) while keeping his arm free of any contact with the desk or paper except through the writing instrument used. This writing is then repeated with the patient blindfolded. Imbalances of the reflexes cause a constant deviation of the characters in the column. This often occurs in the quiescent period of Meniere's disease in the absence of spontaneous nystagmus, past pointing, or Romberg's phenomenon. Fukuda feels that the stepping and vertical writing tests demonstrate that the patient with differences in labyrinth function turn on their longitudinal axis. He therefore modified this test so that the head is held inclined to right and left both anteriorly and posteriorly and so can demonstrate imbalance of individual canals. In attempting this test three difficulties arose. First, it is extremely difficult for a non-Japanese to write in a neat vertical column, even if only numbers were used. Second, it is hard to keep a conscious awareness of the locality of the paper when one is blindfolded and touches the paper only with the writing instrument. Third, to accomplish this writing much cerebral activity is required. It has been shown that accompanying cerebral activity increases cristo-ocular reflexes materially.[23] Hence, by inference there may be exaggeration of the cristo-spinal reflex by a similar mechanism.

ROMBERG SIGN

For gross testing we prefer the Romberg sign test in which the feet are brought together to present a minimal supporting base. The base may be cut in half by having the patient stand on one foot. If the patient has a vestibular impairment, he will be unable to remain erect on this limited support. Analysis of his movements demonstrates first a motion away from the midline in a definite direction due to the labyrinthine impairment. A split second later the righting reflexes take over and return the patient to the erect position. These movements recur cyclically.

SHUSTER'S PELVIC GIRDLE TEST

The Romberg sign is an excellent gross test which was improved by the addition of Shuster's modifications of pelvic girdle resistance. Here the pelvis of the patient in Romberg position is seized by the examiner and pushed in one direction after another until the pelvis has had pressure exerted on it in all directions. Patients with intracranial lesions in the posterior fossa, especially in the midline of the cerebellum, or those with lesions which exert pressure on the pyramidal tracts do not exhibit resistance to the examiner's push in one definite direction and have a "broomstick fall" because of the lack of spinal righting reflexes. It is our opinion, however, that more refined diagnosis will require analysis of either cristo-spinal or of the righting reflex arc alone, while both the Romberg and pelvic girdle resistance tests are summation of both effects.

TIPPING TESTS

Attention was therefore turned to a study of the tipping reaction. Animal work[20,24,25] had indicated that frogs, pigeons, or dogs lost their defensive movement to slow or fast tipping after destruction of their semicircular canals. It was postulated that the vertical semi-circular canal induced muscular defense to rapid tipping and the proprioceptive organs caused the reaction to slower movements. As expected, the cerebellum coordinated the muscular reaction. Tipping tables have been of two main types. The first is a table with an axis on one side used for the tipping; the second is a rotary type on which the patient was placed on hands and knees and the table rotated. Since this introduced rotation as well as a tipping reaction, it was gradually replaced. Gradually a table was evolved in which the tipping is executed about the longitudinal axis in the horizontal plane. The tipping table is provided with U-shaped blocks in which the knees fit to prevent the patient from sliding off the table during the test. On testing, the patient is placed on hands and knees on the table with equal distance between the knees and to the longitudinal axis, so that it coincides with that of the table. The head is held raised, face forward with the eyes covered. The patient is instructed not to be tense, but to let himself go and endeavor to preserve his balance. He is asked not to move his hands from their symmetrical positions. He is first put through slow tipping movements so that he understands what is expected of him. The muscular defenses are measured through the use of a leather harness attached to the shoulder girdles. Light photography, transducers, etc. are used to record the measurements. Rademaker[24] reported that there are three phases to the tipping action (1) A labyrinthine phase inducing muscular defense; (2) a passive phase in which the body, transported by the movements of the table, passes to one side; (3) A proprioceptive phase, characterized by the body's exertion to stabilize its equilibrium. Cerebellar phenomena become apparent in this phase, as do cutaneous and deep sensitivity. Rådmark[26] showed that the second phase could be eliminated if the patient were placed in a very symmetrical position on the table and by avoiding abrupt stops during the tipping. Nyman[14] found that normals always react in the same way to slow tipping. Patients with vertigo showed that the tipping investigation would be weaker on the side with the lesser defense reaction. He pointed out that about 8 per cent of the people with known vestibular spinal disease still would have normal tipping reactions and warns that this must be remembered. He stresses that the vestibular organs are paired and that the tipping only demonstrates the quantitative dissimilarity between the organs. He feels that in studying vestibular spinal disorders, using the tipping action, one must remember physiologic variations and vestibular dissimilarity factors.

LATEROPULSION

In reviewing the various methods of vestibular spinal reflex evaluation, Torok and Kahn[27] developed a device which records the reflexes electrically. They call the resulting movement, lateropulsion. It is our feeling that this is one of the best methods in recording

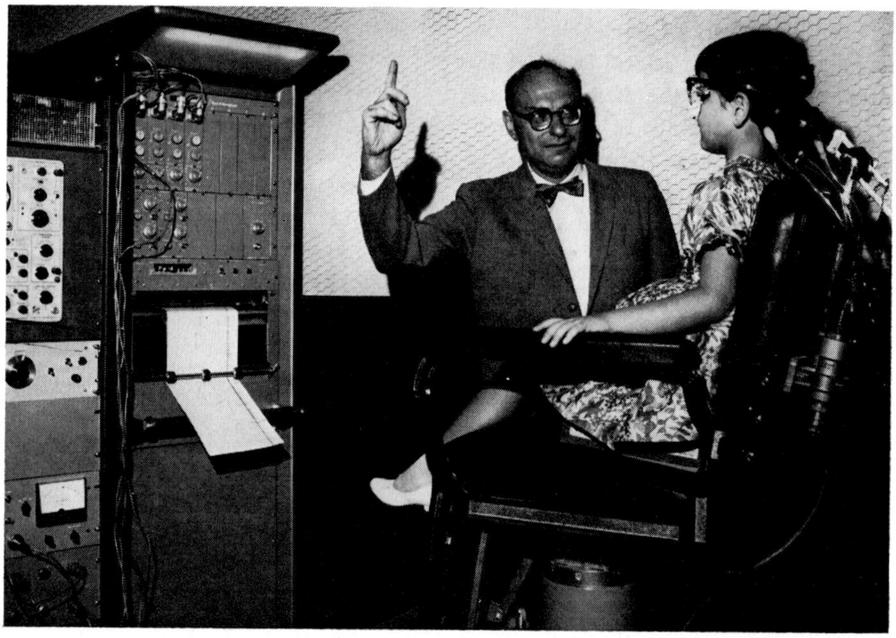

FIG. 1. Simultaneous recording of cristo-ocular and cristo-spinal reflexes.

vestibular spinal reflexes. Patients are placed in a harness in a rotary chair, which records the lateral sway of the patient in a sitting position as he responds to a rotary stimulus. In reviewing the test, however, we felt there was a compensatory movement of the body to prevent falling, and hence, theoretically, the deviation would be diminished. This view was strengthened since the measurements found by Torok[28] were minimal.

In efforts to remove the compensatory movement, the laterotorsion test was developed.[38] Here simultaneous records are made of the cristo-ocular and cristo-spinal reflexes elicited by a single caloric stimulus. This more complete otoneurologic examination was felt to provide more exact information. The person tested is placed in a relaxed, supine position, eliminating the need for cerebral control. Since there is a large base of support, any of the postural compensatory reflexes are felt to be excluded. It is further felt that, since the body remains relaxed during this test, secondary electrical disturbances resulting from the complicated body movements of many tests are eliminated. This is especially important since the nystagmus is recorded simultaneously. Caloric irrigations were found to produce a lateral twist of the head, neck, and body in the direction of the slow phase of the nystagmus in normal individuals.[29] The twist was felt to be the result of the torquelike action of the spinal muscles in twisting the body; therefore, the reflex was named "laterotorsion." Caloric stimulation used in this test employs principles of Fitzgerald and Hallpike, in which water of 30° and 44° centigrade is used to irrigate each ear for 40 seconds. The reclining patient lies on two cylindrical, rubber, air-containing devices which lie between the head and the sponge rubber-covered braces of an ordinary examining chair. Each device has three outlets. One equalizes pressure in the two devices, the second maintains a constant pressure measurement, and the third is used for the recording. The recording outlet may be connected to a water manometer and/or a transducer[30] by means of a Y outlet. The adjusting outlet permits the pumping of air into the system until the predetermined pressure of 30 millimeters of mercury is reached. The pressure must be achieved after the patient has rested his head on the balloon device to compensate for the various weights, size, and shapes of different patient's heads. If this is done, all tests are made at the same pressure levels, eliminating a problem. The third outlet connects the two balloons, equalizing pressure between them until the test is begun when the connection is closed. The torquelike twist of the head and neck produces different weights on the two systems, causing unequal pressure within the pneumatic system. Transducers are adjusted so that a deflection of one millimeter on the recorder corresponds to a difference of one centimeter between the water columns of the manometer. Using weights, one can easily calculate the number of grams that produce the deflection of one millimeter on any given system. By simple calculations, all systems can be reduced to a common denominator. Since it is possible to record simultaneous cristo-ocular reflexes on a second channel of the recorder, the spontaneous optikinetic, gaze, positional, and caloric nystagmus are simultaneously recorded. The quantitative studies have shown that maximum laterotorsion and nystagmus are fairly consistent for any given individual, but vary between individuals.[31] There is a lack of quantitative correlation between nystagmus and laterotorsion, as evidenced by the unequal patterns of behavior and a lack of correlation between the maxima of the two reflexes and unequal time for the development of the maxima and an unequal duration of the nystagmus and laterotorsion. The degree of vertigo and caloric laterotorsion show some correlation, but none could be established for vertigo and caloric nystagmus.

Light has an effect on both nystagmus and laterotorsion, decreasing them. The decrease of the nystagmus is greater than that of the laterotorsion. Peripheral labyrinthine lesions were found to decrease the measured amounts of vertigo, laterotorsion, and nystagmus. In Meniere's disease[32] while the measured nystagmus and vertigo decreased, laterotorsion remained normal in amount. Infection such as meningoencephalitis showed normal nystagmus but an increase in vertigo and laterotorsion. These findings are strengthening our impression that cristo-ocular and cristo-spinal reflexes have different mechanisms modulating them, despite the common origin of their stimulus.

It must be stressed that one must do a complete otoneurologic examination, using every tool and not become so enamored of the cristo-spinal reflexes as to ignore the others. We feel that with the study of laterotorsion and the simultaneous study of nystagmus we are beginning to avoid this pitfall.

REFERENCES

1. Gernandt, B. E., and Gilman, S.: Descending vestibular activity and its modulation by proprioceptive, cerebellar and reticular influences. Exp. Neurol. 1:274, 1959.
2. Mc Cough, G. P., Deering, J. D., and Ling, T. H.: Location of receptors for tonic neck-reflexes. J. Neurophysiol. 14:192, 1951.
3. Lowenstein, O.: Oscillographic analysis of non-acoustic function of vertebrate ear. Nature (London) 161:652, 1948.
4. Lowenstein, O., and Roberts, T.D.M.: The localization and analysis of responses to vibration from the isolated elasmobranch labyrinth; a contribution to the problem of hearing in vertebrates. J. Physiol. 114:471, 1951.
5. Ross, D. A.: Electrical studies on frog's labyrinth.
6. Wersall, J.: Studies on the structure and innervation of the sensory epithelium of the cristae ampullares in the guinea pig. Acta Otolaryng. (Suppl.) 126:1, 1956.
7. Gray, L. P.: Experimental evidence on connections of vestibular mechanism in cat. J. Comp. Neurol. 41:319, 1926.
8. Ramon y Cajal, S.: Histologie du Systeme Nerveux de l'Homne et des Vertebres. Paris, Maloini, 1909.
9. Barany, R.: Weitere unterschungen uber den vom Vestibularapparat des Ohres refleptorisch ausgelosten rhytmeschen Nystagmus und seine Begleiterscheinungen. Msschr. Chrenheilk. 41:4777, 1907.
10. Barany, R.: Vestibularapparat und Zentralnervensystem. Deutsch. Z. Nervenheilk. 43:356, 1911.

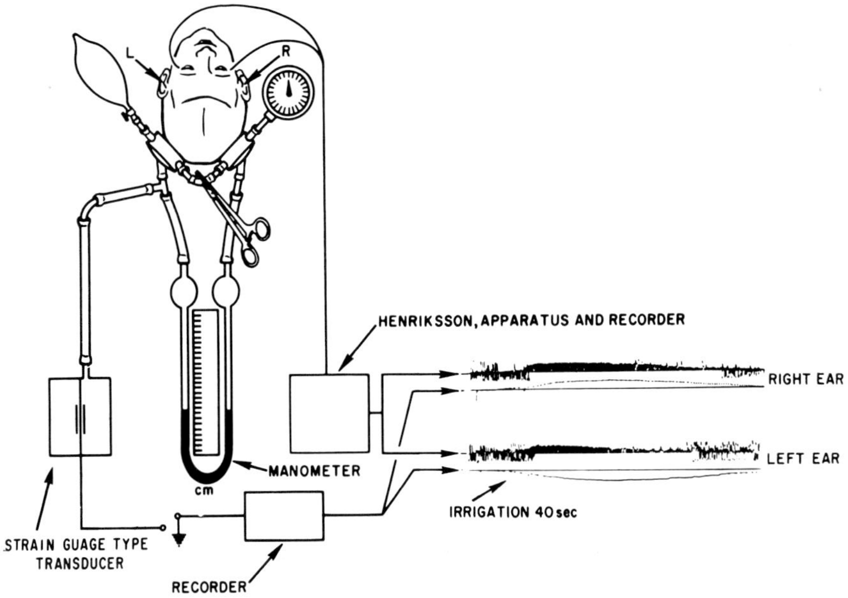

FIG. 2. Diagram of laterotorsion apparatus.

11. Fischer, M. H., and Wodak, E.: I. Beiträge zur Physiologie des menschlichen Vestibularapparates. II. Mitteilung. Die Grundlagen und graphischen Registriermethoden der >>vestibularen Korperreflexe<<. Pflüger Arch. Ges. Physiol. 202:553, 1924.
12. Fischer, M. H., and Wodak, E.: Prinzipielle Betrachtungen zum Probleme des Zeigerversuches. Acta Otolaryng. 10:24, 1926.
13. Wodak, E., and Fischer, M. H.: Eine neue Vestibularisreaktion. Munchen. Med. Wschr 69: 193, 1922.
14. Nyman, H.: A graphic registration of tipping and pointing reaction. Acta Otolaryng. (Suppl.) 60, 1945.
15. Guttich, A.: Beitragzur Physiologie des Vestibularapparates. Beitr. Path. Anat. 7:1, 1914.
16. Unterberger, S.: Neue Objektiv registrierbare Vestibularis-Korperdreaktion, erhalten durch Treten auf der Stelle. Der "Tretversuch." Arch. Ohr. Nas Kehlkopfheilk. 145:478, 1938.
17. Fukuda, T.: The stepping test. Two phases of the labyrinthine reflex. Acta. Otolaryngol. 50:95, 1959.
18. Zilstoff-Pedersen, K., and Peitersen, E.: Vestibulospinal reflexes 1. Arc. Otolarnyg. 77: 237, 1963.
19. Peitersen, E., and Zilstoff-Pedersen, K.: Vestibulospinal reflexes VIII alterations in the stepping test in various intracranial diseases. Arch. Otolaryng. 79:6000, 1964.
20. Peitersen, E.: Vestibulospinal reflexes. Arch. Otolaryng. 79:481, 1964.
21. Fukuda, T., and Topita, T.: A new arrangement of the vestibular examination. Acta. Otolarnyg. 179:178, 1963.
22. Fukuda, T.: Vertical writing with eyes covered. A new test of vestibular spinal reaction. Acta Otolaryng. 50:26, 1959.
23. Mahoney, J. L., Harlan, W. L., and Bukford, R. G.: Visual and other factors influencing caloric nystagmus in normal subjects. Arch. Otolaryng. 66:46, 1957.
24. Rademaker, G. G. J.: Ractions labyrinthiques et Equilibre., Paris, Masson et cie, 1935.
25. De Kleyn, A., and Versteegh, C.: Über Labyrinthäre Gleichgewichtsreaktionen bei Menschen und Tieren nach schnellem Kippen um die longitudinale Achse. Acta Otolaryng. 24:34, 1936.
26. Rådmark, K.: Tipping reaction in cases of vertigo after head injury. Acta Otolaryng. 31: 454, 1943.
27. Torok, N., and Kahn, A.: Vestibular lateropulsion. Ann. Otol. 69:61, 1960.
28. Torok, N.: Recording Vestibular Lateropulsion. Confin. Neurol., 20:266, 1960.
29. Henriksson, N. G., Dolowitz, D. A., and Forssman, B.: Studies of cristo-spinal reflexes (laterotorsion). I. A method for objective recording of cristo-spinal reflexes. Acta Otolaryngol. 55:33, 1962.
30. Dolowitz, D. A., Henriksson, N. G., and Forssman, B.: Laterotorsion, a vestibular-spinal reflex. Laryngoscope 73:893, 1963.
31. Henriksson, N. G. Dolowitz, D. A., and Forssman, B.: Studies of Cristospinal reflexes (laterotorsion). II Caloric nystagmus and laterotorsion in normal individuals. Acta Otolaryngol. 55:116, 1962.
32. Dolowitz, D. A., Forssman, B., and Henrikkson, N. G.: Studies of cristo-spinal reflexes (laterotorsion). III. Patterns of cristo-ocular and cristo-spinal reflexes in clinical oto-neurology. Acta Otolaryngol. 55:496.

Neurological Examination and Symptoms Suggesting Neurological Checkup

NEUROLOGICAL EXAMINATION

J. U. Toglia

The following parts of the neurological examination should be emphasized: nystagmus, past pointing, Romberg, cerebellar tests, gait, and the examination of certain cranial nerves.

NYSTAGMUS

The patient is instructed to follow the examiner's finger as it is slowly moved in his visual field. Nystagmus is considered pathological if it develops within 45 degrees of the visual angle at each side of the midline. However, nystagmus of extreme gaze is also pathological if it develops upon gazing in one direction and especially if it does not disappear after a few seconds.

Central vestibular nystagmus has a great variety of form and direction: purely horizontal, vertical, multiple, oblique, pendular, rotatory, retractorius. It lasts longer than peripheral nystagmus and is not easily altered by caloric nystagmus and by optokinetic nystagmus. Although central nystagmus does not establish an etiologic diagnosis, in some instances specific forms have anatomical diagnostic value:

1. The nystagmus associated with cerebellopontine angle tumors is coarser when looking toward the side of the lesion and may be associated with vertical nystagmus and other forms if the brainstem is compressed by the expanding tumor.
2. Rotatory nystagmus is observed only in cases of bulbar pathology—i.e., posterior inferior cerebellar artery syndrome.
3. Nystagmus retractorius and convergence nystagmus are seen only in patients with pretectal midbrain lesions.

Aubry[1] found among 566 cases of central nystagmus the following incidence of the various forms: 32 per cent horizontal, 30 per cent multiple, 23 per cent positional, 8 per cent rotatory, 4 per cent vertical, and 3 per cent horizontal-rotatory. There were also 11 cases of pendular nystagmus and one of nystagmus retractorius. Of all the cases, 452 were associated with posterior fossa lesions and 109 with supratentorial lesions.

Vestibular nystagmus of peripheral origin is horizontal-rotatory, usually unidirectional, and may be distinguished from central vestibular nystagmus by the characteristics indicated in Table 2.

The relationship between nystagmus and central vestibular lesions was investigated by Leidler and his findings are summarized as follows:

A. Nystagmus and Brainstem Lesions

1. The greater the extent of the lesion, the longer the duration of the nystagmus.
2. Among other factors not understood, the level of the brainstem lesion influences the direction of the nystagmus: caudal lesions induce homolateral nystagmus; rostral lesions induce contralateral nystagmus. The height

TABLE 1. Spontaneous Vestibular Nystagmus

	Peripheral (Labyrinth, Vestibular Nerve)	*Central* (CNS)
Form	horizontal-rotatory	horizontal; vertical; diagonal; rotatory; multiple; retractorius; convergence; pendular; alternating
Frequency	½-6/sec.	any frequency, usually low or variable at long intervals (weeks to months)
Intensity	decreasing intensity	constant
Direction of fast component	towards "stimulated" labyrinth or away from "destroyed" labyrinth	towards side of CNS lesion
Duration	minutes to weeks	weeks to months
Dissociation between eyes	none	possible
Vertigo	present	present or absent
Cochlear signs	frequently present	seldom present
Autonomic nervous system signs	definite	less definite or absent
Past pointing and falling	direction of slow phase	direction of fast phase

of the lesion in the brainstem also determines the nystagmus form: rotatory nystagmus is seen with bulbar lesions, vertical nystagmus with midbrain lesions, and horizontal nystagmus with lesions in the pons.

3. With bilateral lesions the direction of the nystagmus is to the side of the greatest lesion.

4. When lesions in the bulbopontine area spare the arcuate fibers, normal caloric nystagmus can be elicited.

B. Nystagmus and Cerebellar Lesions

1. Lesions of the cortex of the cerebellar vermis induce no nystagmus.

2. Lesions of the vermis in toto cause no spontaneous nystagmus, but influence the nystagmus induced by rotation.

3. Lesions in one-half of the vermis cause increased vestibular response to homolateral stimuli. (Probably the result of loss of inhibition from the cerebellar nuclei.)

4. Lesions of one cerebellar hemisphere cause no spontaneous nystagmus nor influence induced nystagmus.

C. Nystagmus and Cerebral Lesions

1. Lesions of both cerebral hemispheres and thalamus do not cause or influence induced nystagmus.

2. Lesions of one cerebral hemisphere increase the excitability of the contralateral labyrinth and decrease that of the homolateral. Some of Leidler's conclusions have been challenged in the literature; additional studies are necessary to clarify controversial points.

PAST POINTING

The patient keeps his eyes closed and extends both arms forward, laying the index fingers on the examiner's fingers. He then raises (or lowers) both arms and keeping the eyes closed brings both index fingers slowly to the original position. This test is repeated with the patient's head inclined 105 degrees first over one shoulder and later over the other. With peripheral vestibular diseases both arms will miss the original points, being deviated in the direction of the slow phase of the nystagmus. With central vestibular diseases, this deviation may involve one or both arms but is directed toward the side of the fast phase of the nystagmus—that is, toward the diseased side. If past pointing is modified by testing the patient with his head inclined over one or the other shoulder, this indicates peripheral rather than central vestibular pathology. At the other end, past pointing in absence of nystagmus and Rombergism indicates central vestibular pathology.

The above tests have more of a diagnostic value if the past pointing expected after caloric stimulation is absent or has inverted direction.

TABLE 2. Differentiation of Central from Peripheral Vertigo

	Peripheral (Labyrinth, Vestibular Nerve)	*Central* (CNS)
Hallucination of movement	definite	less definite
Onset	usually paroxysmal	seldom paroxysmal
Intensity	usually severe	seldom severe
Duration	minutes to weeks	weeks to months
Influenced by head position	frequently	seldom
Nystagmus	present	present or absent
Autonomic nervous system symptoms	definite	less definite or absent
Tinnitus	frequently present	seldom present
Deafness	frequently present	seldom present
Disturbances of consciousness	seldom present	more frequently present
Other neurological signs	usually absent	frequently present

ROMBERG TEST

Standing with both feet together or on either foot or with one foot in front of the other, and with eyes closed, the patient has a positive Romberg if he has a definite tendency to fall. It is difficult to evaluate this test in patients with central vestibular diseases because of the intervention of other factors such as the frequent association of proprioceptive, cerebellar, or corticospinal lesions. However, with peripheral vestibular disease the direction of the fall is consistently to one side and influenced by changing position of the head and by caloric stimulation. By inclining the head to either side, the direction of the fall changes from lateral to lateral-forward or lateral backward.

In patients with central vestibular lesions, the Romberg may also be negative, or vice versa a positive Romberg may be seen in patients even after nystagmus and vertigo have long disappeared.

It should be recalled that with lesions of the proprioceptive system, the direction of the Romberg changes from one test to the next, and that with cerebellar lesions, if any difficulty of balance exists, it is present whether the eyes are opened or closed.

CEREBELLAR TESTS AND GAIT

Lesions of the cerebellum cause dysmetria, asynergy, static and kinetic tremor, hypotonia, dysarthria, and ataxic gait. The tests usually performed in order to demonstrate these signs include: finger to nose, thumb to fingers, finger to finger, heel to knee, alternating movements of the hands, etc. The differential diagnosis between cerebellar and vestibular disturbances of posture and gait should not be difficult.

With unilateral cerebellar lesions, the head and trunk are inclined to the side of the lesion and are not influenced by closing the eyes; the gait is hemiataxic and the automatic arm swing on the side of the lesion is increased because of hypotonia. With bilateral cerebellar lesions, the patient stands with feet far apart, both arms in abduction, and obviously has difficulty in keeping his balance. Although he walks with ataxic steps, he does not deviate consistently to either side.

Vestibular disturbances of station and gait are more obvious when the subject keeps his eyes closed. They are not the result of poor coordination, but of poor body equilibrium. The subject stands and walks with his feet well separated, the arms abducted to help his balance; if the lesion is unilateral his gait deviates to the side of the lesion without evidence of ataxia. If the lesion is bilateral, the gait will be extremely difficult, the patient falling forward and backward. Gait and balance may be better tested by having the patient walk on rails of various widths.

When testing the gait forward and backward the patient with unilateral vestibular disease outlines on the ground a pattern resembling a star (Babinski-Weil sign). The value of this sign is doubted by many. On changing the position of the head, the direction of the gait will change only if the patient has peripheral and not central vestibular disease.

EXAMINATION OF THE CRANIAL NERVES

The presence of symptoms or signs due to lesions of the cranial nerves indicate that probably the vertigo is of central origin; however, a patient with neurologic disease may also suffer vertigo of labyrinthine origin. Inquiry should be made about diplopia, numbness of the face and tongue, dysphagia, etc. Perhaps the examination of the fifth, the seventh, and the eighth cranial nerves is the most informative. The motor component of the fifth cranial nerve is examined by checking the muscle bulk and power of both temporal and masseter muscles and the movements of the jaw; the sensory component is examined by checking the sensations of the face and the corneal reflexes. The test for corneal reflex is relatively simple: While the patient is looking upwards and to one side, the physician touches the cornea of the opposite side with a piece of cotton. If blinking is absent in both eyes this indicates loss of sensation in the cornea tested; if blinking is absent only in the eye tested, the result indicates that corneal sensation is intact whereas the orbicularis oculi innervated by the homolateral seventh facial nerve is impaired. Absence of the homolateral corneal reflex is frequently noted in cerebellopontine angle tumors.

The seventh cranial nerve is examined by checking the symmetry of the mimic muscles of the face. The patient looks upwards and corrugates the forehead, closes the eyelids tightly and keeps them from being passively opened, smiles, shows his teeth, blows his cheeks or whistles. If the seventh cranial nerve is involved the facial muscles are paralyzed homolaterally. Involvement of the seventh cranial nerve is also frequently seen in cases of cerebellopontine angle tumors.

The eighth cranial nerve is best examined by the audiologist for the cochlear portion and by electronystagmography for the vestibular portion. These examinations will be discussed separately.

The examination of the IX, X, and XI cranial nerves is carried on by checking the pharyngeal reflexes, the movement of the uvula and of the vocal cords, the motor power and bulk of sterno-cleido mastoids and trapezius muscles. When these cranial nerves are involved there is difficulty in swallowing and talking, hoarseness, stridor; with paralysis of the XII cranial nerve the tongue will be protruded towards the side of the paralyzed nerve and show homolateral atrophy and fasciculations.

The neurological evaluation of patients afflicted by vertigo and other vestibular disturbances should include, when necessary, studies such as blood and spinal fluid chemistries, skull and cervical spine x-rays, pneumoencephalography, arteriography, electroencephalography, and electronystagmography. These studies will be discussed separately in other sections of this book.

REFERENCES

1. Arslan, M., and Sala, O.: Fisiopatologia and Clinica delle vie Vestibolari Centrali. Padova, Soc. Coop. Tipografica, 1956.
2. Aubry, M., and Pialoux, P.: Maladies de l'oreille interne et oto-neurologic. Paris, Masson et Cie, 1957.
3. Cawthorne T.: Vertigo. Proc. Roy. Soc. Med. 52: 1-8, 1959.
4. Grinker, R. R., and Bucy, P.: Neurology, Fifth Edit. Springfield, Ill., Charles C Thomas, 1960.
5. Leidler, R.: Wie Weit Kann man aus der vestibularuntersuchung auf art und sitz einer Hirner Kran Kung Schliessen. Prac. Otolaryng. 2:152-190, 1939.
6. Macrae, P.: The neurological aspects of vertigo. Calif. Med. 42:255-259, 1960.
7. Nylen, C. O.: Positional nystagmus. J. Laryng. 64:295-310, 1950.
8. Wechsler, I. S.: Clinical Neurology. Philadelphia, W. B. Saunders Co., 1963.

SYMPTOMS SUGGESTING NEUROLOGICAL CHECKUP

Martin Spector

1. Continuous ataxia between attacks of dizziness.
2. Episodes of unconsciousness.
3. Occipital headaches.
4. Diplopia or dimming of vision.
5. Perioral or lingual numbness and paresthesia. (Numbers 4 and 5 may occur for minutes at a time.)

I. Spontaneous Signs
   1. Vertical or oblique nystagmus.

2. Nystagmus lasting more than two weeks without vertigo.
3. Poor pelvic girdle resistance.
4. Falling with the direction of fall not influenced by change in position of the head with reference to the body.
5. Spontaneous past pointing which cannot be altered by an appropriate vestibular test.

II. After Tests
1. Fixed positional nystagmus lasting more than three months without definite peripheral etiology. Neurologic examination will often be negative here.
2. Central type positional nystagmus—i.e., persistent, direction changing, non-fatigable.

Heath Rails Test

G. O. Proud

On occasions the Romberg test is not sufficiently sensitive to demonstrate the phenomenon of faulty balance. In such instances, the rail-walking test described by Heath[2] may yield much information. Three rails, each measuring 3 inches from top to floor, are used. Rail one is 9 feet long and 4 inches wide. Rail two measures 9 feet by 2 inches, and the third rail is 6 feet by 1 inch. Each bears transverse marks at 12 inch intervals.

The subject is asked to mount rail one barefooted and walk in any manner he may choose (Fig. 1) until the end is reached. Three such "trial runs" are performed to get the "feeling." In actual testing, he walks the length of the rail heel to toe and as far as he

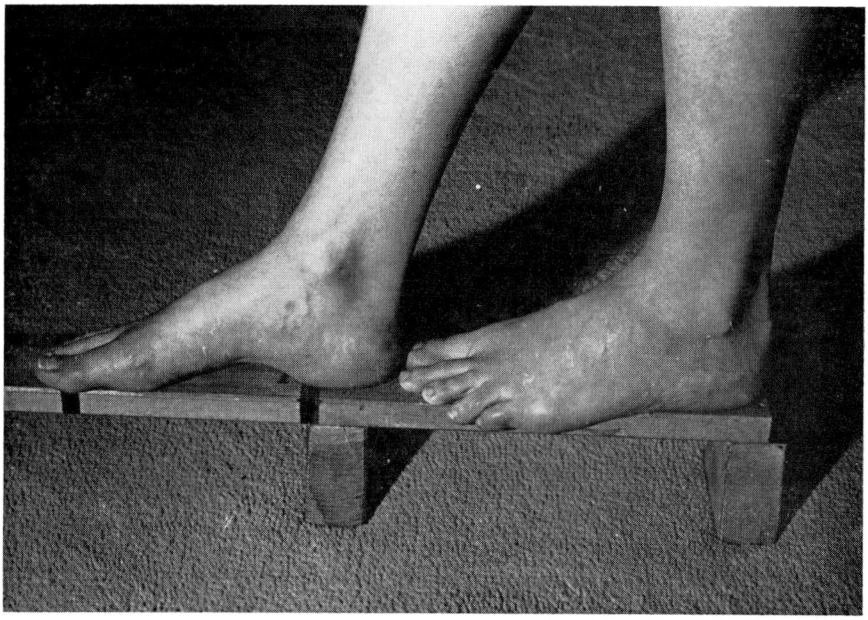

FIG. 1. Patient walking Heath Rails.

is able three times. The identical exercises are repeated on rails two and three and the scores averaged. Norms have been established for performance at various ages[1,2] on the different rails.

In the presence of a recent vestibular paresis, the subject will often fall toward the side of the lesion, while the Romberg response is normal. This test is of special value in the assessment of small children who are frightened by caloric or rotational testing.

REFERENCES

1. Goetzinger, C. P., Ortiz, J. D., Rousey, C. L., and Dirks, D. D.: A re-evaluation of the Heath Railwalking Test. J. Educ. Res. 54:3, 187-191, 1961.
2. Heath, S. R. (quoted by Mykelbust, H. R.): Auditory Disorders in Children. New York, Grune & Stratton, 1954, p. 311.

Roentgen Studies

Marc S. Lapayowker and Henry J. Woloshin

The roentgenographic examination and evaluation of patients whose presenting symptom is vertigo may involve many types of procedures and film studies. Although the percentage of demonstrable roentgenographic pathology found in these patients is not large, the cause of vertigo can and must be sought by these various means. When present, abnormal findings are frequently related to the cause of the patient's difficulty.

In most cases, roentgenographic evaluation begins with the routine examination of the skull. In our department this examination includes stereoscopic views in the postero-anterior projection, the Chamberlain-Towne or half-axial view, and the lateral projection. It is felt that stereoscopy in these projections affords considerable advantage over single views. There is so much anatomic detail within the skull that only by trying to visualize these structures by three-dimensional viewing can overlying anatomic details be separated and assigned their true position. Stereoscopy is imperative for evaluating detail near the bony vault and determining whether a radiographic shadow is indeed within the bony vault or within the scalp. The position of abnormal calcifications near the sella or the base of the skull can be accurately determined by stereoscopy, as can abnormalities which may be superimposed on one projection but are actually widely separated.

The postero-anterior projection, when properly positioned will project the internal auditory canals through the orbits. This is the best routine radiographic view for evaluation of the status of the canals since the beam is perpendicular to the canal. The orbits themselves, as well as the floor of the sella turcica, are also well visualized in this projection.

The Chamberlain-Towne or half axial view was developed in 1926 by Dr. W. Edward Chamberlain in response to a request by Dr. Towne for a radiographic projection which would best visualize the petrous ridges and internal auditory canals of the temporal bone. The petrous ridges are shown to advantage by this view, being projected against the relatively featureless topography of the occipital bone. The internal auditory canals and meati are often shown. In addition, the region of the vestibule and semicircular canals just beneath the arcuate eminence is also well demonstrated. In a properly positioned view the dorsum sella and posterior clinoid processes are projected through the foramen magnum, and early abnormal changes in these structures can be determined. The Chamberlain-Towne view also provides an excellent view of the posterior walls of the maxillary antra and the infra-orbital fissure leading to the pterygo-palatine fossa.

The lateral projection provides the most information about the sella turcica and craniovertebral junction. Calcification of the carotid arteries adjacent to the sella can frequently only be identified in the lateral view.

In addition to the bony vault and other structures of the skull, the presence of calcification in the pineal gland and habenular commissure is vital in determining the possibility of a shift of the midline structures. This is an extremely infrequent occurrence with lesions presenting with vertigo, but, if present, leads to further diagnostic possibilities. Ultrasound for evaluation of midline shift has recently been used almost routinely, since it provides an indication of midline shift in the absence of any demonstrable intracranial calcification and without further diagnostic procedures.

The submentovertex or "base" view of the skull is included in selected cases. This provides information about the basal foramina, the foramen ovale, spinosum, lacerum, and the jugular foramen. Involvement of the cranial nerve exits by an upward growing nasopharyngeal neoplasm is first determined by this projection. In addition, this view is an excellent starting point for evaluation of the mastoid areas. Comparison can be made of the mastoids in terms of their degree of development and state of aeration. Other structures of the temporal bone will be discussed in the pages that follow, but suffice it to say that this view provides certain information not found in other views of the temporal bone.

Certain disease states associated with vertigo can be diagnosed with certainty on the routine skull examination. Paget's disease is a condition characterized by a usually classic radiographic appearance. The "cottonwool" appearance, with softening of the bony vault

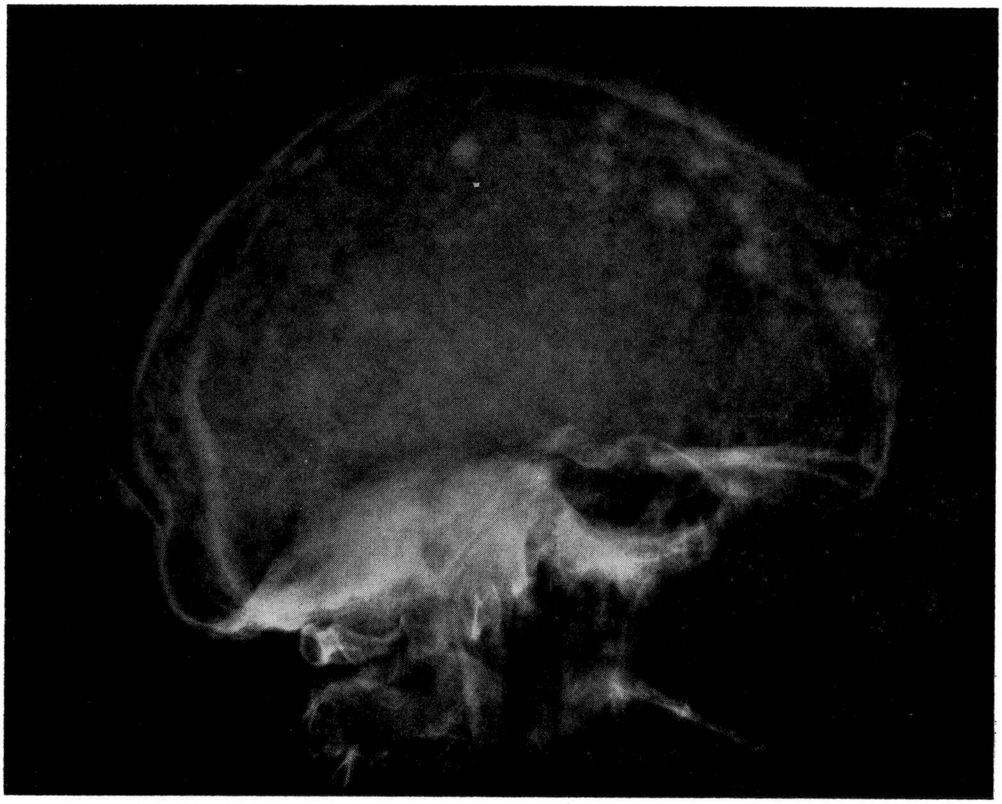

FIG. 1. Paget's disease of skull with "cotton-wool" appearance of vault, increased density of base and basilar invagination.

and acquired basilar invagination, are seen in advanced cases (Fig. 1). Congenital basilar invagination and platybasia are also diagnosed on routine plain films of the skull.

Other conditions which are associated with vertigo are better visualized on special views of various portions of the skull. Most of them are obtained for better visualization of the temporal bone. Our routine examination of the temporal bone ("mastoid study") consists of five views: Runström, Mayer, Base, Stenvers, and Chamberlain-Towne.

The Runström view is a valuable view in the evaluation of mastoid disease. This is taken stereoscopically. The projection is obtained with the patient in a lateral position and with the tube angled 35° caudad. The central beam is centered at the external audi-

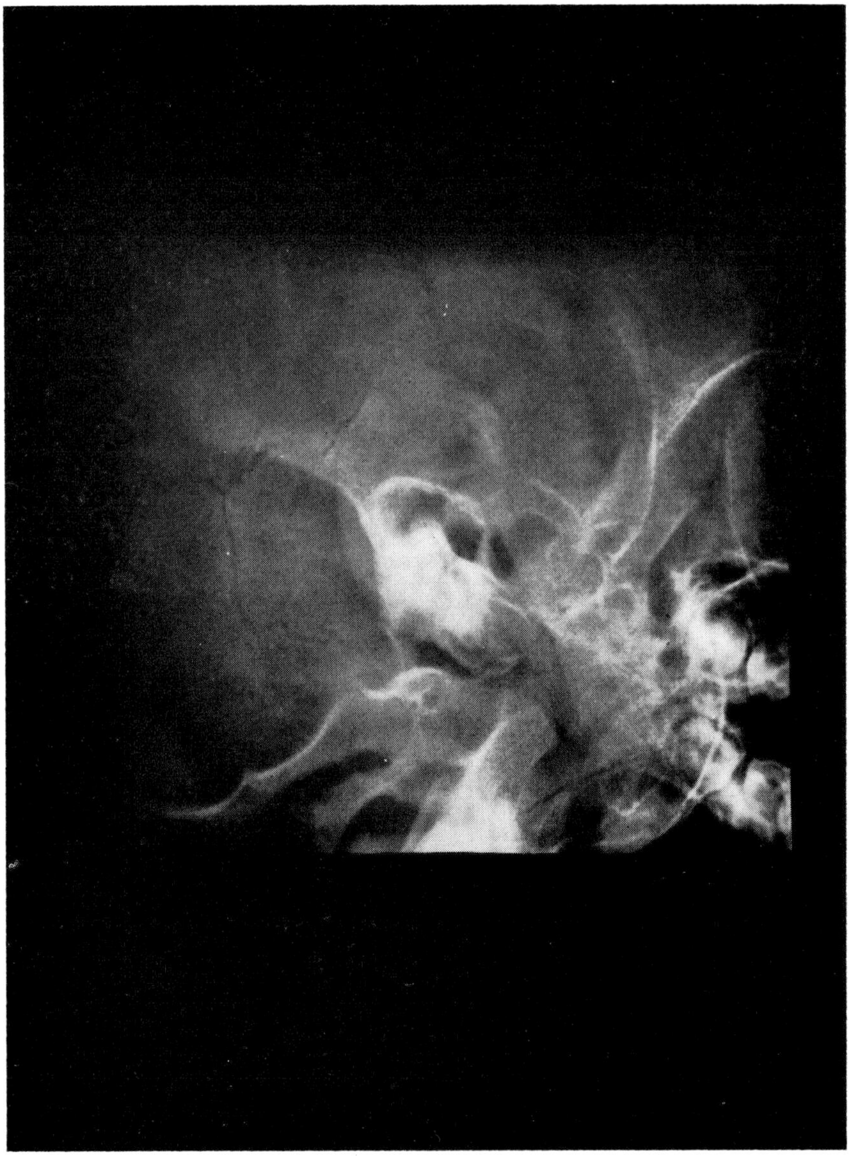

FIG. 2. Cholesteatoma. Radiolucent defect extending from middle ear out into mastoid antrum and process represents bony destruction secondary to cholesteatoma. (Runstrom projection.)

tory canal of interest. Cholesteatoma extending into the mastoid antrum may be demonstrated in this view (Fig. 2). The Mayer projection also provides information about the attic and antral regions. The base view shows both mastoids and middle ears and allows for a good comparative study. Other information revealed by this projection has been previously discussed. The Stenvers projection shows the petrous pyramid with the internal auditory canal, bony labyrinth, and the mastoid cells. The internal auditory canal is foreshortened in this view. The Chamberlain-Towne projection has already been discussed.

Supplementary information about the temporal bone is obtained by tomography. Either single-section or multisection tomography may be used. We have found plesiosectional tomography of considerable value in the study of the region. This method, a refinement of linear multisection tomography, was developed in 1961 by M. J. McGann, R. T., and has found considerable application in the evaluation of temporal bone disease since that time. The advantages are the availability of linear tomography to many American radiologists, the limitation of radiation exposure since only two exposures are needed for each

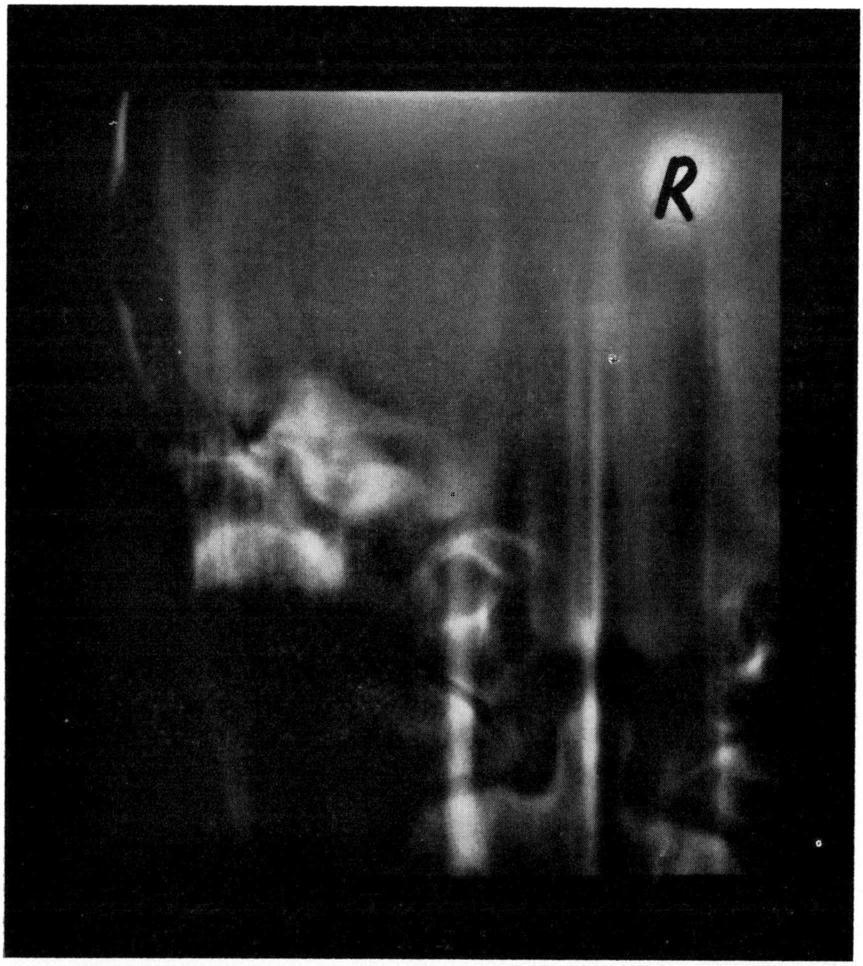

FIG. 3. Normal temporal bone as disclosed by plesiosectional tomography. Ossicular mass within middle ear demonstrated. Detail of bony labyrinth is evident. Note the vertical and lateral semicircular canals, vestibule, promontory of cochlea and internal auditory canal.

temporal bone, and the ease with which technicians can do the study. The resultant visualization of radiographic anatomy compares quite favorably with that obtained by the use of multimotion tomographic apparatus. The ossicles and oval window can be satisfactorily visualized in over 75 per cent of cases with this study (Fig. 3). Occasionally, additional exposures are made if visualization of anterior structures such as the carotid canal or posterior ones like the jugular fossa are desired.

Cerebellopontine angle tumors of all types are not uncommon as a cause of vertigo. Diagnosis of these lesions is considerably aided by radiographic examination. Routine skull films frequently show evidence of erosion of portions of the internal auditory area and the apex of the petrous pyramid. The specialized views of the temporal bone have improved upon our diagnostic ability to demonstrate minute changes of bone erosion (Fig. 4). When no bony abnormalities are evident or when the diagnosis is in question, partial pneumoencephalography may provide the answer. Small amounts of air placed in the spinal subarachnoid space can, with proper positioning of the head, give excellent visualization of the cerebellopontine angle cistern, the subarachnoid space overlying the internal auditory meatus. A space-taking lesion in this region can often be outlined by air in this manner. Recently the use of contrast encephalography has been described for evaluation of this region.

Petrous bone fractures are best seen by tomography. Otosclerosis has been suspected on plesiosectional tomograms of the temporal bone when there is sclerosis in the region of the bony promontory with obliteration of the oval window.

Vertigo can also be caused by space-taking lesions in the posterior fossa, particularly acoustic neurinomas. In addition to diagnostic findings on plain radiographs of the skull, special procedures are most valuable. Radiographically contrasting substances can be used to opacify the subarachnoid cisterns, the

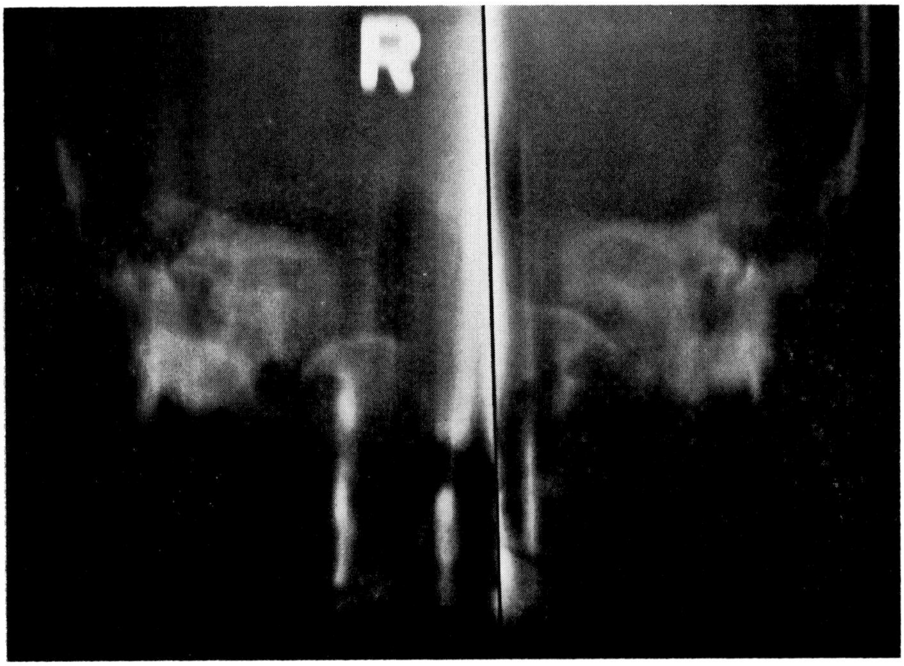

FIG. 4. Left internal acoustic neuroma. Plesiosectional tomogram of left temporal bone shows enlargement of internal auditory canal with erosion of posterior wall. Right side is normal.

ventricular system, and the vasculature of the posterior fossa.

The subarachnoid cisterns and ventricles are most often examined by partial pneumoencephalography if no obvious increase in intracranial pressure is evident. We, however, usually proceed with arteriography as the initial examination. The risks of arteriography are considerably less and the procedure does not have to be immediately followed by surgery, as ventriculography often does, and, to a lesser extent, pneumoencephalography. The description of changes in the posterior fossa vessels due to tumor or other space-

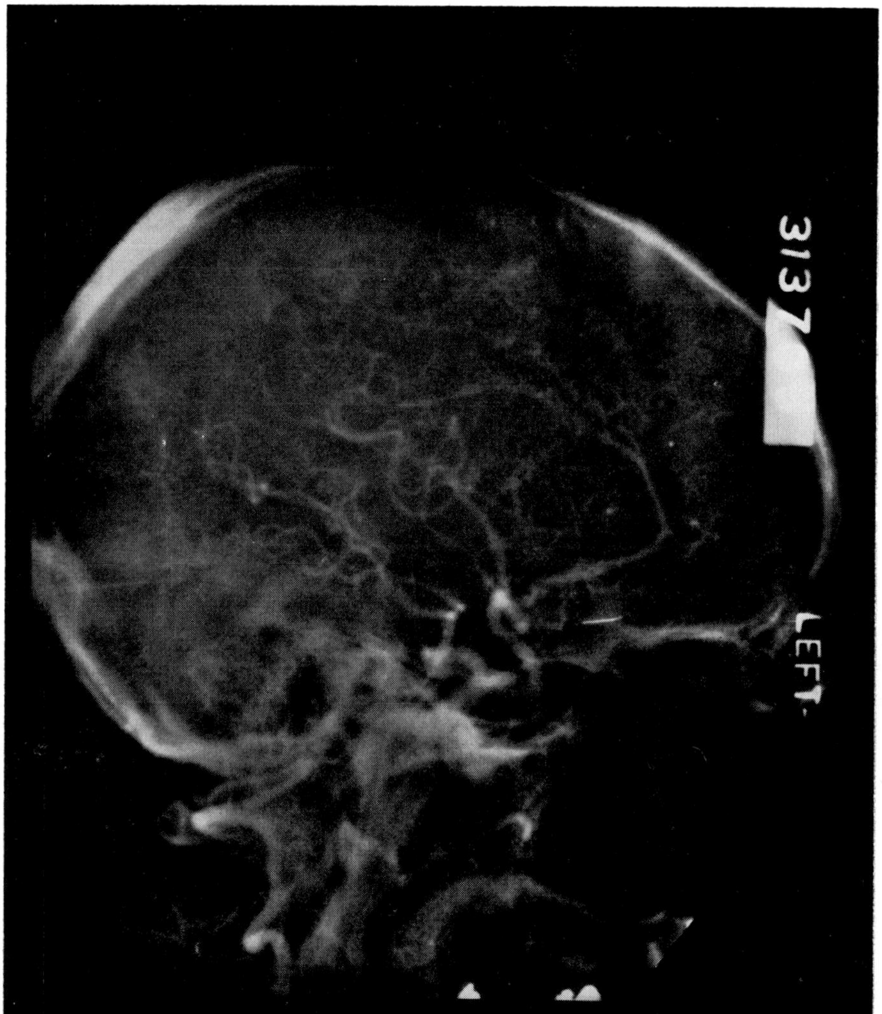

Fig. 5A. Right cerebellar tumor. Right retrograde brachial arteriograms. The lateral view shows depression of the right posterior inferior cerebellar artery below the level of the foramen magnum. The basilar artery is pressed against the clivus. Incidentally, a carotid-basilar anastomosis is present.

taking lesions is beyond the scope of this treatise. The vessels are usually visualized by the injection of iodinated contrast material in an antegrade manner into the vertebral arteries or by retrograde injection of the brachial arteries. This latter is preferable because it is done under local anesthesia and there is no direct trauma to the vessels in the neck (Fig. 5, A and B).

Cisternal visualization can be accomplished by the introduction of small amounts of air through a lumbar puncture needle and obtaining proper films with the patient in the erect sitting position. Ordinarily, 15 cc. of air will be satisfactory for examination of the posterior fossa. In the face of slight elevation of cerebrospinal fluid pressure, air can be injected without removal of any significant

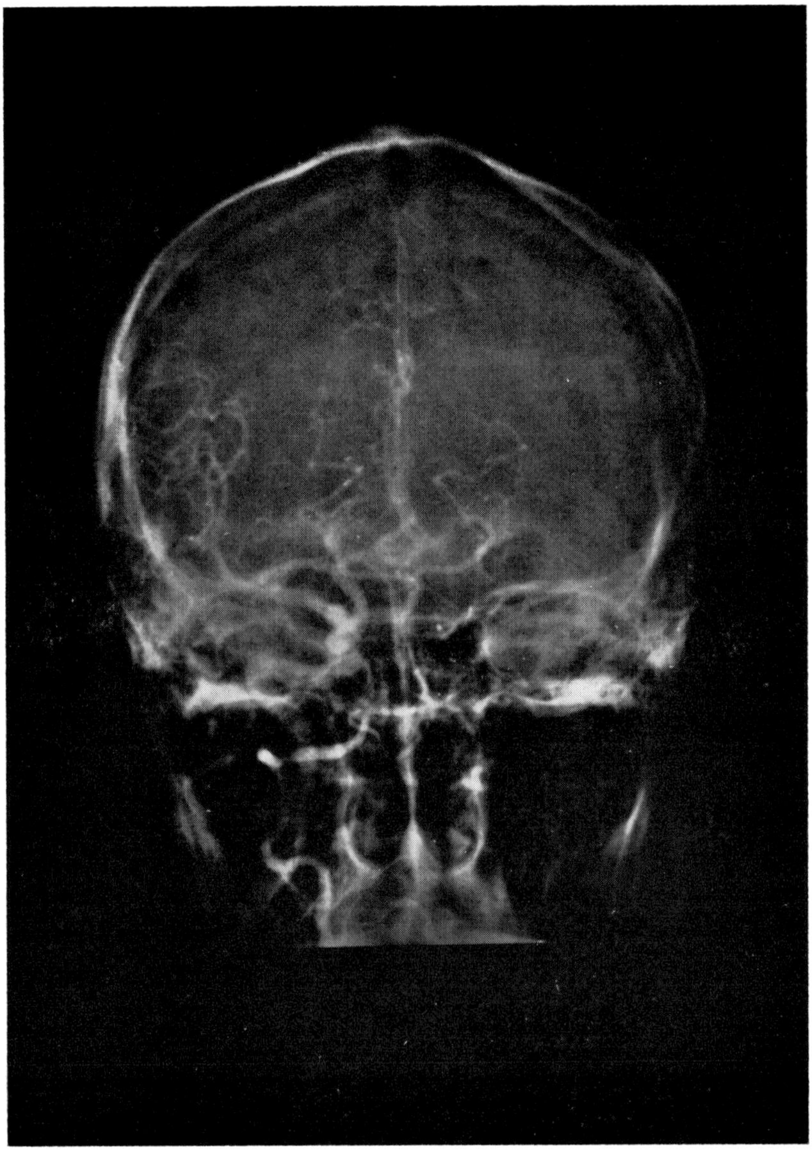

FIG. 5B. Right cerebellar tumor. The PA projection shows displacement of the distal portion of the right posterior inferior cerebellar artery across the middle.

amount of cerebrospinal fluid, thus lowering the chance of disturbance of cerebro-spinal dynamics.

Radiographically, the use of autotomography can be an aid in visualization of the fourth ventricle and aqueduct of Sylvius if stereoscopy is not employed. We feel that stereoscopy is of more value for reasons already mentioned. Autotomography is the term applied to a selective blurring of the overlying mastoid areas when obtaining a film in the lateral projection. With the head slightly flexed, the axis of rotation passes through the fourth ventricle and aqueduct of Sylvius. Slow rotation of the head during a relatively long exposure of 2 to 3 seconds provides adequate blurring of the overlying structures (Fig. 6).

The use of ventriculography is generally limited to cases with increased intracranial pressure, and ordinarily these patients do not present primarily with vertigo. Ventriculography is invaluable for cases of obstruction of the aqueduct of Sylvius from whatever cause.

More recently, the opacification of the basal cisterns has been performed by contrast encephalography. This procedure is an extension of pantopaque myelography. The contrast material is placed in the spinal canal in the

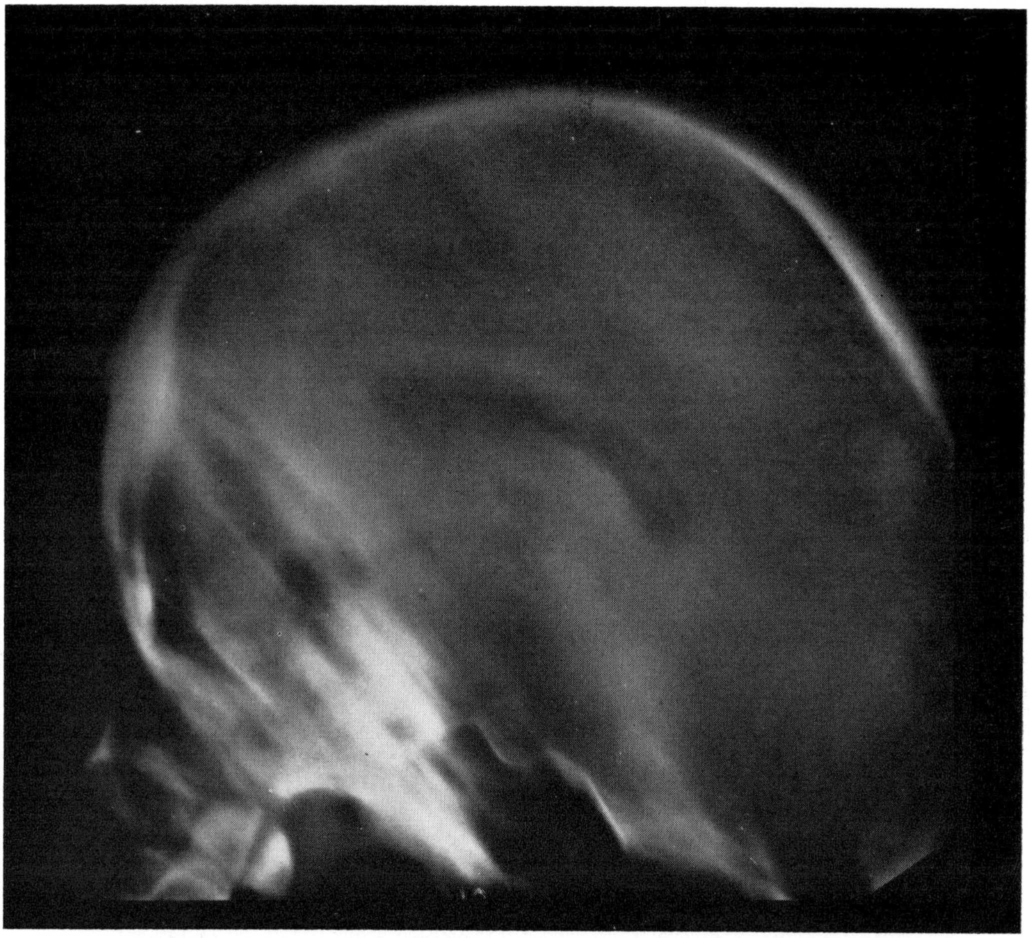

Fig. 6. Automography. Rotation of the head during a long radiographic exposure in the lateral view causes blurring of all structures away from axis of rotation. Gives good visualization of the back of the 3rd ventricle, aqueduct and 4th ventricle.

usual manner for myelography and guided into the cervical region. When the head is slowly flexed, the contrast rises onto the clivus. Slight rotation of the head then causes the contrast to fill the cerebellopontine cistern, visualizing the internal auditory meati and canals. A few workers feel that this method is superior to partial pneumoencephalography for diagnosis of lesions of the eighth nerve. These examinations are more fully reviewed in various neuroradiologic texts, but are frequently involved in the evaluation of vertigo.

Vertigo can also be caused by posterior fossa tumors of varying types. Radiographic findings on plain films are usually scarce. Special examinations are needed for visualiza-

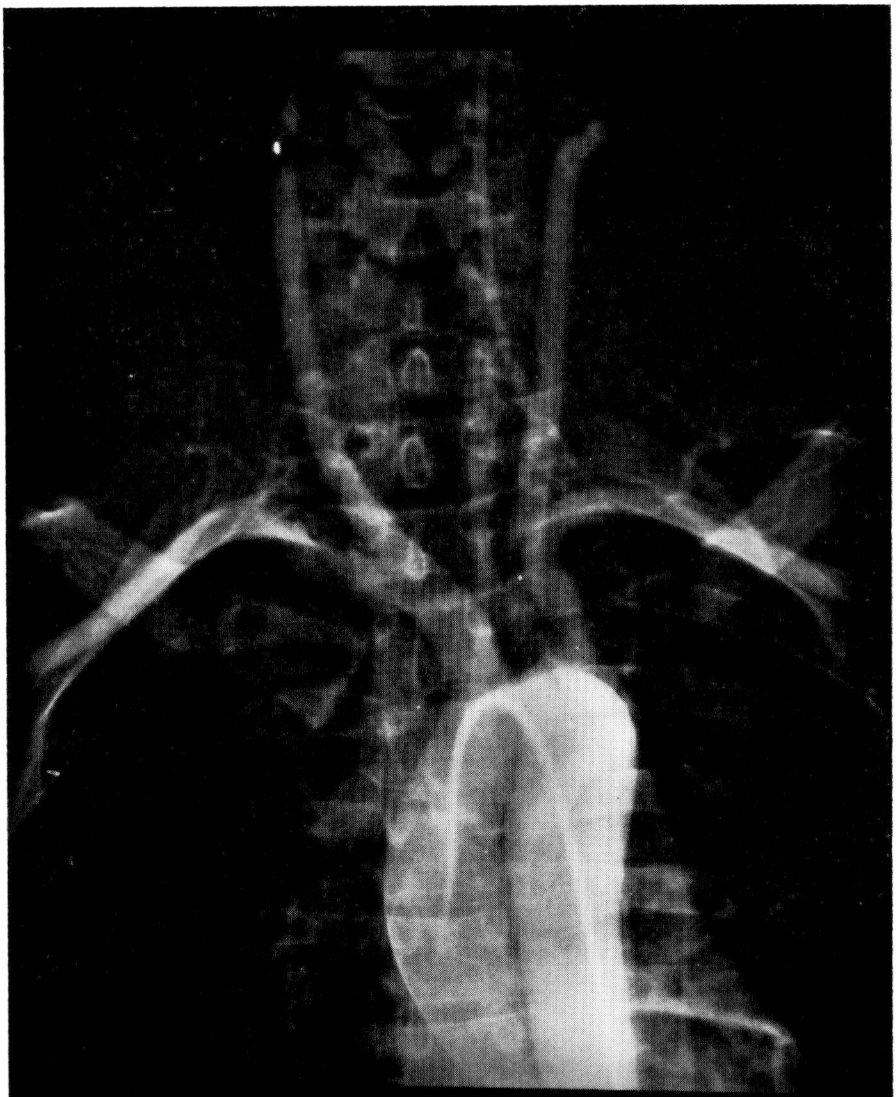

FIG. 7. Aortic arch study done by retrograde passage of catheter using Seldinger technique of percutaneous introduction of catheter. Arrow points to site of obstruction of right vertebral artery.

tion of the vascular structures of the posterior fossa. The ventricular and cisternal system evaluation is usually more reliable.

Vascular disease of the vertebrobasilar system may also cause vertigo. Occlusion or insufficiency of any of the vessels supplying contents of the posterior fossa of the skull must be evaluated by opacification studies. Visualization of these vessels may be obtained in a variety of ways. Our usual method is by retrograde brachial arteriography. This is performed almost exclusively by the percutaneous placement of a 17- or 18-gauge Cournand needle into the brachial artery just above the antecubital fossa. A pressure injector is necessary with this type of study in order to cause enough retrograde flow of the contrast material to reach the origins of the vertebral arteries in sufficient quantity for opacification of these vessels in the neck and within the skull. On the left, only the vertebrobasilar system is ordinarily visualized, while on the right, the usual picture shows the carotid and vertebrobasilar system. Serial films are obtained on the Chamberlain-biplane stereoscopic device through the entire arterial phase if extracranial vessels are being studied. If intracranial problems are suspected, films are obtained every 0.7 seconds during the entire arterial and venous phase of intracranial circulation.

Stereoscopic films have a great advantage in that individual vessels may be delineated with more accuracy and separated from overlying vessels. These vessels may also be studied by direct percutaneous puncture of the vertebral arteries. This procedure frequently requires anesthesia and is often not as successful as retrograde brachial arteriography.

The entire aortic arch and its branches may be studied by means of a percutaneously introduced catheter. This may be done via the axillary or femoral arteries by means of the Seldinger technique. The individual branches of the aortic arch can then be selectively catheterized by the use of various curves on the catheter tips if any disease or areas of suspicion are encountered (Fig. 7).

The effect by hypertrophic bony changes on the vertebral arteries has been rare. Tortuosity may cause slowed circulation within the vessels but actual authentic cases of obstruction or diminution of flow by the effect of spurs on these extracranial vessels has rarely been proved.

The so-called "subclavian steal" syndrome, in which blood from one vertebral artery is shunted across to the other vertebral artery and down in a retrograde fashion, has been frequently associated with basilar insufficiency syndromes and vertigo. Obstruction of the proximal subclavian artery causes this reversal of blood flow with diminution in the amount available for intracranial circulation. These cases have been most often found involving the subclavian and vertebral arteries, although the carotid arterial systems have been implicated in other cases of occlusion with varying degrees of collateral circulation. These patients frequently present with vertigo as one of the main symptoms (Fig. 8, A and B).

Cervical nerve root irritation has also been suspected as a cause of vertigo. Compression and pressure on these roots most often occurs as they pass through the neural formina between the pedicles of the cervical vertebral bodies. An en face view of the neural foramen is only visualized in the oblique projection of the cervical spine. The beam is angled approximately 20 degrees toward the head when an anteroposterior oblique view is obtained. This projects the central beam of radiation perpendicular to the neural foramina on the same side.

Hypertrophic degenerative changes involving the border of the foramina are frequently the cause of encroachment upon the space available for the passage of nerve roots. These bony spur formations most often occur with advancing age and affect primarily the uncovertebral joints (or joints of Luschka). These joints are present between the rimlike lip of the superior portion of the vertebral body along its posterolateral aspect and the body of the vertebra immediately above. While the normal neural foramen allows considerable extra room for the passage of nerve roots, small bony spurs as seen on the radiographs may actually be pushing considerable soft tissue in front of their advancing edges, thus compressing the exiting nerve roots. The lip continues across the entire posterior portion of the superior aspect of the cervical vertebra, and hypertrophic changes here may cause a series of ridgelike impressions on the ventral aspect of the spinal canal. The ridges

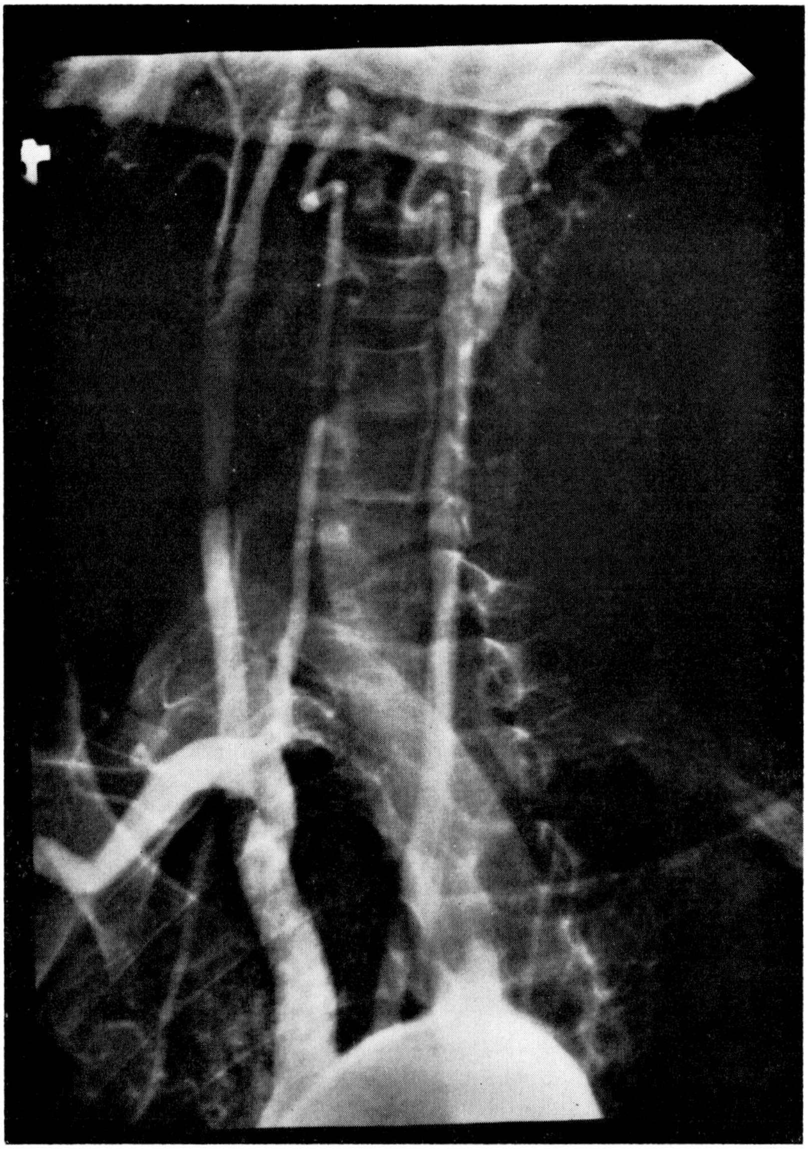

FIG. 8A. Subclavian steal syndrome. Aortic arch study by retrograde Seldinger catheter technique. The right innominate, carotid and vertebral arteries are normal. The left carotid artery is normal. The left subclavian artery is blocked 2 cm. above its origin. Retrograde flow of contrast is seen in the left vertebral artery.

may actually cause pressure on the spinal cord itself and can be demonstrated by myelography causing an extradural compression of the canal, and in advanced cases the ridges may cause flattening and widening of the spinal cord with the production of symptoms.

In addition to these cervical spondylitic changes the presence of any benign neurogenic tumor involving a nerve root or a malignant lesion in the area can also cause irritative symptoms. Collapse of the vertebral bodies from metastatic disease or infection may also cause encroachment on the neural foramina. The usual roentgenographic method of demonstrating lesions in this area, there-

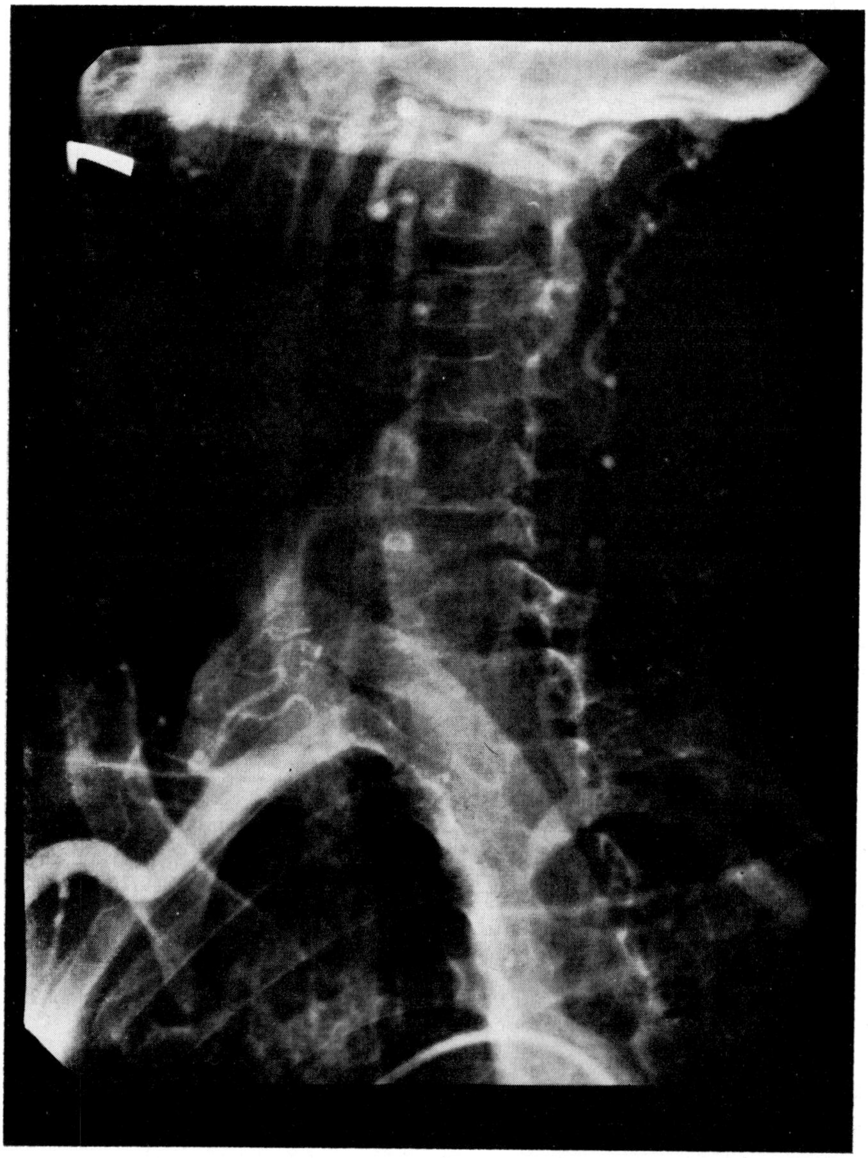

Fig. 8B. Subclavian steal syndrome. Aortic arch study by retrograde Seldinger catheter technique. Delayed film. Retrograde flow of contrast through left vertebral artery fills the subclavian artery and causes diminution of blood available to the posterior fossa.

fore, must include oblique views in addition to the anteroposterior and lateral projections. Our routine study is stereoscopic views in these four projections as well as an open-mouth view for visualization of the odontoid process. Flexion and extension films are often obtained for evaluation of extent of motion. We feel that cineradiography of the cervical spine is more worthwhile for determination of motion and limitation of movement since flexion deformities and sharp angulation at various levels may be readily apparent when the patient is examined while carrying out routine motion of the head and neck.

Contrast and air myelography, of course, are used to diagnose the presence of intraspinal pathology which could be the cause of vertigo.

SUMMARY

The initial roentgenographic study of the patient with vertigo is usually the conventional skull examination. Other examinations are utilized for study of specific areas. The temporal bone examination ("mastoid study") can yield considerable information in mastoid disease. Plesiosectional tomography has proved of value, particularly in detection of internal acoustic neuromas. Partial pneumoencephalography is employed when one is searching for cerebellopontine angle tumors. Arteriography has been performed during investigation of space-taking lesions of the posterior fossa. Retrograde brachial arteriography is preferred to direct vertebral arteriography in this respect. Posterior fossa lesions are often best studied by partial pneumoencephalography or ventriculography. Retrograde brachial arteriography is utilized in study of vascular disease of the vertebrobasilar system. Further study of the aortic arch and branches may be made by the Seldinger catheter technique.

If the cervical spine is suspected as the cause of vertigo, radiographic study including oblique views affords information relative to the intervertebral foramina. The proper selection of roentgenographic studies can yield valuable information in the work-up of the patient with vertigo.

REFERENCES

1. Baird, R. M., Lapayowker, M. S., Murtagh, F., and Scott, M.: Percutaneous retrograde brachial arteriography: a nonoperative, noncatheter technique. Amer. J. Roentgen. 94: 19-29, 1965.
2. Brünner, S., Petersen, Ø., and Stoksted, P.: Laminagraphy of temporal bone. Amer. J. Roentgen. 86:281-281, 1961.
3. Becker, J., and Woloshin, H. J.: Mastoiditis and cholesteatoma: a roentgen approach. Amer. J. Roentgen. 88:1019-1031, 1962.
4. Camp, J. D., and Cilley, E. I. L.: Significance of asymmetry of pori acoustici as aid in diagnosis of eighth nerve tumors. Amer. J. Roentgen. 41:713-718, 1939.
5. Castellanos, A., and Pereiras, R.: Countercurrent aortography. Rev. Cubana Cardiol. 2:187, 1939.
6. Chamberlain, W. E., and Stauffer, H. M.: New device for stereoscopic cerebral and cardiac angiography. Trans. Coll. Physicians Phila. 148:19-20, 1951-1953.
7. Collins, W. F., Jr., Slade, H. W., and Lockhart, W. G.: Brachial vertebral angiography in adults. J. Neurosurg. 14:466468, 1957.
8. Gass, H.: Pantopaque anterior basal cisternography of the posterior fossa. Amer. J. Roentgen. 90:1197-1204, 1963.
9. Gould, P. L., Peyton, W. T., and French, L. A.: Vertebral angiography by retrograde injection of brachial artery. J. Neurosurg. 12: 369-374, 1955.
10. Hodes, P. J., Pendergrass, E. P., and Young, B. R.: Eighth nerve tumors; their roentgen manifestations. Radiology 53: 633-665, 1949.
11. Kuhn, R. A.: Brachial cerebral angiography. J. Neurosurg. 17:955-971, 1960.
12. Lapayowker, M. S., Carter, Barbara L., and McGann, Margaret J.: The use of plesiosectional tomography in the diagnosis of eighth nerve tumors. Amer. J. Roentgen. 88:1187-1193, 1962.
13. Lapayowker, M. S., Woloshin, H. J., and Ronis, M. L.: The use of plesiosectional tomography in otology. Laryngoscope 75:1837-1846, 1965.
14. Lindgren, E.: Radiologic examination of brain and spinal cord. Acta Radiol. Suppl. 151: 1-147, 1957.

15. Marshall, T. R., and Ling, J. T.: Direct percutaneous noncatheter brachial angiography (left panarteriography-right cerebral angiography). Radiology 80:258-260, 1963.

16. McGann, Margaret J.: Plesiosectional tomography of the temporal bone: a new multiscreen cassette. Amer. J. Roentgen. 88: 1183-1186, 1962.

17. Olsen, A., and Horrax, G.: Symptomatology of acoustic tumors with special reference to atypical features. J. Neurosurg. 1: 371-378, 1944.

18. Ostrowski, A. Z., Hardy, W. G., Lindner, D. W., Thomas, L. M., and Gurdjian, E. S.: Retrograde brachial vertebral-basilar angiography. A.M.A. Arch. Neurol. Psychiat. 4: 608-616, 1961.

19. Runström, G.: Roentgenological study of acute and chronic otitis media. Acta Radiol. Suppl. 17, 1933.

20. Scanlan, R. L.: Roentgen diagnosis of acoustic neuroma with particular reference to the use of Pantopaque. Laryngoscope 74:999-1003, 1964.

21. Schinz, H. R., Baensch, W. E., Friedl, E., and Uehlinger, E.: Roentgen Diagnostics. New York, Grune & Stratton, 1951.

22. Schmitz, A. L., and Haveson, S. B.: Roentgen diagnosis of eighth nerve tumors. Radiology 75:531-543, 1960.

23. Scott, M. T., Murtagh, F., Lapayowker, M., and Baird, R. M. Vertebral basilar and carotid angiography by injection of brachial artery: a cannula (non-catheter) technique. Am. J. Roentgen. 90:546-553, 1963.

24. Siqueira, E. B., Karras, B. G., Cannon, A. H., and Bucy, P. C.: Percutaneous brachial cerebral angiography. J. Neurosurg. 19: 1050-1057, 1962.

25. Shambaugh, G. E., Jr.: Surgery of the Ear. Philadelphia, W. B. Saunders Company, 1959.

26. Tarp, O.: Tomography of temporal bone with polytome. Acta Radiol. 51:105-116, 1959.

27. Towne, E. B.: Erosion of petrous bone by acoustic nerve tumor: demonstration by roentgen ray. A.M.A. Arch Otolaryng. 4: 515-519, 1926.

28. Young, B. R.: The Skull, Sinuses, and Mastoids: A Handbook of Roentgen Diagnosis. Chicago, Year Book Publishers, 1948.

29. Zegelaar, F.: Spot-film radiography of skull by means of fluoroscopy with 5″ image intensifier. Mesicamundi 2:54-65, 1956.

30. Zimmer, J.: Planigraphy of temporal bone. Acta Radiol. 37:419-430, 1952.

Part II. Clinical Syndromes of Otologic Origin

CHAPTER 5

Incidence of Various Types of Dizziness

MARTIN SPECTOR

There is a wide divergence of opinion as to the causes of dizziness and their relative frequency. The same case may easily be given different labels by different observers. Even from the limited viewpoint of one specialty, such as otology, the reports on incidence vary greatly. Some statistics on incidence have been culled from the literature. Hugh Barber reported that in a series of more than 1000 dizzy patients, he diagnosed vestibular neuronitis in 27 per cent and positional nystagmus in 18.8 per cent. In 28 per cent, no diagnosis was reached. Nicholas Torok reported that the largest group of patients with organic dizziness was that with postural vertigo. He added that the majority of these patients exhibited osteoarthritic cervical spine alterations. He also emphasized that a goodly percentage of dizzy patients will be found to have no objective evidence of organic disease. McNally and Stuart labeled 78 out of 200 cases as endolymphatic hydrops, 47 as cardiovascular disease, and 29 as organic disease of the central nervous system. The difficulties in diagnosis were indicated by a 5-year review in which the diagnosis of Meniere's syndrome was reduced to 55 patients from 78 after the 5 years. Only 12 cases were considered psychosomatic. It was pointed out that both cardiovascular disease and Meniere's disease were often present in the same patient. Cawthorne and Hewlett reported that among 1900 cases of vertigo, 61 per cent were due to Meniere's disease and about 10 per cent were of intracranial origin. Several other authors concurred in the figure, about 10 to 15 per cent for intracranial causes. Wastenson studied 178 cases by multiple disciplines. He found 37 cases of Meniere's disease, 7 due to trauma, 30 due to cerebrovascular disease and 5 due to cardiovascular disease. He pointed out that several factors may be causing the vertigo in one case. The editor asked a general practitioner, Louis Castor, to classify the cases of dizziness who came through his office in a 6-month period. Castor considered that 50 per cent of all the dizzy patients he saw were functional. Above the age of 40, he considered 20 per cent as associated with the menopause. Donald Macrae reported that in 7723 patients referred for neurologic consultation, the chief complaint was dizziness in 6 per cent. He reported that 25 per cent were functional. Aantaa reported that in spite of a long followup period of 6 years, a definite diagnosis was still impossible in almost one-half of their patients.

The reader will thus understand that there is no unanimity of opinion as to definite diagnosis. It is hoped that Part II of this volume will aid in his categorizing of each case.

REFERENCES

1. Aantaa, E.: Vertiginous attacks in the light of followup studies. Acta Otolaryng. 53:455-460, 1961.
2. Cawthorne, T., and Hewlett, E.: Meniere's disease. Proc. Roy. Soc. Med. 47:663-670, 1954.
3. Macrae, D.: The neurologic aspects of vertigo. Calif. Med. 92:255, 1960.
4. McNally, W. S., and Stuart, E. A.: An additional five-year review of some cases of vertigo. Ann. Otol. 64:519-536, 1955.
5. Torok, N.: Classification and pathologic conditions responsible for vertigo. Laryngoscope 74:528-535, 1964.
6. Wastenson, N.: Aspects of otoneurologically examined cases of vertigo. Svensk. Lakartidn. 54:697-703, 1957.

CHAPTER 6

Meniere's Disease and Its Pathology

Meniere's Disease (Endolymphatic Hydrops)

Maurice Saltzman

The designation "Meniere's disease," in a clinical sense, implies the presence of the classical triad of symptoms—episodic vertigo, tinnitus and deafness. Pathologically, it has become identified as endolymphatic hydrops. If the patient has only cochlear hydrops, he has the incomplete form of Meniere's disease —fluctuating deafness and tinnitus. In the course of time, he is apt to add vertiginous attacks to his symptom complex. On the other hand, he could begin with episodic vertigo while the cochlear symptoms would appear months or years later.

Through the years, sufficient histopathologic data have accumulated to prove that the hydrops does not affect the several parts of the inner ear uniformly and not to the same degree. In a study of the reports of Hallpike and Cairns,[1] Altmann and Fowler,[2] Lindsay,[3] and Kristensen,[4] the cochlear duct was dilated in all cases, the saccule in most, the utricle in some, and the semicircular canals in none. It follows that if the static labyrinth was not involved, there would be no vertiginous attacks. Furthermore, according to the hypothesis of Schuknecht,[5] fistulization of the membranous labyrinth that occurs sometimes after rupture may give prolonged remissions and even total subsidence of vertiginous attacks.

Rupture and fistulization has no effect on the hearing loss which is slowly progressive. According to Williams,[7] the hearing loss is due to physical and chemical changes of the endolymph, while, by the theory of Lawrence and McCabe[6] and Schuknecht,[5] the vertiginous attacks are brought about by ruptures in the membranous labyrinth.

ETIOLOGY

Endolymphatic hydrops is a disease of middle age or older. It is rare before age 20. In Cawthorne and Howlett's[8] series of 900 cases, the average age at onset was 44 years. It was slightly more prevalent in the male. It followed the fenestration operation in a few cases, and it was associated with a blocked Eustachean tube in only one case. Less than 5 per cent of the patients showed any evidence of allergy. Endolymphatic hydrops is unilateral in most patients. It is generally held that bilateral involvement occurs in about 10 per cent of the cases. However, the disease does not necessarily begin synchronously in the two ears. In an occasional case, there is a lapse of months or even years before the second ear becomes affected.

The disease has been described as "idiopathic Meniere" because of the obscurity of its causation. To be sure, there are numerous documented case reports with a cause and effect implication. However, most of them were not evaluated by modern methods, and the reports do not contain the strict criteria for the diagnosis of endolymphatic hydrops. A notable exception is the case of VerMeulen and Saunders.[9] A resumé of their report follows:

On 4-2-60, a 33-year-old man accidentally grounded a wire carrying 440 volts. The resulting explosion left him dazed and with second degree burns of the arms and face. "Vertigo" and a buzzing sound in the left ear appeared immediately after the accident and they subsided within a week.

One month later, vertigo and nausea reappeared, the attack lasting 3 hours. Tinnitus returned and the patient became cognizant of a hearing loss in the left ear. During the 7 months that followed, there were 30 to 40 crises with increased tinnitus and hearing loss. He had no pain or loss of consciousness at any time. Next came a period of freedom from vertiginous attacks for about 6 months, but the tinnitus persisted and the deafness grew worse. Music sounded discordant. In June 1961 vertiginous crises began to recur with increased frequency, each attack lasting about 3 hours. He was no longer able to work. In August 1961 he was admitted to the University Hospital. A complete medical and neurological work-up disclosed nothing abnormal. Audiologic and otoneurologic studies established the diagnosis of Meniere's disease in the left ear. There was sensorineural deafness in the left ear. Recruitment was present and the discrimination score was reduced in the left ear. The caloric test showed a difference in reaction between the two ears.

Since medical therapy was ineffective and since the left ear had no longer any serviceable hearing, a destructive labyrinthectomy was done. When seen 10 months later, he reported there was no recurrence of vertiginous attacks.

How did an electric explosion cause endolymphatic hydrops in one ear? Hyslop[10] ascribes secondary circulatory and vasomotor reactions to accidental electric shock. "The current pathway did not reach the brain if there was no loss of consciousness." He agrees with Scheinker,[11] who states, "Profound circulatory disturbances may be seen in regions remote from the direct influence of the irritant stimulus. The transmission is by the way of the neurovascular network. The accumulation of carbon dioxide, which is an active vasodilator, results in further vascular dilation and increased permeability of the vessel wall."

Williams[7] states that allergy is the etiologic factor in Meniere's disease. (This theory is discussed at length in the section on "Allergy.")

A violent psychic upheaval is an etiologic factor in Meniere's disease according to Fowler and Zeckel.[12] They studied 23 patients who had their first vertiginous seizure soon after severe emotional upsets. The experimental introduction of noxious thoughts brought on an attack in some cases. The injection of procaine intravenously was effective in alleviating or altering the tinnitus. Pharmacologically, procaine increases the speed of circulation and prevents the clumping of red cells in small vessels. Within hours after a vertiginous attack, the small blood vessels of the conjunctivae were studied in several patients. Narrowing of the blood vessels and blood sludging were found. Microhemorrhages were seen in a few. Therefore, it was inferred that the Meniere attacks in these patients were due to the disrupted function of the labyrinth as a result of the psychic storm. This usually happens in predisposed personalities. All of the 23 patients were disturbed people. It was hypothesized that the emotional upheaval would cause narrowing of the blood vessels from spasm, that there would be sludging of the red cells and slowing of the circulation, and that hydrops would result from the augmented osmotic pressure.

Vertebral artery insufficiency plays a role in the etiology of Meniere's disease in some cases. Kristensen[16] cites the case report presented by Golding-Wood at a meeting of the Royal Society of Medicine in February 1962. The patient was middle-aged, with severe attacks of vertigo, a hearing loss of the perceptive type and sensitivity to noise. When he came to autopsy, a very small vertebral artery and a correspondingly small internal auditory artery were present on the side where endolymphatic hydrops was also found. Neither the brain stem nor the opposite ear showed pathologic changes.

SYMPTOMS AND SIGNS

The onset is usually insidious. Frequently, there is a sensation of dullness or fullness in one or both ears and the patient becomes cognizant of a hearing loss that comes and goes. He becomes sensitive to sounds, and music appears discordant. One or both ears begin to buzz. Sometimes the head noise is of a double nature—a whistling sound which is comparatively not troublesome, and a roaring that is most disturbing. Then suddenly the ground beneath his feet seems to become loose. Visible objects appear to turn in front of his eyes. When he closes his eyes, he feels that he is whirling. He is seized with nausea and vomiting. He becomes prostrate, finding some relief when lying on the healthy side with the head slightly raised and the affected ear uppermost. Any movement of the head aggravates the condition. Throughout the attack and for sometime afterwards, there may be pain and numbness in and about the affected ear. More often, it is a feeling of pressure and discomfort.

In most cases, the vertiginous seizure goes on for several hours, but a few patients are subject to recurrent fleeting attacks, each lasting but a minute or two. Occasionally, the duration of an attack may be a week or longer, and after the subsidence of vertigo it may take a month before the patient regains his normal equilibrium. Occasionally, the vertiginous attack causes the patient to lose momentary control of his legs, and he falls suddenly. This has been termed "otolithic catastrophe" by Tumarkin.[18] There is no loss of consciousness.

Recurrences of vertiginous attacks take place at irregular intervals — days, weeks, months or years apart. Most often, the patient gets a warning of an impending attack. There may be a change in the character and intensity of the tinnitus; he may become alarmed by a sudden increase in his deafness; he may have momentary sensations of fleeting dizziness. The character of one attack may vary from another in the same individual. Between the attacks, the patient has no vestibular symptoms.

During the attack, spontaneous nystagmus is a constant finding. It is usually rotary, but it may be horizontal or combined, and it is rarely vertical. It is directed toward the diseased or healthy ear, and the direction may change from side to side during a prolonged attack. Aschan and Stahle[19] made a nystagmographic study of 21 Meniere patients during episodes of vertigo. Nystagmus was always present but it varied in character. The most common findings were true spontaneous nystagmus and direction-fixed positional nystagmus. In about 25 per cent of the cases, direction-changing positional nystagmus was found. When the vertiginous attack was of long duration, the character of the nystagmus changed from one form to another.

In the quiescent period in Meniere's disease, spontaneous nystagmus is rarely detectable. Following a vertiginous attack, when some residual symptomatology lingers on, critical positioning may bring out fleeting nystagmus in some cases. This is due to residual imbalance between the two labyrinths. The nystagmus is more readily detectable by nystagmography.

In the affected ear, the caloric reaction is abnormal in the overwhelming majority of patients. The results were normal in only 51 of a series of 900 consecutive cases reported by Cawthorne and Hewlett.[8] In this series, canal paresis was present in 640, combined canal paresis and directional preponderance in 108, directional preponderance in 75.

An outstanding feature of Meniere's disease is the fluctuation in the auditory acuity—a diminution of hearing with each vertiginous attack and an improvement during the intermission. Serial audiograms show fluctuations of 10-30 db. for the various frequencies. The hearing deterioration grows greater as time goes on.

The Meniere patient with bilateral involvement presents a characteristic deafness pattern. His hearing of speech is poor in spite of a favorable audiogram and an up-to-date hearing aid. He has a 40-60 db. impairment and his hearing loss curve is usually, more or less, flat across the board. Without a hearing aid, he cannot hear. With a hearing aid and lip reading, he makes out the gist of a conversation when speaking to one person. The setting of the volume is critical to him. At 75 db. intensity a word becomes intelligible, and at 80 db. it is too loud and intolerable. Intelligibility is diminished in group conversation. He gets confused when several sounds come through his hearing aid. From time to time he has to change over the wearing of his hearing aid from one ear to the other because of fluctuations in cochlear function. At various intervals, the ears take turns in becoming unreceptive to meaningful sounds. The poor speech intelligibility is accounted for by the fact that the Meniere patient is encumbered with numerous pathologicophysiologic disabilities. According to Saltzman,[20] these include the following: (1) recruitment and hyperrecruitment, (2) diplacusis, (3) low threshold of discomfort, (4) fluctuations, and (5) reduction in capacity for selective hearing.

DIAGNOSIS

The audiologic findings are the mainstay in the diagnosis of endolymphatic hydrops. These include a sensation of fullness in the ear, fluctuating low-tone perceptive deafness, roaring low-tone tinnitus, diplacusis, recruitment, sensitivity to loud sounds, low discrimination score, and no marked tone decay.

A history of episodic vertiginous attacks completes the clinical picture. An abnormal caloric response constitutes confirming evidence. Abnormal findings referable to the central nervous system are ruled out. The audiometric pattern may include a high-tone loss due to premature presbycusis, acoustic trauma, or neural degeneration. Significance is to be attached to the impressive low frequency loss. The tinnitus may have a ringing component, but significance is to be attached to its low-tone buzz which measures 100-300 cycles, according to Day.[21] Diplacusis may not be elicited across the board. It may be shown in the low-tone segment only, or in the high frequencies only. Recruitment may be partial or complete. Frequently, there is also hyperrecruitment.

The typical vertigo in Meniere's disease is the spinning or turning variety. It is not associated with unconsciousness and it is not followed by undue somnolence. Spontaneous nystagmus is a constant finding during the vertiginous attack. It is usually rotary, but it may be horizontal, oblique, vertical, or combined. During the intermission, no spontaneous nystagmus is elicited, as a rule. The sensitivity of the Meniere ear is an important diagnostic feature. A jarring effect is produced by any loud sound, especially if it is high-pitched. Jerger and associates[22] developed the SISI test (short increment sensitivity index). They found that patients with end-organ lesions are able to detect a one decibel increase in the loudness of a tone, 20 decibels above threshold. The discrimination score is usually only moderately lowered. Parker and associates[23] reported an average discrimination score of 72 per cent in 118 Meniere cases. Less than 3 per cent of the group showed a 0 per cent discrimination score.

Differential Diagnosis

The present-day rigid diagnostic criteria serve to isolate endolymphatic hydrops from other clinical entities with some resembling features. The other conditions have some distinctive symptoms and signs of their own. These will be described in order to facilitate the differential diagnosis.

Psychogenic Vertigo

The background is revealed in the history. Personality traits are detected in the interview. In anxiety neurosis, the complaint is usually a disturbance of balance. If there are hallucinations of sound, it is "high-pitched" or musical, and it is in "the head." A sensation of "spinning" is rarely complained of. If there is nausea or vomiting, it is usually not tied up with an attack of vertigo. If there is a hearing loss, it may be traceable to some causative factor in the past. The audiologic findings would be characteristic. The vestibular tests would not only reveal nothing abnormal, but would also give evidence of vasomotor instability. Upon minimal calorization, the reactions would be hyperactive with marked vegetative disturbances.

However, a psychoneurotic individual may also have an organic disease. He may be the rare patient who has both Meniere's disease and neurosis. This can be uncovered only by a thorough work-up.

Acoustic Neuroma

In the early case, the symptoms and signs are mainly auditory and vestibular. They frequently simulate the findings in Meniere's disease. In the report of Pulec and House,[24] episodic vertigo was present in 5 out of 53 patients who were operated upon, and eighth-nerve tumors were found. In the same group, complete recruitment was present in 3 cases and partial recruitment in 5, according to Johnson and House.[25] However, the clinical pictures and the results of the tests show many points of difference between the two conditions. At the outset, the history in acoustic neurinoma will reveal a long period of unsteadiness which would be aggravated by sudden head movements. Nystagmus is usually horizontal. The caloric reaction is markedly depressed. This was impressive in 96 per cent in the series of Pulec and House.[24] The hearing loss does not show any fluctuations. Audiometry reveals a high-tone deafness pattern in the great majority of cases. Recruitment and diplacusis are usually absent. The tinnitus is usually high-pitched. In the series of Parker and associates,[23] 8 of 13 cases with retrocochlear lesions showed a discrimination score of 2 per cent or less. The average for the group was 25 per cent. The SISI score is low in individuals with retrocochlear lesions. Tone decay, causing a marked shift in threshold, is a most frequent finding in retrocochlear lesions. This finding carries much weight in the differential diagnosis. The Bekesy pattern is Type III or Type IV in 70 per cent of the cases.[25] Directional preponderance is present in most patients with acoustic neuroma who show depressed reactions to caloric stimulation in the affected ear, whereas in the 900 Meniere cases of Cawthorne and Hewlett,[8] directional preponderance was present in only 20.3 per cent.

Vestibular Neuronitis

The sudden onset with vertigo, nausea and vomiting and spontaneous nystagmus resembles a Meniere crisis. However, the duration of the disability due to an attack of vestibular neuronitis is lengthy, 4 to 8 weeks. Cochlear symptoms are absent and an infection frequently precedes the onset of an attack. An abnormal caloric reaction is the important criterion in the diagnosis of vestibular neuronitis. In a series of 40 cases, Lumio and Aho[26] found canal paresis in 38 cases and directional preponderance in 2 cases. A high incidence of diminished galvanic excitability was reported by Dix and Hallpike.[27] They are of the opinion that the lesion in vestibular neuronitis is retrolabyrinthine. In a follow-up study 2 years after the onset of the disease, Lumio and Aho found that all the patients had been cured of vertigo, that 20 per cent experienced a slight sensation of dizziness in connection with sudden movements, and that in 70 per cent the caloric reaction was hypoactive in the affected ear.

Cerebellar Tumor

In a child with a midline tumor, the clinical picture comprises headache, vomiting without nausea, staggering gait, dysmetria, dyssynergia, dysarthria, and choked disc. These classical symptoms and signs are frequently absent in an adult with an astrocytoma in one cerebellar hemisphere. His main complaint would be vertigo, and on examination a unilateral hearing loss may be discovered. Accordingly, a suspicion of Meniere's disease might be aroused. However, the unsteadiness would prove to be unremitting; his hearing loss might be traced to an attack of mumps in childhood; his gait would show a veering to one side and past-pointing with one arm might be elicited; positional nystagmus—

Table 1.

Disease	Onset	Nystagmus	Clinical Features
Endolymphatic Hydrops	Fullness in ears. Some roaring and impaired hearing, or attack of vertigo	During attack, rotary, horizontal or combined During intermission, no nystagmus	Ear sensitive to sound. Fullness and discomfort in ear. Episodic attacks of vertigo, nausea and vomiting, not followed by somnolence. No unconsciousness
Acoustic Neuroma	Long period of unsteadiness. High pitched tinnitus	Horizontal (Coarse)	Incoordination—unilateral deafness and tinnitus—facial pain and numbness — facial weakness— corneal anaesthesia
Cerebellar Tumor	Staggering gait, vomiting, headache	Coarse horizontal, spontaneous and positional	Ataxia, dysmetria, dyssynergia, dysarthria, past pointing
Head Injury	Following trauma, headache, vertigo on movements	Positional	Vertigo or rising headache associated with dizziness
Occlusion of posterior inferior cerebellar artery	Violent vertigo	Coarse, horizontal	Dysphagia, hoarseness, Horner's Syndrome, numbness of side of face and contralateral side of body
Acute suppurative Labyrinthitis	Complication of an ear infection	Rotary, horizontal, vertical or combined	Vertigo, fever, headache, vomiting, tinnitus, deafness. Relief in a specific position
Peri-Labyrinthitis	Complication of chronic otitis media	Horizontal, if present	Cholesteatoma or fistula
Luetic neuro-labyrinthitis	Insidious	Positional	Vertigo, deafness, incoordination
Toxic Vertigo	After taking an ototoxic drug	Horizontal, rotary, vertical	Vertigo and incoordination. Also, tinnitus and deafness in some cases
Benign positional vertigo	Ear disease, toxins, concussions or idiopathic	Positional Rotary, horizontal or combined	Vertigo and nystagmus with a latent period of about 5 sec. and duration of 20-30 sec. and fatigueability
Cervical Vertigo	Associated with trauma or a spinal lesion	Positional	Vertigo on sudden head movements — occipital headache. Stiffness and tenderness of neck
Epilepsy	Aura heralding an oncoming seizure	Rotary, vertical	History of epilepsy—period of unconsciousness
Vestibular Neuronitis	After an infection frequently	Rotary, horizontal or combined	Vertigo, nausea and vomiting
Arteriosclerosis	Insidious	Fleeting, horizontal	Dizziness on stooping and on rising in morning
Multiple Sclerosis	Insidious or sudden	Spontaneous and positional	History of alleviation and recurrence — neurologic defects and parasthesias
Psychogenic Vertigo	After an emotional storm	None	History of psychoneurosis. Complaints are vague

TABLE 1 (*continued*).

Vestibular Tests	Audiologic Tests	Special Tests	Course
Canal paresis in 70%. Directional preponderance in 20%	Fluctuating low-tone perceptive deafness. Displacusis, recruitment, high SISI score. Moderate reduction in discrimination score	Bekesy Audiometry Nystagmography	Attacks prone to become more frequent and severe. Profound deafness ensues Lengthy intermissions may occur
Canal paresis in 96%. Directional preponderance in most cases	High tone deafness. Marked tone decay. Low discrimination score	X-Ray of Internal acoustic meatus Sp. Fl. protein Bekesy	Progressive deterioration without operative intervention
Exaggerated caloric responses. Marked directional preponderance	Do not contribute	Ventriculography	Progressive deterioration without surgery
Directional preponderance in some cases	High tone deficit, mostly at 4000 cycles	X-Ray of Skull	Variable
Canal paresis and directional preponderance in some cases	Do not contribute	Medical and Neurological surveys	Recovery in most cases
Canal paresis	Perceptive deafness	Lumbar puncture	Recovery in most cases. Antibiotics are helpful
Dundas-Grant	Mixed deafness	Fistula test X-Ray Mastoids	Depends on results of surgery
Bizarre sometimes. There may be active responses to turning and not to caloric or vice versa	Progressive sensori-neural deafness	Wassermann	Antileutic therapy may influence outcome
Canal paresis	High tone deafness in some cases	None	Recovery from vertigo in 4-6 weeks. Deafness, if present, is apt to persist
Normal caloric in most cases. Canal paresis and directional preponderance in some cases	Do not contribute	Positioning Nystagmography	Recovery in eight weeks May recur May last years
Do not contribute	Do not contribute	X-Ray of cervical spine	Depends on response to orthopedic measures
Do not contribute	Do not contribute	EEG	Slow deterioration
Canal paresis in all cases and directional preponderance in some	Do not contribute	Galvanic	Recovery in about two months, usually
Do not contribute	Presbycusis, frequently	Medical survey	Some improvement under medical management
Directional preponderance in some cases	Do not contribute	Neurologic survey	Variable—poor prognosis in most cases
Hyperactive responses	Do not contribute	Psychiatric	Depends on success of psychiatric measures

coarse and repeatable—might be present. In a case reported by Saltzman,[28] the bithermal test of Hallpike was most revealing. It showed unusual hyperexcitability and marked right-sided directional preponderance. Ventriculography showed a space-taking lesion in the posterior fossa, and at operation a cystic astrocytoma was removed from the right cerebellar hemisphere.

Epilepsy

McKenzie[29] reported a case of vertiginous epilepsy that resembled Meniere's disease. The patient, aged 25, complained of having had 3 rotational attacks which were associated with "pounding" and deafening of the left ear. The history uncovered that the patient was an epileptic and that each of his seizures was preceded by a vertiginous attack as an aura. In the differential diagnosis, epilepsy is featured by a period of somnolence following an attack, and the encephalogram shows a characteristic pattern.

The Infections

The primary form of acute neurolabyrinthitis may be of viral etiology. The onset is with violent vertigo, which is associated with tinnitus and deafness. Some relief is obtained when lying on one side. Subsidence is gradual in the course of a few weeks. Special studies with antigen sera are helpful to the diagnosis. Complete recovery may ensue. Some cases go on to profound deafness. The hearing loss shows no fluctuation. In some cases, there is also loss of function of the static labyrinth. When both ears are involved, the individual will have poor balance on closing the eyes.

Acute neurolabyrinthitis is more frequently of bacterial etiology as an extension of a middle ear infection or cerebrospinal meningitis. Its clinical course will be influenced by the use of antibiotics and chemotherapeutic agents.

The secondary form of acute neurolabyrinthitis constitutes a complication of chronic middle ear disease. The otologic examination will disclose a fistula or a cholesteatoma.

Chronic neurolabyrinthitis may be of syphilitic etiology. The Wassermann test will clarify the diagnosis. The course shows no fluctuations. It may be amenable to antiluetic therapy.

Focal infection may give Meniereform symptoms. Its elimination might free the patient of his complaints, thereby being helpful in the differential diagnosis.

Toxic Vertigo

In the report of Thomas,[30] vertigo was present in 31 per cent of 66 patients treated with streptomycin. Caloric reactions were reduced or absent in 70 per cent of the individuals with an untoward effect to the drug. Differential diagnosis from Meniere's disease will revolve around the occasional individual who has deafness and tinnitus in addition to vertigo. The distinguishing features will include the history and the audiogram, which invariably shows a high-tone loss.

Meniere-like symptoms may be produced by salicylates and quinine, according to Mygind.[31] Here again, the history will be helpful in the differential diagnosis.

Thrombosis of Posterior Inferior Cerebellar Artery

The attack—with severe vertigo, nausea, and vomiting—resembles a Meniere crisis, but the telltale signs of posterior inferior cerebellar artery occlusion appear soon. These include a change in voice and difficulty in swallowing, marked incoordination, numbness of one side of the face and numbness of the opposite side of the body, and Horner's syndrome. In one case, the patient's audiogram showed marked sloping at both ends, with preservation of the middle tones.

Head Injury

The symptomatology in some cases of concussion of the inner ear is Meniereform. As described by Schuknecht and Davison,[32] the findings include transient attacks of vertigo, a hearing loss, and tinnitus. However, the significant feature in head injury is the fact that the nystagmus is positional. It is demonstrated more readily by moving the patient from a sitting to a head-low position, with the affected ear undermost. In my experience the positional nystagmus is direction-changing in some cases, but it is direction-fixed more frequently. The audiogram usually shows a high frequency defect, but a hearing loss may be present in the entire tonal range.

Postural Vertigo

The so-called "benign paroxysmal" type may present difficulties. A case reported by Citron and Hallpike[33] had to be differentiated from Meniere's disease and acoustic neuroma. The final diagnosis was arrived at after a craniotomy. The symptoms and signs included progressive nerve deafness and tinnitus in the left ear, ablation of the left caloric responses, positional nystagmus with the left ear undermost, and absence of recruitment. At operation, no cerebellopontile angle tumor was found. The eighth nerve was divided and the patient was cured of his postural vertigo and positional nystagmus. Citron and Hallpike concluded that the symptom complex was due to a derangement occurring somewhere within a sensory-neural circuit, and that the defective circuit included the otolith organs.

Paroxysmal positional nystagmus is due to a peripheral disturbance in most cases. In the series of Dix and Hallpike,[27] middle ear disease was present in two-thirds of the patients. The nystagmic reaction was initiated when the diseased ear was placed undermost. The characteristic features of this condition include (1) a latent period of 2 to 5 seconds, (2) nystagmus—rotary, horizontal, or combined—of the duration of 20 to 30 seconds, (3) fatigueability, (4) no progressive hearing loss, and (5) a normal caloric response in most cases.

Central causes of paroxysmal positional nystagmus include brain tumor, according to Nylen,[34] toxic and infectious lesions in the central nervous system, as reported by Aschan and associates,[35] and cerebral concussions, as described by Harrison.[36]

From the foregoing, it must be inferred that the causes of paroxysmal positional nystagmus are variable. This would account for the differences in the clinical picture in this condition. Periodic dizziness occurs on change of position or on sudden turning of the head by some people past middle age. In most cases, it is associated with arteriosclerosis; in others, an attack is brought on by a sudden drop in blood pressure on changing from the supine to the upright position. Droller and Pemberton[37] made a survey of elderly people in home surroundings. Complaints of vertigo were registered by 47 per cent of the men and 61.2 per cent of the women.

If deafness and tinnitus are present, they are usually high-pitched. As the vertigo is positional and is initiated by movements of the head, there is little difficulty in the differential diagnosis.

Positional vertigo is a frequent complication of disease or trauma of the cervical spine. Ryan and Cope,[38] who observed the occurrence of vertigo associated with nystagmus in individuals with neck injury and therapeutic traction, considered this condition a clinical entity. They named it "cervical vertigo" and ascribed it to pathologic neck reflexes. It may also be due to disc pathology. X-ray would be helpful in the differential diagnosis.

Multiple Sclerosis

The unique feature in this disease is the dissociation of vertigo and nystagmus. While vertigo is a less frequent symptom, nystagmus —horizontal or vertical—is the commonest finding. It is due to involvement of the medial longitudinal fasiculus, according to Schumacher.[39] The diagnosis is confirmed when separate lesions in several parts of the nervous system are discovered. This finding is useful in the differential diagnosis when deafness and tinnitus are present coincidentally.

Barany's Syndrome (Arachnoiditis of the Posterior Fossa)

This syndrome is featured by attacks of severe headaches, intense vertigo, and auditory disturbances. A remission is ushered in by a sensation of "something bursting in the head." It has been ascribed to a precerebellar cyst and it frequently involves the side in which a labyrinthectomy had been done previously. In the case reported by Watkyn-Thomas,[40] the attack terminated with the discharge of clear fluid from the operation cavity and the ductus endolymphaticus could be traced into the cyst.

The Lermoyez Syndrome

The dramatic restoration of hearing by an episodic attack of vertigo was described by Lermoyez.[41] "There is a period of progressing deafness; then, an attack of vertigo and good hearing; the repetition of the cycles occurs over and over again." It is generally held that the Lermoyez Syndrome is a rare variant of Meniere's disease. The dramatic phenomenon at the vertiginous attack may be explained by the hypothesis of Lawrence and McCabe.[6] The rupture of the membranous labyrinth releases the basilar membrane from the deleterious effect of the hydrops.

PROGNOSIS

Meniere's disease is never fatal by itself. The vertiginous attacks are apt to become more frequent and more severe as time goes on. Total deafness, the so-called "burned out Meniere," is uncommon, but a severe hearing loss develops in the affected ear in the course of time. The disease remains unilateral in about 90 per cent of the patients. However, in a given case there is no way to predict whether the other ear will not become involved.

In Wright's statistical survey,[42] spontaneous cure occurred in 20 per cent of the cases. This might have resulted from a favorable turn in the disease, such as the fistulization of the membranous labyrinth after a rupture.[5] Lengthy intermissions of the duration of months or even years may occur. These could be accounted for by favorable changes in the secretion or absorption of the endolymph. Another plausible explanation would be the intermittent discontinuation of the causative or contributing factors. These would include allergens, emotional stress, or a faulty diet.

Good results from therapy may be predicted for most patients. Some proponents of medical methods have reported that about 80 per cent of their patients were favorably affected.[14,16] Surgery offers relief to the patient who becomes demoralized or incapacitated as the result of unmanageable vertiginous attacks. The various procedures with their advantages and hazards are presented in the section "Surgery for Vertigo."

REFERENCES

1. Hallpike, C. S., and Cairns, H.: Observations on the pathology of Meniere's syndrome. J. Laryng. 53:625, 1938.
2. Altmann, F., and Fowler, E. P., Jr.: Histologic findings in Meniere's symptom complex. Ann. Otol. 52:52, 1943.
3. Lindsay, J. R.: Hydrops of the labyrinth. A.M.A. Arch. Otolaryng. 71:500, 1960.
4. Kristensen, H. K.: Histopathology in Meniere's disease. Acta Otolaryng. (Stockh.) 53:237, 1961.
5. Schuknecht, H. F.: Meniere's disease: a correlation of symptomatology and pathology. Laryngoscopy 73:651-665, 1963.
6. Lawrence, M., and McCabe, B.: Inner ear mechanics and deafness. J.A.M.A. 171: 1929-1932, 1959.
7. Williams, H. L.: Allergy of the Inner Ear. A.M.A. Arch. Otolaryng. 56:24-44, 1952.
8. Cawthorne, T., and Hewlett, A. B.: Meniere's disease. Proc. Roy. Soc. Med. 47:663-670, 1954.
9. VerMeulen, V., and Saunders, W. H.: Eye, Ear, Nose and Throat Monthly 42:56, 1963.
10. Hyslop, G. H.: Distant secondary circulary and vasomotor reactions to accidental electric shock. Bull. N. Y. Acad. Med. 21:302, 1945.
11. Scheinker, I. M.: Vasoparalysis of the central nervous system: a characteristic vascular syndrome. Arch. Neurol. Psychiat. 52:43, 1944.
12. Fowler, E. P., Jr., and Zeckel, A.: Psychosomatic aspects of Meniere's disease. J.A.M.A. 148:1265, 1952.

13. Mygind, S. H., and Dedering, D.: The pathogenesis of Meniere's disease and of kindred conditions in the ear and the rest of the body. Ann. Otol. 47:938-946, 1938.
14. Falbe-Hansen, J., quoted by Dederding, D.: Our Meniere treatment. Acta Otolaryng. 16:404, 1931.
15. Furstenberg, A. C., Richardson, G. and Larthrop, F. D.: Meniere's Disease, Arch. Otolaryng. 34:1083, 1941.
16. Kristensen, H. K.: Meniere's disease, pathology and pathogenesis. Acta Otolaryng. Suppl. 188:149, 1963.
17. Petersen, W. F., with the technical assistance of Milliken, M. E.: The Patient and the Weather: Autonomic Disintegration. Ann Arbor, Mich., Edwards Bros., 1934.
18. Tumarkin, A.: Otolithic catastrophy: a new syndrome. Brit. Med. J. 2:175-177, 1936.
19. Aschan, G., and Stahle, J.: Nystagmus in Meniere's disease during attacks: a nystagmographical study. Acta Otolaryng. 74:189-201, 1957.
20. Saltzman, M.: Meniere's disease, cochlear type. A.M.A. Arch. Otolaryng. 62:59-61, 1955.
21. Day, K. M.: Twenty-five years experience with Meniere's disease. Laryngoscope 73:693-98, 1963.
22. Jerger, J., Shedd, J. L., and Hartford, E.: On detection of extremely small changes in sound intensity. A.M.A. Arch. Otolaryng. 69:200-211, 1959.
23. Parker, W., Decker, R. L., and Gardner, W. H.: Auditory function and intracranial lesions. Arch. Otolaryng. 76:425-435, 1962.
24. Pulec., J. L., and House, W. F.: Vestibular involvement and testing in acoustic neuromas. Arch Otolaryng. 80:677, 681, 1964.
25. Johnson, E. W., and House, W. F.: Auditory findings in 53 cases of acoustic neuronomas. Arch. Otolaryng. 80:667-676, 1964.
26. Lumio, J. S., and Aho, J.: Vestibular neuronitis. Ann. Otol. 74:264-70, 1965.
27. Dix, M. R., and Hallpike, C. S.: The pathology, symptomatology and diagnosis of certain common disorders of the vestibular system. Proc. Roy. Soc. Med. 45:341, 1952.
28. Saltzman, M.: The bithermal test of Hallpike. Arch. Otolaryng. 77:484-490, 1963.
29. McKenzie, W.: Aural vertigo: an account of certain cases resembling Meniere's disease. J. Laryng. 65:70-88, 1951.
30. Thomas, J. A. N.: The toxic effect of streptomycin on the VIII cranial nerve. J. Laryng. 65:472-476, 1951.
31. Mygind, S. H.: Experimental-histological studies on the labyrinth. XI. Correlation of our histological and clinical experiments and observations. Conclusive review. Acta Otolaryng. 35:108-129, 1947.
32. Schuknecht, H. F., and Davison, R. C.: Deafness and vertigo from head injury. A.M.A. Arch. Otolaryng. 63:513-528, 1956.
33. Citron, L., and Hallpike, C. S.: a case of positional nystagmus of the so-called benign paroxysmal type and the effects of treatment by intracranial division of the VIIIth nerve. J. Laryng. 76:28: 1962.
34. Nylen, C. O.: The otoneurologic diagnosis of tumors of the brain. Acta Otolaryng. Suppl. 33, 1939.
35. Aschan, G., Bergstedt, M., and Stahle, J.: Nystagmography recording of nystagmus in clinical neuro-otologic examinations. Acta Otolaryng. Suppl. 129, 1956.
36. Harrison, M. S.: Notes on clinical features and pathology of post-concussional vertigo, with special reference to positional nystagmus. Brain 79:474, 1956.
37. Droller, H., and Pemberton, J.: Vertigo in a random sample of elderly people living in their homes. J. Laryng. 67:689-694, 1953.
38. Ryan, G. M. S., and Cope, S.: Cervical vertigo. Lancet 269:1355-1358, 1955.
39. Schumacher, G. A.: Multiple sclerosis. J.A.M.A. 143:1059, 1950.
40. Watkyn-Thomas, F. W.: Diseases of the Throat, Nose and Ear. Springfield, Ill., Charles C Thomas, 1953, p. 669.
41. Lermoyez, M.: Le Vertigue qui fait entendre (Angiospasme labrenthique). Ann. Areille Larynx 48:575-583, 1929.
42. Wright, A. J.: Meniere's disease. Proc. Roy. Soc. Med. 41:801. 1948.

Pathology of Meniere's Disease

John R. Lindsay

The term "Meniere's disease," as it is presently in general use, refers to the clinical entity of sensorineural hearing impairment beginning with low tones, fluctuating in severity from time to time, associated with vertigo in the form of recurring spells with usually rapid onset and recovery, therefore described as episodic. The classical description was first given by Meniere[9] about 1860, but the term "Meniere's disease" was applied only after the histopathology found in the inner ear was demonstrated to be a dilatation of the endolymphatic system, or "hydrops" of a characteristic type. The term "idiopathic" is applied to this type to distinguish it from hydrops commonly found in a variety of diseased states of the inner ear in which the hydrops has occurred secondary to a hyperplastic pathologic process in the perilymphatic labyrinthine spaces.

The hydrops found in Meniere's disease is therefore characterized by a lack of evidence of abnormality in the perilymphatic spaces or of associated disease of the labyrinthine capsule. The pathology has been found only within the endolymphatic system. It has consistently involved the cochlear duct and saccule and usually the areas of junction of the utricle with one or more semicircular canal ampullae.

The existence of a hydrops of the endolymphatic system of this type had already been observed in the occasional specimen in some laboratories for several years, but it was the report by Hallpike and Cairns[3] in 1938 which established its relationship to the clinical syndrome now known as Meniere's disease. The observers reported the finding of hydrops of the labyrinth in two cases presenting the clinical syndrome which had been described originally by Meniere, which terminated fatally after sectioning of the vestibular nerve.

Hydrops has also been found to be restricted to the cochlear duct[8] in which there have been associated auditory disturbances characteristic of Meniere's disease, but without a history of attacks of vertigo. The similarity of the pathology in the cochlea and the associated auditory symptoms and findings to those in Meniere's disease suggests that this represents an early stage of the same disease. Hydrops limited to the vestibular labyrinth

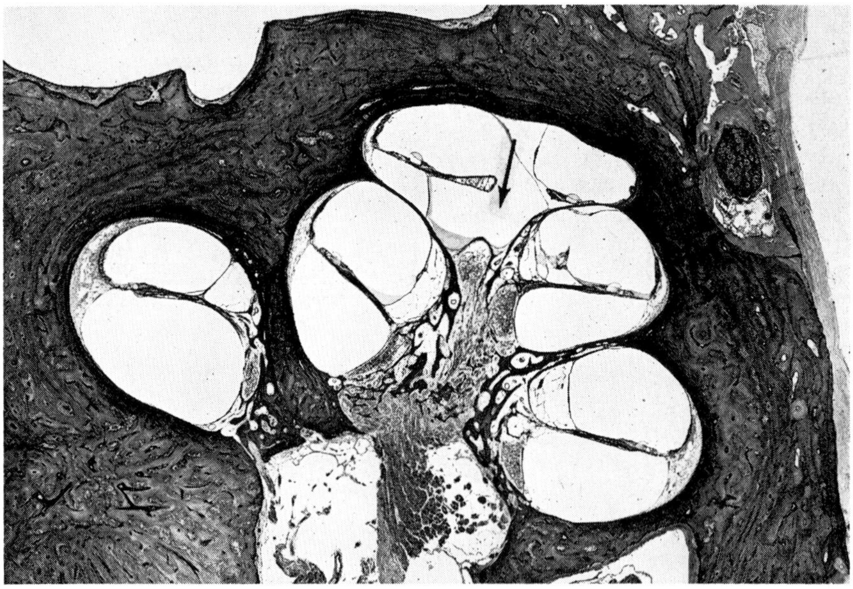

FIG. 1A. Midmodiolar section of a cochlea of a 66-year-old male illustrating dilatation or hydrops of the cochlear duct to an extreme degree, with projection through the helicotrema (arrow) into the scala tympani. Ganglion cells, nerve fibers and organ of Corti are well preserved. The stria vascularis showed moderate degeneration in the upper basal coil.

has not yet been reported as an explanation for recurring spells of vertigo.

HISTOPATHOLOGY

The description of histopathology which follows is based on the findings in eight temporal bones in which there was no evidence of disease in the perilymphatic spaces or in the labyrinthine capsule bordering the intralabyrinthine spaces, which might have been the cause of the hydrops, and upon findings reported by others.

The term "idiopathic" in reference to these ears is used to distinguish them from several other human specimens and several experimental animals' ears, each of which also presented a hydrops, but of a different type. In each of these the dilatation of the endolymphatic spaces was associated with, and obviously secondary to, hyperplastic pathologic changes in the perilymphatic spaces, each representing a different etiologic disorder.

Cochlea

Dilatation of the scala media or cochlear duct has apparently been a constant finding in the cases so far described in which the auditory findings have been characteristic of Meniere's disease. The degree of dilatation varies and may extend to occupy all of the scala vestibuli in some coils, usually the middle or upper (Fig. 1). The cochlear duct also increases to a limited degree in length and may bulge through the helicotrema into the scala tympani.

The stria vascularis has shown a moderate degree of atrophy in ears with hydrops of long duration (Fig. 2); whether the atrophy is related to the hydrops is not definite. A moderate degree of atrophy of the stria has been found to be compatible with normal hearing.[1]

The tectorial membrane varied in its appearance in this series but was considered to be within normal range in all except two cases. The tectorial membrane in the living animal cochlea has been observed to be in contact with the hairs of the hair cells and to extend onto the cells of Hensen which border

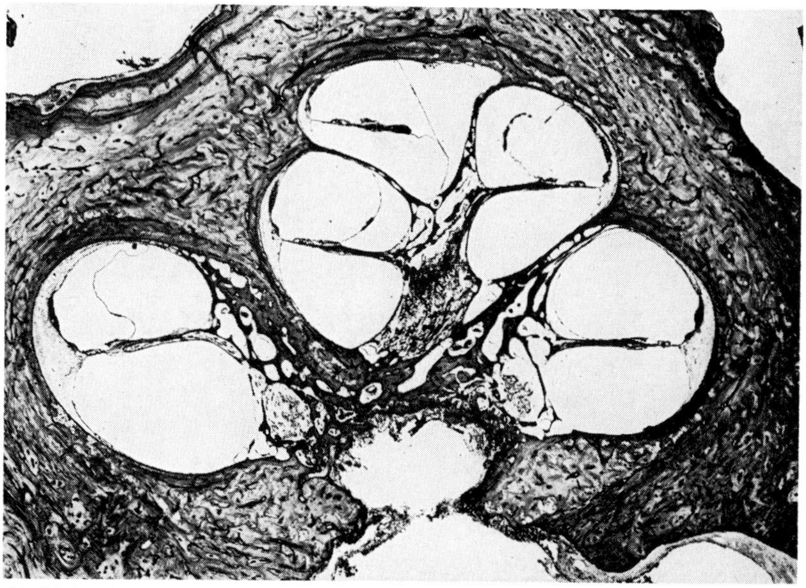

FIG. 1B. Midmodiolar section of a cochlea from a middle-aged patient showing hydrops of the cochlear duct. Ganglion cells, nerve fibers, and hair cells were approximately equal in number to those in the uninvolved ear. The stria vascularis showed moderate degeneration in the basal coil. (The collapse of Reissner's membrane in the helicotrema and its displacement in the basal coil are attributed to artifact.)

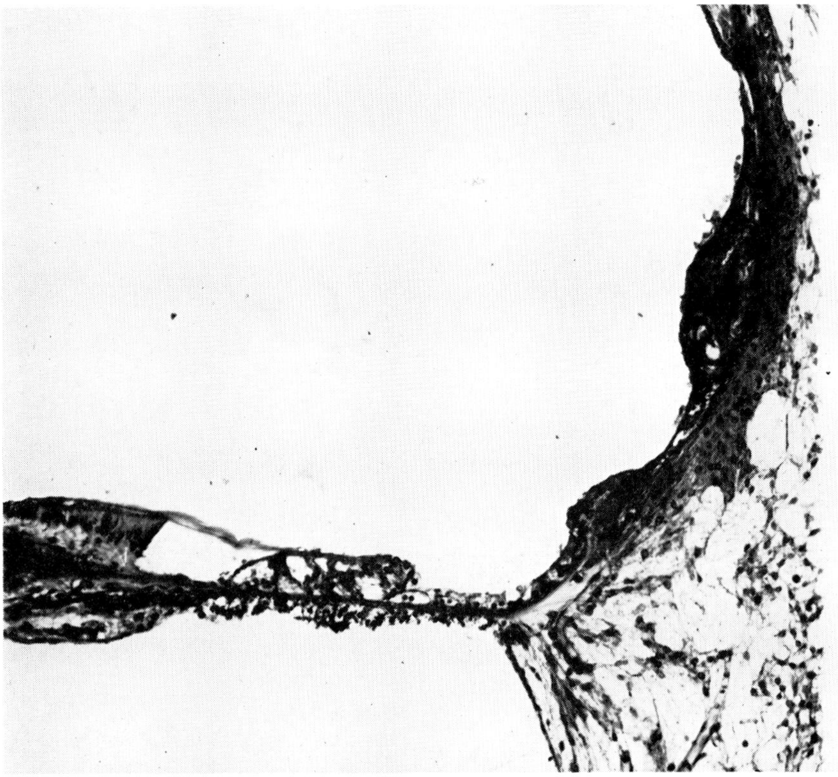

FIG. 2. Higher magnification of Corti's organ and the stria vascularis in the basal coil of Figure 1B. The stria shows a degree of degeneration frequently seen in the presence of advanced hydrops.

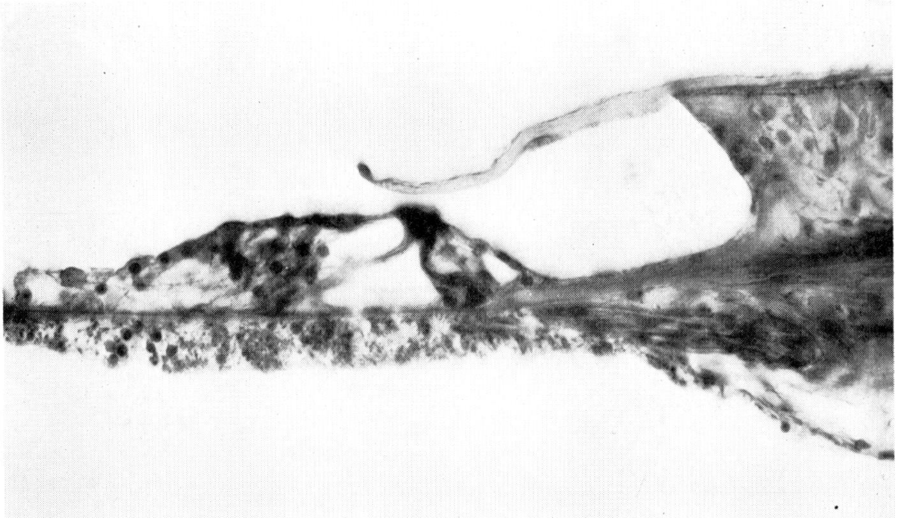

FIG. 3A. Photomicrograph of Corti's organ illustrating types of artifact in preparation: Corti's organ from a normal ear. The tectorial membrane appears thinned and retracted from its normal position in contact with the hair cells. The pillars and supporting cells are distorted and deviated toward the limbus. The hair cells show distortion but can be distinguished.

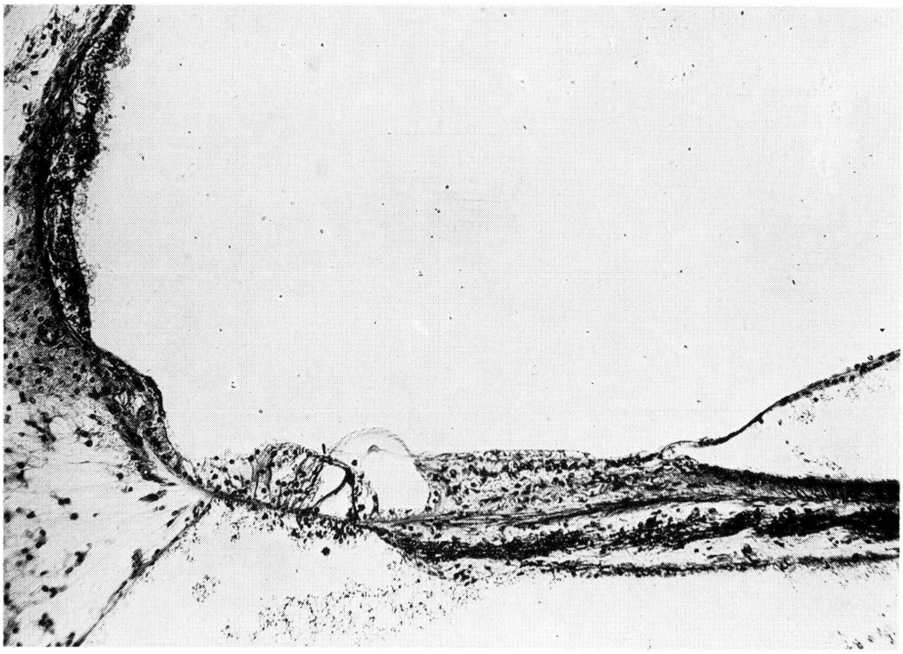

FIG. 3B. Photomicrograph of Corti's organ illustrating types of artifact in preparation: Corti's organ from the basal coil in a case of idiopathic hydrops of the cochlear duct. Hair cells are well preserved. The tectorial membrane is retracted and the stria vascularis of about normal extent. Early postmortem autolytic changes are present.

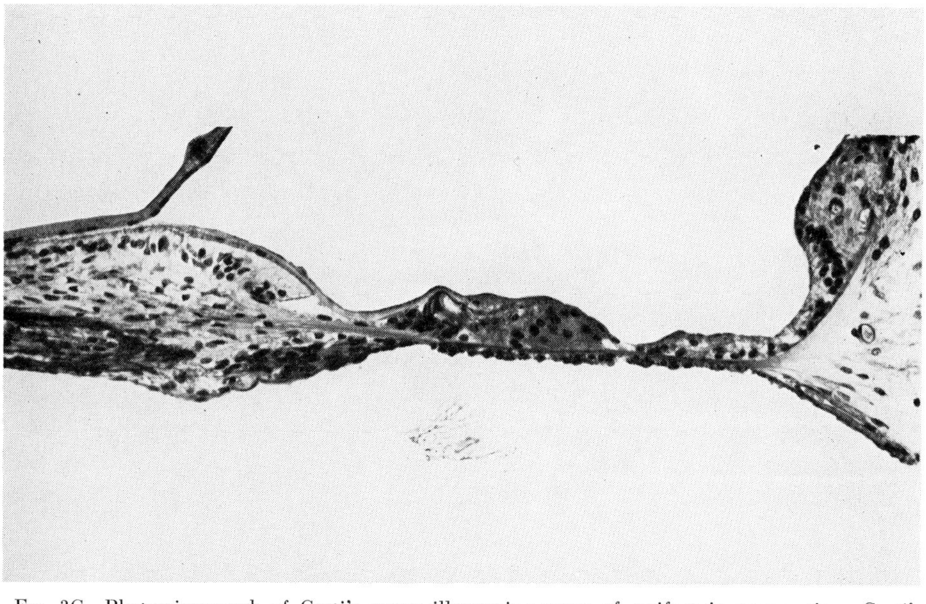

FIG. 3C. Photomicrograph of Corti's organ illustrating types of artifact in preparation: Corti's organ from a normal hearing ear showing compression. The tectorial membrane is thinned and lies in contact with inner sulcus cells and Corti's organ. Hair cells, pillars, and supporting cells appear compressed. The limbus is compressed so that the inner sulcus is almost obliterated. This "compression" phenomenon is attributed to artifact in preparation.

on the outer hair cells.[4] The method of processing temporal bones for study by light microscopy usually disturbs this relationship, and the tectorial membrane is seldom found in contact with the hair cells. It usually shows signs of shrinkage to different degrees or may sometimes appear edematous (Fig. 3, A and B).

In some specimens from normal as well as impaired-hearing ears the tectorial membrane may be flattened out, lying on the surface of Corti's organ which is also compressed on the basilar membrane. This "compression phenomenon" is thought to be an artifact not yet explained (Fig. 3C).[2]

In two of the eight ears in the University of Chicago collection the tectorial membrane and Corti's organ presented an unusual appearance. The first of these showed an extensive hydrops with the tectorial membrane separated from the limbus and compressed onto Corti's organ in the basal and middle coils with an apparent layer of flattened cells extending from Hensen's cells over its surface. This condition indicated that it had been a vital phenomenon, but it appears unlikely that these changes could be compatible with function.

The second ear was also a case of extensive hydrops and was similar to the first case (Fig. 4). In the basal and lower middle coils the tectorial membrane was separated from the limbus and projected into the space between the outer pillar and the first row of outer hair cells displacing and distorting these cells. A layer of cells extending from Hensen's cells laterally and from the inner sulcus cells medially seemed to have grown over to envelop the tectorial membrane.

Several tests of hearing had been made during the course of illness. Two threshold tests made in 1957 and 1962, two months before death, showed a severe sensorineural deafness on the left, and the right ear was

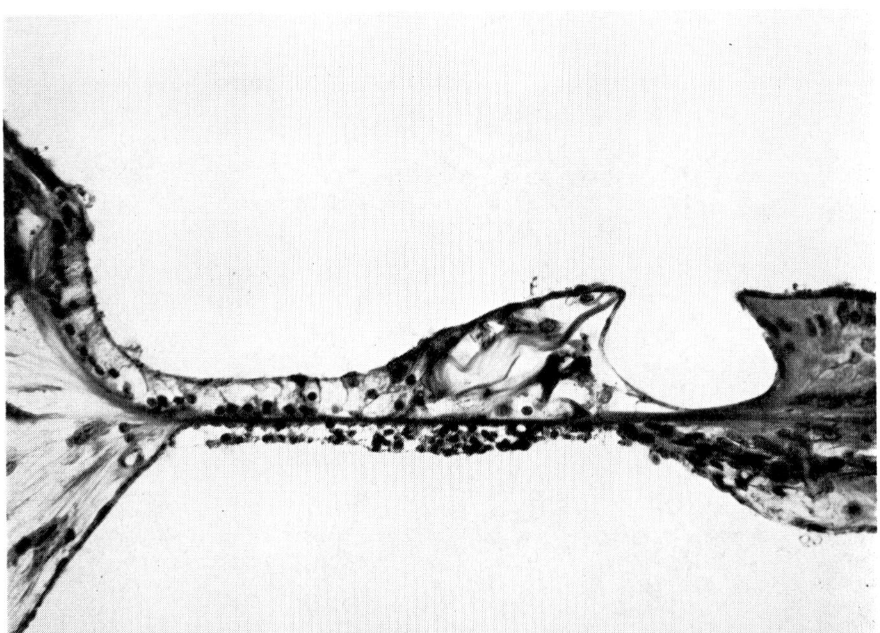

FIG. 4. Photomicrograph of Corti's organ in the basal coil of a case of idiopathic hydrops with profound deafness. The tectorial membrane has separated from the limbus and has extended into the space between the external pillar and the first row of hair cells. The external hair cells are present but distorted and displaced. A layer of flattened cells covered the projecting part of the tectorial membrane.

profoundly deaf on both examinations. The left ear, in which a hydrops was also present and in which the stapes had been dislodged during removal, showed a well-preserved Corti's organ. Although the interpretation is not positive, the evidence indicates that the unusual appearance of Corti's organ in this ear was a vital phenomenon and incompatible with hearing function.

Hair Cells

The number of hair cells in the two ears in the unilateral cases in which an estimate was possible showed no definite asymmetry. In the two ears of the bilateral case just described (see Fig. 4), the abnormal appearance of one Corti's organ did not preclude an accurate estimate of hair cell population.

The peripheral nerve fibers and ganglion cell count were approximately symmetrical bilaterally in all except one case. In that case,[8] there was degeneration of ganglion cells and nerve fibers to the apical region in the diseased ear, with a well preserved organ of Corti, including the hair cells (Fig. 5).

Vestibular Labyrinth

The saccule was found to be dilated in four out of the eight ears with "idiopathic" hydrops. In two the saccule was ruptured. In the one postoperative ear the vestibular labyrinth showed extensive changes, including the saccular wall, utricle and canals, due to the surgical procedure. In the one ear with hydrops of the cochlear duct only,[8] the saccule was found to be normal.

Dilatation of the saccule was common also in cases of hydrops secondary to perilymphatic labyrinthine pathology. In one of these cases, however, a dilated cochlear duct occupied the perilymphatic cistern instead of the usually dilated saccule.

The thickened outer portion of the wall of the saccule described by Perlman[10] usually retained its normal position although the remainder of the wall had expanded to occupy the perilymphatic cistern completely, thereby coming into contact with the outer bony wall of the vestibule, part of which consists of the stapes footplate (Fig. 6).

The rupture of the saccule in one case[6]

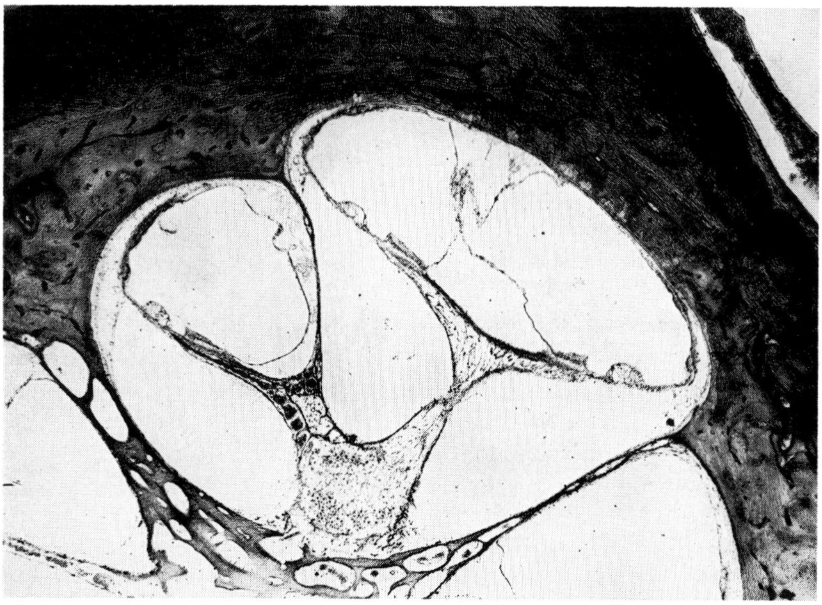

Fig. 5. Photomicrograph of a section through the middle and upper coils of a case of idiopathic hydrops showing degeneration of the spiral ganglion cells and nerve fibers to the apical coil, but normal-appearing hair cells and Corti's organ.

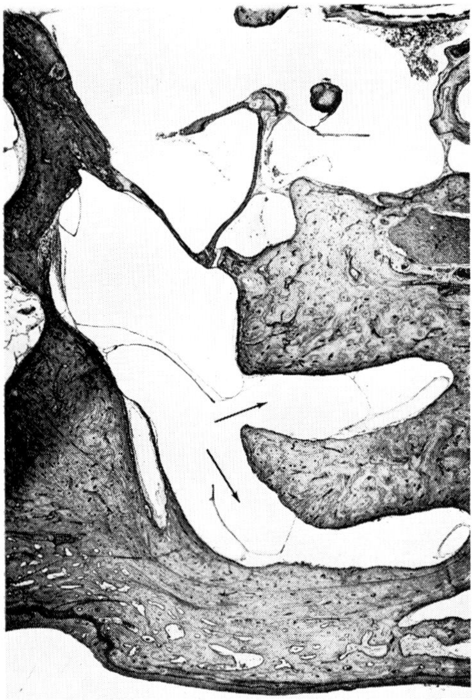

FIG. 6. Photomicrograph of a horizontal section through the vestibule of an ear with idiopathic hydrops showing a dilated saccule in contact with the stapes footplate. The utricle shows two localized herniations of its wall, one extending into the perilymphatic space of the common crus and one into the small end of the horizontal canal (arrows).

obviously occurred before the membranes had been fixed by the formalin solution, because of the retracted and wrinkled appearance of the margins of the torn membrane (Fig. 7). Whether the rupture had occurred during life could not be definitely stated.

The rupture of the saccule in the second ear[7] presented a similar appearance. The tear had been more extensive and irregular with margins similar to the former case. However, the stapes had been driven into the vestibule along with bone dust in the process of removal of the bone before fixation. The rupture of the saccule had obviously occurred before fixation of the membranes, but whether it had been a vital phenomenon was not definite.

In summary, therefore, the eight ears with idiopathic hydrops include one ear with hydrops confined to the cochlear duct, two ears with hydrops of the cochlear duct plus a ruptured saccule of questionable etiology, four ears with hydrops involving the cochlear duct, saccule and the utricle at its junction with canal ampullae, and one ear in which the vestibular contents had been disorganized and destroyed by a surgical procedure.

In four of the ears the saccule was dilated to occupy the available perilymphatic space in the vestibule. However, the cochlear duct was dilated in one case[6] of labyrinthine hydrops of the secondary type to occupy the perilymphatic cistern. The rupture of the saccule in two ears remains of undetermined etiology. Hearing is known to have been present in both of these ears until the final

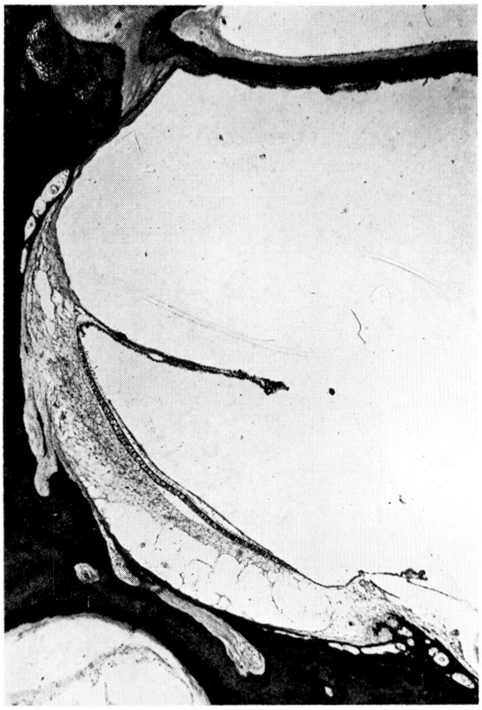

FIG. 7. Photomicrograph of a section through the saccule in a case of idiopathic hydrops. The edges of the torn membrane appear retracted and wrinkled, indicating that rupture occurred before the membrane had been fixed by the fixative solution. Whether it had been a vital phenomenon could not be determined.

acute terminal illness. When present, the characteristic changes in the utricle and canals consisted in dilatations of the membranes at the weakest points, which were at the junction of the utricle and the ampullae, and in some instances at the small end of the canals (Figs. 8-10). Rupture of the membranes at these points have been described by others;[3,5,11,12] however, in the cases described here the presence of a complete rupture, except those that were obviously due to artifact, could not be demonstrated.

FUNCTIONAL SIGNIFICANCE OF HISTOLOGIC CHANGES

Auditory Disturbances

The characteristic auditory disturbances requiring explanation are threshold shift for low tones as compared to high tones in the early stages, fluctuation in threshold, recruitment of loudness, diplacusis, and dysacusis or hypersensitivity to loud sounds.

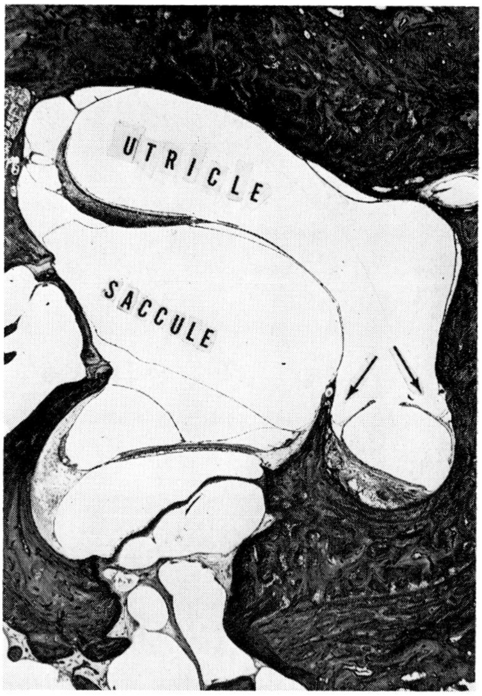

FIG. 9. Vertical section of another ear in a plane passing through the utricle and posterior canal ampulla showing beginning herniation of the utricular walls between the walls of the ampulla and the bone.

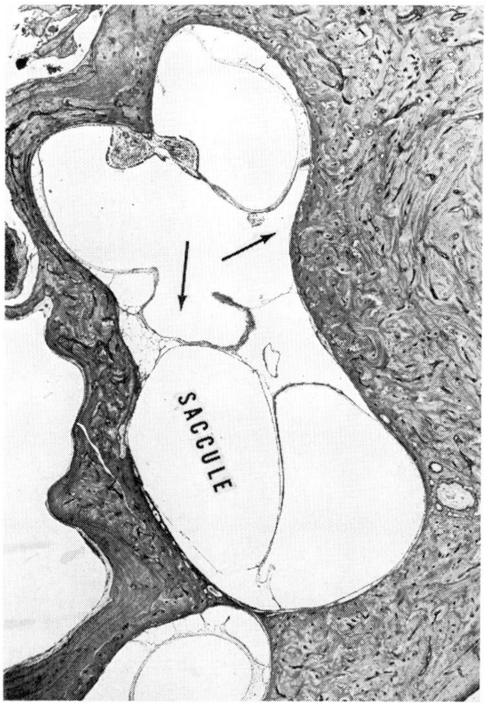

FIG. 8. Vertical section showing areas where herniations (arrows) have been characteristically found in advanced cases in relation to the horizontal and vertical canal ampullas.

One explanation for the low-tones loss and fluctuating threshold has been offered on the basis of an inner ear conduction impairment due to either a temporary increase in pressure or impedance of the traveling waves. This fails to explain the consistent finding of recruitment and the frequent diplacusis and dysacusis. An alteration in the constitution of the endolymph offers a plausible basis for these latter characteristics and could also explain the threshold fluctuations. A mixing of perilymph and endolymph due to rupture of Reissner's membrane has also been suggested to explain these auditory characteristics. This theory does not seem tenable in view of the fact that extreme dilatation of the cochlear duct with extension through the helicotrema is common in these advanced

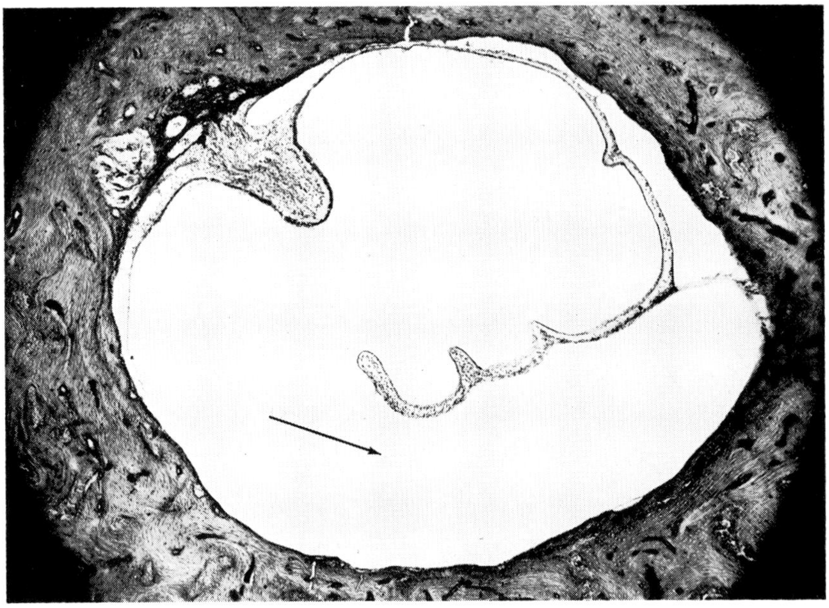

FIG. 10A. Horizontal section from another ear showing a herniation of the utricle between the ampullary wall of the posterior canal and the bone (arrow).

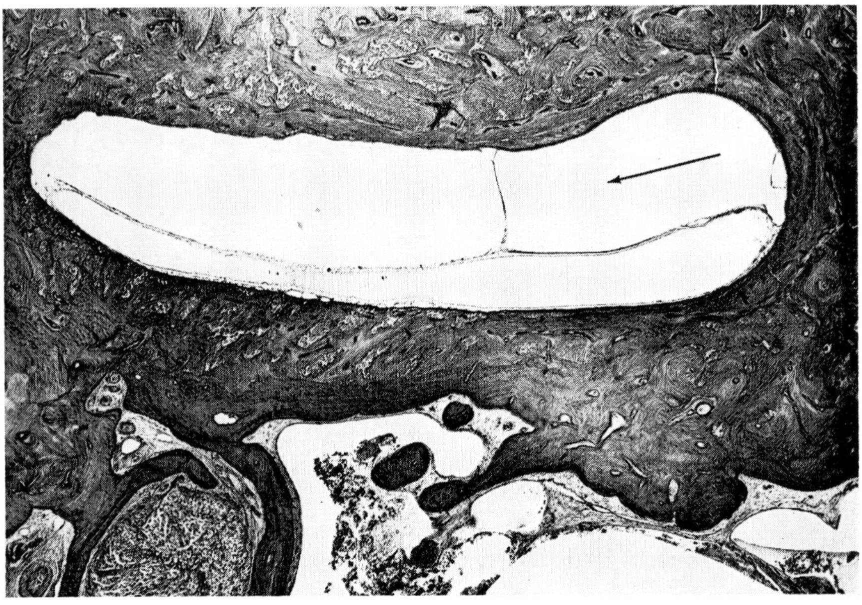

FIG. 10B. Section showing the extension of the herniation shown in Figure 10A into the perilymphatic space beyond the ampulla.

cases, yet rupture of Reissner's membrane other than those obviously due to artifact has not been clearly shown. Also, a mixing of fluids would fail to explain the rapid improvement in auditory symptoms a feature of Lermoyez's syndrome, a variant of Meniere's disease. It seems possible also that more than one factor may contribute to these auditory disturbances.

Vestibular Disturbances

The explanation for the clinical characteristics of the vestibular attacks—namely, the rapid or sudden onset and a rapid cessation —is suggested by the histopathology. The distortions in the regions where the canals join the utricle suggest a basis for a shift in the physical relationship. The weaker areas in membranous walls permit expansion in areas where a disturbance of the contour of the wall of an ampulla is produced, or may account for asymmetrical movement of endolymph. A rupture of the membrane would explain a sudden onset of vertigo, but neither a rupture nor the consequent mixing of the labyrinthine fluids gives a plausible explanation for a sudden or rapid cessation of the vertigo which is a frequent occurrence.

The essential feature of the histologic findings is that they support an explanation of the disturbances of equilibrium on the basis of a mechanical or physical disturbance of the ampullary mechanism in one or more canals. The occasional observation of a purely vertical nystagmus in an acute attack is evidence that an attack of vertigo may be caused by a disturbance of a single semicircular canal.

Pathogenesis

The pathogenesis of idiopathic hydrops remains in question. Proposed theories have included impedance of absorption of endolymph from the endolymphatic duct and sac, increased secretion of endolymph, and a disturbance in the chemical constituents of endolymph. It is usually assumed that the dilatation of the saccule and utricle represent a spread from the cochlear duct; however, the vestibular organs are older in the phylogenetic scale and have separate sources of endolymph. It is possible that the changes in these structures may be independent of the cochlear duct.

REFERENCES

1. Crowe, S. J., Guild, S. R., and Polvogt, L. M.: Observations on the pathology of high-tone deafness. Bull. Hopkins Hosp. 54:315-379, 1934.
2. Fernandez, C.: Postmortem changes and artifacts in human temporal bones. Laryngoscope 68:1586-1615, 1958.
3. Hallpike, C. S., and Cairns, H.: Observations on the pathology of Meniere's syndrome. Proc. Roy. Soc. Med. 31:1317-1336, 1938.
4. Hilding, A. C.: Studies on the otic labyrinth. I. On the origin and insertion of the tectorial membrane. Ann. Otol. 61:354-370, 1952.
5. Lawrence, M., and McCabe, B. F.: Inner-ear mechanics and deafness. Special consideration of Meniere's syndrome. J.A.M.A. 171: 1927-1932, 1959.
6. Lindsay, J. R.: Labyrinthine dropsy. Laryngoscope 56:325-341, 1946.
7. Lindsay, J. R., and Sciarra, P. A.: Meniere's disease: pathology and manifestations. *In:* Proceedings of the International Vestibular Symposium. Philadelphia, University of Pennsylvania Press (in press).
8. Lindsay, J. R., and v. Schulthess, G.: An unusual case of labyrinthine hydrops. Acta Otolaryng. 49:315-324, 1958.
9. Meniere, P.: Memoire sur des lésions de l'orielle interne donnant lieu à des symptômes de congestion cérébrale apoplectiforme. Gaz. Med. Paris 3, 16:597-601, 1861.
10. Perlman, H. B.: The saccule. Observations on a differentiated reenforced area of the saccular wall in man. Arch. Otolaryng. 32:678-691, 1940.
11. Rollin, H.: Zur Kenntnis der Labyrinthhydrops und des durch ihn bedingten Meniere. Hals-, Nasen- u. Ohrenarzt (Teil 1), 31:73-109, 1940.
12. Schuknecht, H. F., Benitez, J. T., and Beekhuis, J.: Further observations on pathology of Meniere's disease. Ann. Otol. 71:1039-1053, 1962.

CHAPTER 7

Labyrinthitis

MARTIN SPECTOR

Labyrinthitis is second in frequency only to hearing loss as a complication of otitis media.

CLASSIFICATION

Lund divided labyrinthitis into four groups:

1. Serous labyrinthitis—in which there are vestibular symptoms with diminished function which later returns.
2. Circumscribed labyrinthitis—in which there is a fistula.
3. Acute diffuse destructive labyrinthitis—in which all function is lost permanently within a few days. This group corresponds to the so-called acute purulent labyrinthitis.
4. Chronic destructive labyrinthitis—in which there has been complete absence of acoustic and vestibular function. This group also has been called diffuse purulent latent labyrinthitis.

Shambaugh distinguished two groups: (1) localized or circumscribed with serous labyrinthitis, and (2) diffuse purulent with permanent total destruction. We divide labyrinthitis into (1) serous, with fistula as a subgroup, and (2) diffuse suppurative.

SEROUS LABYRINTHITIS

Pathology

Inflammation of the labyrinthine contents is rarely hematogenous; that is, it is rarely indirect through the blood vessels and is nearly always a result of an extensive infection with osteitis of the labyrinthine capsule or temporal bone. Extension of inflammation to the labyrinth by preformed pathway may occur in early acute suppurative otitis media through the annular ligament of the oval window or the secondary tympanic membrane of the round window. This may result in a serous, uncommonly a suppurative, labyrinthitis. Labyrinthine inflammation arising during a primary otitis is a rare infection which even in preantibiotic times was reported only occasionally. It was most frequent with scarlet fever. The infection of the labyrinth occurs much more often in chronic middle ear suppuration, especially with cholesteatoma. Circumscribed inflammation of the labyrinth may spread over the entire labyrinth after an exacerbation of a chronic middle ear infection. Stapes luxation may occur during mastoid or middle ear surgery, or even after paracentesis, and open a pathway for infection of the labyrinth. According to Shambaugh, aural polyps accompanied 52 of 129 cases with labyrinthitis. Removal of aural polps by snare may also precipitate labyrinthitis. Serous labyrinthitis is the usual cause of hearing loss in congenital syphilis and also may occur in tuberculosis of the middle ear.

Symptoms

The symptoms of serous labyrinthitis are the result of disturbed vestibular and cochlear function. Nearly always there is a depression rather than hyperexcitability of vestibular function. The vestibular symptoms precede the cochlear by a few hours to several days. They consist of a spontaneous nystagmus to the opposite ear, nausea and vomiting, vertigo, ataxia, pastpointing, and loss of hearing. In mild serous labyrinthitis, definite retention of labyrinthine function can be demonstrated by the caloric test. In severe serous labyrinthitis, there may be a temporary suppression of all labyrinthine response. It is impossible to differentiate such a severe serous labyrinthitis during an acute stage from an acute suppurative labyrinthitis. Differentiation can be made by tests weeks later when definite recovery occurs with serous labyrinthitis. Proud reports that the hot caloric response is later to leave and earlier to return than is the cold caloric response. If serous labyrinthitis is a possibility, it is advisable to examine labyrinthine function to make sure there is no involvement. Tests advised are for spontaneous nystagmus, positional nystagmus, fistula test, and Dundas Grant caloric test.

Prognosis

As long as labyrinthitis is of the serous type as indicated by definite labyrinthine response, there is no danger of intracranial invasion. However, it may progress to the suppurative type. Lund reported that among 102 patients with serous labyrinthitis, 15 developed intracranial infection and there were 3 deaths. This statistic was gathered in the preantibiotic era. When the stapes is avulsed or the oval window opened, the prognosis depends upon whether suppuration in the internal ear ensues.

Treatment

Treatment of the serous labyrinthine inflammation is directed toward the etiologic factor. In early suppurative otitis media, myringotomy and antibiotics will suffice. If it be a chronic perilabyrinthine osteitis, mastoidectomy with removal of diseased bone should be combined with antibacterial medication. Vertigo may disappear after removal of cholesteatomatous masses from the ear either by office treatment or operation. Supportive and palliative medication for the vertigo is indicated. Chemotherapy should be used as a prophylactic measure when the stapes is avulsed in an infected field.

Fistula of the Labyrinth

A fistula into the labyrinth denotes an abnormal opening through the labyrinthine capsule into the perilymphatic space. A fistula may be considered a major subdivision of the group labeled serous labyrinthitis.

Site of Occurrence

Politzer stated that the order of frequency of fistulas of the labyrinth is, first, in the horizontal canal; secondly, the framework of the oval and round windows; less frequently, the promontory; and rarely, the anterior and posterior vertical semicircular canals. Permin reported that out of 62 patients with fistulas, 59 had a fistula in the lateral semicircular canal, one in the vestibule and one in the posterior semicircular canal, and one on both the lateral and posterior semicircular canals. Twelve patients in Permin's series had no fistular reaction before operation, but a fistula was found at operation. These 12 did have preserved vestibular function as determined by caloric tests. In some the fistula was microscopic in size.

Etiology

Shambaugh wrote: "A spontaneous fistula of the labyrinth is in the great majority of cases due to bone erosion by cholesteatoma. In fact, the development of a spontaneous labyrinthine fistula is so characteristic of cholesteatoma as immediately to suggest the presence of the latter in a case of chronic suppurative otitis media or attic perforation. Rarely, a spontaneous fistula of the labyrinth may arise in a gummatous syphilitic osteitis of the labyrinthine capsule, in a tubercular otitis media, in a chronic perilabyrinthine osteomyelitis, or with a neoplasm such as carcinoma or glomus jugulare tumor." In Permin's series, two-thirds of the cases of labyrinthine fistula had cholesteatoma; one-third had osteitis alone. Permin reported an incidence of 13 per cent of fistulas among a large series of chronic suppurative ears; Nylen reported an incidence of 7 per cent. The finding of vertigo in the presence of a discharging ear almost invariably indicates the presence of a cholesteatoma and labyrinthine fistula. It may be mentioned that today a fistula into the labyrinth is also commonly due to stapedectomy.

Pathology

The bone in the neighborhood of a fistula of the semicircular canals always shows inflammatory changes. The fistula itself may be covered with granulations or cholesteatoma. The semicircular canal may contain pus or granulation tissue or, conversely, it may appear to be uninvolved by disease. The annular ligament of the footplate of the stapes may be perforated. The cholesteatoma may seem to protect the labyrinthine contents from an inflammatory involvement, or a cholesteatoma may erode into the labyrinthine cavity through the fistula.

Symptoms

The initial symptoms may be severe and sudden in onset with loss of equilibrium and with lateropulsion. Sometimes there is only one attack but more often there is a continuous series of vertiginous attacks. Buzzing in the ears, decreased audition, nausea, and vomiting are frequently observed with a fistula. Permin reported that before operation, one-third of his cases exhibited spontaneous nystagmus. Sometimes it was towards the affected ear but more often it was away from it. The outstanding and diagnostic sign of a fistula is a positive fistula test. (See Chapter IV, "Examinations," for details of the fistula test.) A patient with an active fistula of the labyrinth often complains of dizziness if he presses against the tragus, manipulates the auricle, or turns his head quickly. Rarely, he may have momentary vertigo when exposed to a loud noise (the Tullio phenomenon). A fistula into the vestibule through the footplate is not always accompanied by the usual nystagmus of a positive fistula test. In this situation, vertigo with nausea without nystagmus may be elicited due to stimulation of the utricular macula.

Treatment

Lederer stated: "A fistula with circumscribed labyrinthitis can heal spontaneously after conservative treatment of otitis media even in the presence of a cholesteatoma. In practice, however, since no one can tell whether circumscribed labyrinthitis may change to a diffuse labyrinthitis with subsequent meningitis, it is obvious that surgery is the lesser risk." Shambaugh also stated: "Spontaneous fistula of the labyrinth due to cholesteatoma is a positive indication for a radical mastoidectomy to exteriorize the cholesteatoma sac and prevent the retention of infected debris. Conservative management with a fistula has the danger that acute labyrinthitis may develop with a dead labyrinth and even meningitis. A fistula of the labyrinth occurring in chronic perilabyrinthine osteomyelitis also requires surgical intervention." The operation of choice formerly was a radical mastoidectomy, but the tendency today is toward a more conservative operation, particularly if cholesteatoma is absent. An attempt is often made to preserve or improve hearing. Most operators do not advise special measures to close the fistula, nor do they advise disturbance of the membranous covering of the fistula which would entail opening the perilymphatic space.

Prognosis

Both Permin and Nylen in their separate series of cases reported that the fistula reaction persisted in one-third of the patients following radical mastoidectomy. Fifty per cent in Permin's series had no serviceable hearing after operation; his series included cases with impaired hearing prior to operation. Permin reported that the fistula reaction disappeared or persisted, independently of whether suppuration continued, in his series of 108 cases. It has been reported that a fistula may close even with conservative treatment.

In the preantibiotic era, Lund reported that among 112 patients with circumscribed labyrinthitis or fistula, 4 developed intracranial infection and 13 more developed extinction of function. Two of this group died. All 112 patients underwent radical mastoidectomy.

Perilabyrinthitis

This condition has been described extensively by Cawthorne. The typical patient has had one or more mastoid operations resulting in a clean ear without active infection, but the patient continues to complain of severe disturbances of equilibrium and some vertigo on walking. A loud sound may cause vertigo (the Tullio phenomenon) in which a fistula of the labyrinth allows unaccustomed movement in the labyrinth because of the mobile stapes. In Cawthorne's series, very often the patients had active responses to the fistula test, and all responded to caloric stimulation. Some hearing was always present, but their gaits were bizarre. Cawthorne postulated that irregular and unaccustomed fluctuations of vestibular activity might be the cause of this disturbance. Destruction of the offending end-organ was required, and a course of balancing exercises played an important part in restoring balance. In this regard, Proud states: "When any patient with chronic otitis media complains of vertigo for more than 3 months, one is wise, regardless of audiologic findings, to do labyrinthectomy at the time of surgery, be it radical mastoidectomy or tympanoplasty, for vertigo will persist and second stage labyrinthectomy will be necessary otherwise."

DIFFUSE SUPPURATIVE LABYRINTHITIS

In suppurative labyrinthitis, pus is found in all parts of the labyrinth without any effective localization. The same etiology and pathways of invasion apply to diffuse suppurative labyrinthitis as to serous. Rupture of the pus into the labyrinth takes place most frequently through the fenestra vestibulae, less often through the fenestra cochleae, or through a fistula in the horizontal semicircular canal. An exception is the rare involvement of the labyrinth secondary to generalized meningitis, in which purulent labyrinthitis usually occurs without a prodromal period of serous labyrinthitis. It may occur with generalized purulent meningitis via the internal auditory meatus and less often via the cochlear aqueduct or the endolymphatic sac and duct. The usual sequence is the rupture of pus into the labyrinth during an acute exacerbation of chronic middle ear suppuration. Another initiating factor may be an intratympanic operative measure with inadvertent opening of the labyrinth in the presence of suppuration.

Diffuse suppurative labyrinthitis complicating acute suppurative otitis media was attended by a high mortality, but it is rarely seen since the advent of antibiotics.

Symptoms

During an acute exacerbation of a chronic middle ear suppuration, violent symptoms suddenly arise. The symptoms are vertigo, spontaneous nystagmus, disturbances of equilibrium, and vomiting. The characteristic onset of purulent labyrinthitis is abrupt and violent. The onset of severe vestibular symptoms is accompanied by a complete loss of cochlear response. Nystagmus is usually spontaneous of first degree toward the healthy side. The caloric reaction is absent from the diseased ear. Lund, in an extensive series, emphasized that labyrinthine suppuration alone does not cause an elevation of temperature. Headache, pain, malaise, or fever do not occur from a labyrinth filled with pus without some other complication. The total pus contained in the labyrinth is small in quantity and the opportunity for systemic absorption of toxic products is extremely limited from the bony walls of the intact labyrinthine capsule. The development of deafness helps to diagnose a suppurative process. In the uncommon case with gradual progression, there may be no more than a slight sense of unsteadiness.

Differential Diagnosis from Cerebellar Abscess

The differential diagnosis between labyrinthine suppuration and cerebellar abscess may be most difficult. Often the latter is caused by the labyrinthine process. Spontaneous nystagmus occurs when the patient looks toward the healthy side in labyrinthine suppuration and toward both sides in cerebellar abscess, but actually one sees oculomotor asthenia rather than true nystagmus with a cerebellar abscess. In Proud's experience, the patient falls toward the side of the diseased labyrinth in both conditions, and Proud has not found this to be a localizing sign for a cerebellar abscess. Choked disc is present with cerebellar abscess. Other cerebellar signs would help establish the diagnosis of cerebellar abscess. Nystagmus and disturbances in equilibrium arising during the early stages of meningitis may indicate that inflammation of the meninges has taken place from the labyrinth.

Prognosis

After subsidence of acute vestibular symptoms, there is no recovery of cochlear or vestibular responses in the diseased ear. Three to 5 weeks are required for compensation and recovery from vertigo and nystagmus. However, residual ataxia may persist forever. Compensation occurs more rapidly in the young than in the aged.

Shambaugh wrote:

> Today with careful observation of the patient to detect the earliest evidence of meningeal invasion permitting prompt drainage of the labyrinth, combined with antibacterial medication, the relatively high mortality rate of suppurative labyrinthitis should be a thing of the past, and with few exceptions, the patient should recover to good health. The labyrinthine function cannot be recovered. In a dead labyrinth, the labyrinth may continue to harbor viable microorganisms. Unfortunately, there are no symptoms or tests to differentiate a dangerous latent labyrinthitis from a harmless healed labyrinth following suppurative labyrinthitis. If the patient does not die of a cerebellar abscess or meningitis due to intracranial extension, healing eventually occurs by fibrosis followed by an obliterative osteitis. In untreated suppurative labyrinthitis, pus may remain trapped in the bony labyrinth for a week to months before it finally makes its way intracranially or is replaced by fibrous tissue. Such a latent labyrinthitis may exist with no symptoms to betray its presence until the patient suddenly develops meningitis.

Lund reported in the preantibiotic era that with acute diffuse destructive labyrinthitis, all but 43 out of 130 patients developed meningeal infection. According to Lund, meningeal irritation was evidenced by more than two cells per cubic millimeter in the spinal fluid. With acute traumatic labyrinthitis following an operation on the ear, meningeal invasion almost always occurred. The signs indicating spread of labyrinthitis were an increased number of cells in the spinal fluid or facial paralysis. Suppurative labyrinthitis may extend to basilar meningitis through the internal auditory canal. In the chronic form, there is only a slight tendency toward spontaneous recovery through the formation of connective tissue, and before the antibiotic era cerebral complications and death were frequent. The prognosis is more unfavorable in suppurative labyrinthitis of tuberculous origin.

Treatment

In 1959, Shambaugh wrote:

> The most important treatment of suppurative labyrinthitis is to keep the patient in bed and to keep close observation for signs of beginning intracranial extension. Antibacterial medications should be given to prevent extension. The symptoms and signs to watch for hourly are: headache, usually occipital; stiffness of the neck, even very slight; Kernig's sign (rarely present without stiffness of the neck); elevation of temperature above normal, even though slight; and facial paralysis. At the first appearance of any of these symptoms, a spinal fluid examination should be made. If there are increased cells, spread of the infection intra-

cranially is certain; then the labyrinth should be drained surgically. With the help of antibacterial medication, drainage of the labyrinth should arrest further advancement of infection to the meninges or cerebellum.

There has recently been some tendency to be more conservative, and some operators merely rely on a radical mastoidectomy with extensive chemotherapy. However, it may still be maintained that labyrinthectomy is advisable when either manifest meningitis or diabetes complicate a suppurative labyrinthitis; drainage of the labyrinth by labyrinthectomy is an additional safeguard to avoid intracranial spread of the infection. The rare form of suppurative labyrinthitis secondary to meningitis does not require drainage of the labyrinth.

Shambaugh described the technique of labyrinth drainage as follows:

After preliminary radical mastoidectomy, the horizontal semicircular canal is fenestrated far forward toward the ampulla. The vestibule is entered from above. The cochlea and vestibule are then opened from below the facial nerve by extracting the stapes and burring away the promontory until the oval and round windows are connected. A small hook may then be passed into the vestibule under the bony ridge of the facial canal from above and below.

Sequestration of a part or all the bony labyrinth may occur in extensive perilabyrinthine osteitis usually associated with a dead labyrinth. The presence of a sequestrum of the bony labyrinth may be suspected when a patient following a suppurative labyrinthitis develops a facial paralysis. In most cases, sequestration of the labyrinth is an unexpected finding in the course of a radical mastoidectomy in a patient with a dead labyrinth and chronic otorhea. The treatment of a sequestrated labyrinth is simply to lift out the loose bone from the bed of granulations in which it lies, with great care not to injure the facial nerve. If necessary, the sequestrum should be broken in several pieces to permit this removal without facial nerve injury. Remnants of the labyrinthine capsule not loose or without obvious osteitis should not be disturbed.

REFERENCES

1. Cawthorne, T.: Perilabyrinthitis Laryngoscope 67:1237, 1957.
2. Lederer, F. L.: Diseases of the Ear, Nose and Throat. Philadelphia, F. A. Davis Co., 1943, pp. 232-242.
3. Leegaard, T., and Rohrt, T.: Artificial covering of a labyrinthine fistula. Acta Otolaryng. 50:42-46, 1959.
4. Lund, R.: Indications for the labyrinth operation. J. Laryng. 51:425-452, 1936.
5. Nylen, C. O.: Labyrinthitis. Acta Otolaryng. 31:223, 1943.
6. Permin, P.: Fistular labyrinthitis. Acta Otolaryng. 45:416-424, 1955.
7. Politzer, A.: Diseases of the Ear. London, Bailliere, Lindall & Cox, 1909, pp. 604-622.
8. Proud, G.: Personal communication.
9. Shambaugh, G. E., Jr.: Surgery of the Ear. Philadelphia, W. B. Saunders Co., 1959.
10. Williams, H.: The dizzy patient. Trans. Penn. Acad. Opthal. (May), 1962.
11. Zwergius, E.: The mechanism of labyrinthine fistular reactions. Acta Otolaryng. 46:74-79, 1956.

CHAPTER 8

Stapedectomy and Otosclerosis in Relation to Vertigo

MARTIN SPECTOR

VERTIGO AFTER STAPEDECTOMY

Usual Course

Routine observation has indicated that most patients exhibited spontaneous nystagmus immediately after stapedectomy. The duration varies from hours to a day; the intensity, from first degree to third degree. The fast component of the nystagmus is sometimes directed to the side of the operation, sometimes to the opposite side, and often is a gaze nystagmus to either side. The intensity and duration of this spontaneous nystagmus seems proportional to the trauma to the vestibule sustained at operation. Many patients will have no vertigo whatsoever until they are moved off the table and then nausea and even vomiting may ensue. By the following day, most patients will have no vertigo, except on head movement, and no nystagmus or nausea. The great majority of patients will require no palliative medication past the second day. Within 2 weeks after operation, the great majority will have returned to their usual occupations.

Shambaugh reported that following the classical semicircular canal fenestration operation, vertigo was a constant sequel. Severe vertigo rarely lasted more than a few days but noticeable vertigo of varying degree sometimes lasted for a longer period of time. Good hearing results were reported even after severe and prolonged postoperative vertigo.

Excessive Postoperative Vertigo

Vertigo and nystagmus past the second postoperative day may be considered an undue reaction, although not a cause for alarm. Rarely, vomiting may be so severe as to require intravenous fluids. Vertigo and ataxia may persist for several weeks following stapedectomy and occasionally the disability is permanent. This problem may be merely an annoyance but uncommonly it can be incapacitating. This labyrinthosis may take the form of persistent labyrinthine symptoms such as loss of balance, episodic vertigo, or rotatory vertigo as seen in a typical Meniere's syndrome. In most cases, the vertigo is similar to the benign paroxysmal positional vertigo with nystagmus. This incidence of prolonged vestibular disturbance lasting for many weeks probably runs about 2 to 5 per cent. A vestibular disturbance is more commonly immediate in onset but may be delayed for many months after operation. Although vertigo and sensorineural hearing loss may be concomitant, this is not necessarily so. It is not uncommon for vestibular disturbance to be found with an excellent hearing result, just as a profound hearing loss may occur in the absence of any vestibular disturbance whatsoever. On the whole, a severe prolonged vestibular disturbance arouses a fear that the ultimate hearing result will not be ideal. In those with an associated hearing loss, tinnitus, depression of bone conduction, and loudness recruitment are generally present. Persistent vertigo may be accompanied by a depressed discrimination score in the presence of improved air and bone conduction.

Pathology

Four types of inner ear vestibular reaction to stapes surgery were listed by Hohman from his animal experiments. A fifth type, acoustic trauma, is not important in our discussion of vertigo and is omitted here. The four are (1) endolymphatic hydrops, (2) hypotonic atrophy, (3) serofibrinous labyrinthitis, and (4) suppurative labyrinthitis.

Hohman performed stapes surgery on 64 cats. Surgical procedures were purposely performed to provoke labyrinthine reactions by making fistulas into the footplate, implanting metal prostheses into the vestibule, and instillation of blood or cerebrospinal fluid into the vestibule. Among the total, 29 per cent developed hydrops, 14 per cent developed hypotonic atrophy, 12 per cent developed serofibrinous labyrinthitis, and 3 per cent developed suppurative labyrinthitis. More than one type of reaction occurred in some ears.

Endolymphatic Hydrops

Hydrops was the earliest and most common form of labyrinthine reaction to stapes surgery. It occurred after 17 per cent of footplate fractures, after 26 per cent of stapedectomies, and after 45 per cent of stapedectomies when blood or cerebrospinal fluid was instilled into the vestibule. It must be pointed out that this hydrops was found early and was transient in most cases.

Hypotonic Atrophy

Hypotonic atrophy was the second most common abnormal labyrinthine response. This appeared to be the result of biochemical alterations in perilymph and endolymph with disturbance of the fluid pressure balance. The histopathological changes were directly opposite to those of hydrops. All structures of the scala media were shrunken; in severe stages, they appeared compressed. There appeared to be a decreased volume of endolymph. The atrophy involved the saccule severely and the cristae and utricle less severely. It most often occurred when cerebrospinal fluid was inserted into the perilymph.

Shambaugh and Takahara studied monkey ears after classical fenestration of the lateral semicircular canal, and they found that 86 per cent in the first 14 days had some evidence of serous labyrinthitis. In most, there was a bulging of Reissner's membrane indicating hydrops. Where labyrinthitis was severe, there was some atrophy.

Serofibrinous Labyrinthitis

It was demonstrated 40 years ago by Zange and Steurer that opening or traumatizing the labyrinth of animals without grafting frequently resulted in degeneration of the membranous labyrinth because of invasion of proliferating connective tissue. Serofibrinous labyrinthitis occurred in 12 per cent of Hohman's animals and was accompanied by endolymphatic hydrops. The earliest inflammatory reaction was a serofibrinous exudate which was replaced by connective tissue. Serofibrinous labyrinthitis always resulted in severe degeneration of the membranous labyrinth. The cause of this lesion was most likely an inflammatory granulomatous response to trauma with exudation and exuberant repair. The fibrous tissue proliferation is an end result of the unhealed serofibrinous type of labyrinthitis. The latter is readily produced in animals by trauma or by creating a perilymphatic fistula in the oval or round window. This reaction can usually be avoided in human beings and animals by covering surgical fistulas in the otic capsule with viable soft tissue grafts and by refraining from excessive surgical trauma. Occasionally, however, a granulomatous reaction can occur with a graft, which is characterized by connective tissue proliferation with destruction of the graft and invasion of the inner ear.

Growth of a granulomatous mass from a covering membrane is thought to be due to inflammation or infection of the middle ear.

Suppurative Labyrinthitis

In the presence of an oval window fistula, subsequent middle ear suppuration may lead to suppurative labyrinthitis. Hohman reported that in 2 of his 64 cats, fistulas persisted for 2 and 6 months, respectively, before the onset of massive suppurative labyrinthitis. Of course, suppurative labyrinthitis could result from surgery performed in the presence of middle ear infection.

Fistulas of the Footplate

Failure of growth of a membrane to completely cover the fossa ovalis may be listed under pathology.

Preoperative Portents

Certain symptoms preoperatively may foretell the development of vestibular disturbances. These symptoms, according to Shambaugh, include preoperative vertigo, fullness in the ear, and roaring tinnitus. Henry Williams stated that endolymphatic hydrops will develop later in a portion of patients who have vertigo from minor irritations of the end-organ. Such an ear seems much more susceptible to injury from ordinary operative trauma than does an ear with footplate otosclerosis alone. Otosclerosis, which involves other portions of the labyrinth as well as the footplate, seems to render the labyrinth easily hurt by ordinary operative trauma. The labyrinthine otosclerosis and the attending increased fragility may be revealed by preoperative sensorineural hearing loss.

Great care should be exerted in a revision operation if there is a history of vertigo at the first operation. There may be an advantage in waiting a year or more for such a revision to allow complete healing after the first operation. This is particularly true where exposure of the perilymph is contemplated in the second operation.

Clinical Causes for Immediate Vertigo

Damage or Rupture of the Saccule or Utricle

Removal of a Floating Footplate. The footplate should not be removed as a whole. The suction and compression effect of removing the intact footplate, or the injury inflicted by the edge of the footplate rotating into the vestibule, may be disastrous. If the whole footplate becomes mobile, a pothole is created posteriorly and inferiorly through which is inserted a 0.3 mm. hook for cautious removal. This maneuver is not without danger. It is advisable always to break the footplate in half or into smaller portions with straight picks or a bur before removal of the fragments.

Direct Injury with Instruments. According to Anson and Bast, the distance separating the footplate from the saccule, utricle, and scala media varies from 0.57 to 2.0 mm. The saccule lies anteriorly. The macula utriculi is white and shiny and usually lies beneath the facial ridge. Luckily, the membranous labyrinth seems to have some resistance to contact just as a balloon will bounce away from a moderate blow. It is a good dictum to desist from any motion which induces vertigo. The portions of the footplate should be removed atraumatically with 0.3 to 0.5 mm. hooks, using slow, careful motions and inserting the hook just under the fragment and not into the depths of the vestibule. Binocular vision must be maintained at all times and the field should be cleared by discrete suction at a distance from the open oval window. Surgical trauma produces immediate vertigo and often nausea and vomiting while the patient is still on the operating table. Direct injury to the utricle or compression rupture of the utricle or saccule is a probable injury inflicted.

It has been stated that, rarely, the saccule may be attached to the underside of the footplate, but this statement requires further corroboration.

Drilling or Burring. Schuknecht reported that extensive drilling was a very common factor in his cases of severe sensorineural hearing loss—that is, in 11 of 20 cases. Thus, among cases with obliterative otosclerosis, there is a distinctly higher incidence of vertigo than in cases with a blue footplate. To reduce drilling in cases with a distinct annulus, a bony footplate merely need be burred into two pieces and each half removed by a relatively strong hook, such as a Hough Hoe. Many operators feel it is less traumatic to pick away at the footplate, and they have completely dispensed with drilling. A danger with the use of picks alone is that a floating footplate may result from the pressure required. In the use of the bur, the footplate should be thinned until blue and the final cracking of the footplate should be performed by picks. The revolving bur in the perilymph may create a whirlpool of the perilymph, and this can readily damage the membranous labyrinth.

Piece of Free or Depressed Footplate Pressing on Utricle. Damage to the utricle may also result from partial or total dislocation of the footplate into the vestibule as exemplified by the following case:

J. K., male, aged 49, underwent a right stapedectomy, Shea type, on November 6, 1959, for otosclerosis. A vein graft was inserted and a 4 mm. polyethylene strut was used. At operation, the footplate broke around the periphery, and almost the entire footplate bobbed around in the vestibule like a cork. Cautious attempts at removal failed. From the experience of others, I had learned that the trauma of removing such a piece could ruin cochlear function, so the piece was permitted to remain and was covered with a vein graft. On November 16, positional tests for nystagmus and vertigo elicited no reaction in the left supine position, but in the supine position with head hanging there was a rotatory nystagmus to the right and there was vertigo. In the supine position with head turned to the right, there was a violent rotatory nystagmus to the right plus vertigo. When the patient sat up after each of these positions, there was nystagmus to the right. Follow-up examination on December 12, 1959, March 19, 1960, and May 21, 1960, revealed rotatory nystagmus to the right with pronounced vertigo in both the supine position and in the right lateral position. At reexamination on September 23, 1960, the patient reported that the dizziness had disappeared about July. No positional nystagmus and vertigo could be elicited. He was able to work on ladders and at heights. He added that he had sustained a concussion on September 1, 1960, but this had in no way affected his ear. Incidentally, he had achieved and maintained an excellent hearing result, with speech reception threshold at the 5 decibel line and a discrimination of 96 per cent.

Bleeding. Excessive bleeding has been mentioned as a cause of disturbance, but the bleeding may only be important as it obscures vision and permits instrumental trauma. Blood has been instilled into the vestibule in cats and did not cause degenerative changes or fibrosis in the inner ear (Bellucci). Anyway, good hemastasis should be secured before the footplate is opened. Clinically, the types of trauma that caused most harm were pressure into the vestibule and excessive suction. Blood in the vestibule and careful burring over the footplate did not instigate vertigo as much as did mechanical manipulation, in the author's experience.

Excessively Long Prosthesis. Pressure from an excessively long prosthesis is a prominent cause for persistent vertigo. The distance from the incus to the footplate should be measured routinely to ascertain the exact length of prosthesis required. In the following case, vertigo was due to an extralong prosthesis:

A. U., female, aged 53, had a unilateral otosclerosis. On February 15, 1960, a fenestration of the left oval window was performed, with removal of the sclerotic footplate. Here, a vein graft was not used but gelfoam was placed and a 5 mm. strut was fitted onto the lenticular process of the incus. In fitting it onto the incus, the strut was pushed rather deeply into the vestibule. This maneuver precipitated vertigo and vomiting on the table. The patient developed third degree nystagmus to the other side. However, she progressed to a speech reception threshold of between 5 and 10 and a discrimination test of 94 per cent. Tests for positional nystagmus and vertigo on March 16 and again on April 13, 1960, disclosed a rotatory nystagmus to the right in the supine position but nothing in the side positions. On April 13, the supine position caused a left rotatory nystagmus and vertigo, but the side positions elicited no response. There was no spontaneous nystagmus. Positional vertigo continued for 2 years; therefore, in October 1962 the long strut was replaced by a 3.75 mm. polyethylene strut. This relieved her complaints.

Fistula through the Oval Window

After a stapedectomy with removal of mucosa, it is normally expected that the endosteum and mucosa will regrow and cover the oval window within 2 days. Scheer pointed out that fistulas were most likely to occur in the shallow, very broad oval window niche with very thin mucosa. Another possible factor hindering regrowth of mucosa is old age.

Proud, Lewis, and others emphasized the importance of a well-seated oval window cork, be it absorbable cellulose or tissue. Some operators state, however, that the usual blood clot is sufficient cover for the opened oval window.

Fistulas in the footplate can produce immediate or delayed symptoms. The patient with a through-and-through fistula of the footplate may have continuous imbalance, roaring tinnitus, and fluctuating hearing. This is more likely to result when there is a tilt of a fragment of the footplate.

Farrior reported submucosal fistula of the oval window. These patients complained of fluctuating hearing with change in position, fluctuating dizziness, and fluctuating tinnitus. The polyethylene strut gradually had worked its way into the inner ear so that the perilabyrinthine fluid escaped submucosally up the polyethylene tube. Farrior stated, "It is my present belief that some of the immediate postoperative vertigo and fluctuation of hearing is the result of the escape of perilabyrinthine fluid." (Fistulas are further discussed in the section "Delayed Vertigo.")

Infection

Infection has been incriminated as a factor but clinically, gross infection is surprisingly rare. Most cases of gross infection may be traced to operation in the presence of an incompletely healed external otitis. In this regard, a hearing aid mold should not be worn in the operated ear for at least 3 weeks prior to operation.

Serous Labyrinthitis

Serous labyrinthitis may begin on the day of operation or it may be delayed for 2 weeks. It is manifested by a constant roaring tinnitus, postural vertigo, ataxia, nausea, and vomiting. Most patients recover over a period of weeks and are left with good hearing. Some sustain a permanent sensorineural loss of hearing at the 4000 cycles frequency. Recurrent vertigo may be similar to the clinical picture of endolymphatic hydrops. A similar picture can be produced by a fistula in the footplate.

Delayed Vertigo

Serofibrinous Labyrinthitis with a Fibromatous Mass

One cause for vertigo delayed for some weeks is the development of a fibromatous mass into the vestibule. This is an end result of unhealed serous labyrinthitis. Invasion of the vestibule by a fibromatous mass can occur with the vein graft, gelfoam, and even with partial removal of the stapes footplate. The earliest warning sign of a fibromatous mass is persistent vertigo and deafness. The vertigo may begin immediately or 3 to 4 weeks after surgery. The vertigo is persistent rather than paroxysmal and is aggravated by positional changes. Later, these symptoms involve a sensation of falling or unsteadiness. A marked depression of air and bone conduction accompanies the vertigo; there is also poor speech discrimination as well as loudness recruitment. In contrast to a patient suffering from serous labyrinthitis alone, these patients do not improve spontaneously; they steadily worsen. At surgery, a large white fibrous mass occupying the oval window niche is found. The fibromatous mass which invades the vestibule is rarely adherent to the membranous labyrinth. Adhesions would be manifested by vertigo upon removal of the fibromatous mass. It was advised by Pratt that the fibromatous mass be removed.

Falling of a Prosthesis from the Incus

Perforation of a strut through the oval window cover is usually precipitated by lifting a heavy object, violent sneezing, airplane rides, descent in an elevator, diving, mountain travel, necrosis of the incus, or some other factor which causes an abrupt air pressure change in the middle ear.

Lewis pictured an onset, after months or years, with violent vertigo, nausea, loss of hearing, and roaring tinnitus. He considered this an emergency. He ascribed it to a violent inward movement of the incus caused by barometric change in the middle ear and leading to rupture of the membrane covering the oval window. On surgical exploration, one could readily demonstrate the strut lodged deep within the vestibule. Perforation of a strut into the vestibule can cause an irreversible loss of cochlear function very suddenly and may take place years afterwards. Immediate surgery for removal of the perforating strut should be performed for this type of complication in order to relieve the vestibular symptoms and minimize the cochlear impairment.

The use of the polyethylene strut has been largely abandoned on account of this possibility. Where the polyethylene strut has been dislodged violently, it may penetrate the footplate cover and cause direct injury to the membranous labyrinth. In other cases, the mere weight of the polyethylene strut on a thin membrane was sufficient to cause intermittent dizziness.

Viral Labyrinthitis

Viral labyrinthitis may also be a cause of delayed vertigo. Usually an upper respiratory infection occurs about the time of the onset. Air and bone conduction thresholds are depressed, but if the discrimination score remains normal, within a few days as the infection subsides, the vertigo gradually diminishes and the hearing recovers.

Fistula through the Oval Window

Schuknecht reported that fistulas of the footplate can persist for long periods of time without serious morphological or functional alterations. Fistulas into the labyrinth are potentially dangerous in that they provide a direct route for infection from the middle ear to the meninges.

Rutledge and Lewis reported a case in which the footplate had been fragmented and a polyethylene prosthesis inserted. Six months later, while the patient was traveling in the mountains, several brief attacks of vertigo occurred. Audiometry and tests for fistula response were normal then. Two years later, after an acute upper respiratory infection, pain in the ear began with fever, headache, and ataxia. A myringotomy was performed, but meningitis, coma, and death ensued. Pneumococci were cultured from the middle ear. At postmorten examination, the strut actually penetrated the footplate and there was a labyrinthine fistula, probably created by infection. These authors advise sealing the oval window at the initial operation, surgical reexploration of any patient with evidence of labyrinthine fistula, and prompt vigorous therapy of middle ear infections which occur at any time after a stapes operation.

Late Endolymphatic Hydrops

Shambaugh reported that 10 per cent of patients after classical fenestration of the lateral semicircular canal, months or years later, developed endolymphatic hydrops which was mostly transitory.

Destruction of Labyrinthine Response

Groves reported that after a stapedectomy with an excellent hearing result, there was a complete absence of caloric response on that side. The patient had had vertigo for 1 week postoperatively with vomiting. The other ear did have a good caloric response.

Treatment

The average patient after stapedectomy will require no antivertiginous medication on the day following surgery. It does seem preferable to enforce complete bed rest for 24 hours following surgery, and the patient should be cautioned against rapid head movements and strong blowing of the nose with the nostrils closed. Elevation of the head of the bed is believed helpful. Occasional cases will have such severe vertigo as to require antivertiginous medications and even require intravenous fluids.

Myers reported that in about 10 per cent of patients with severe vertigo after stapedectomy, a spontaneous remission took place leaving the auditory acuity at a practical level. Myers believed that a patient with a labyrinthine complication should be treated conservatively for a period of time in order to allow the inner ear an opportunity to recover. Poor results were usually obtained when attempting to revise operations in patients who developed postoperative labyrinthosis. In most cases, the attempt at revision often left a further irreparable damage to the inner ear. Should revision be attempted and no abnormality encountered, the graft and prosthesis should be left undisturbed. In those cases in which the discrimination score remained good in spite of a loss of hearing, conservative treatment should be tried. The inner ear does have a capacity to recover if left undisturbed in these cases. However, in those cases in which a mechanical lesion is suspected, such as fistula or falling off of the prosthesis, surgical intervention is indicated.

REFERENCES

1. Ali, S. Y., and Groves, J.: Vestibular disorders after stapedectomy. Lancet 2:995, 1962.
2. Anson, B. J., and Bast, T. H.: The surgical significance of stapedial and labyrinthine anatomy. Arch. Otolaryng. 71:188-206, 1960.
3. Bellucci, R. J., and Wolff, O.: Tissue reactions following reconstruction of the oval window in experimental animals. Ann. Otol. 69:517, 1960.
4. Bergstrom, J., and Ivstam, B.: Vestibular disturbances after stapediolysis. Acta Otolaryng. (Suppl.) 158:328-334.
5. Harris, I., and Weiss, L.: Granulomatous complications of oval window fat grafts. Laryngoscope 72:870, 1962.
6. Hohmann, A.: Inner Ear Reactions to Stapes Surgery (Animal Experiments). Henry Ford Hosp. Int. Symposium on Otosclerosis. Boston, Little, Brown & Co., 1962, 305-319.
7. House, H.: Stapes surgery—complications. Arch. Otolaryng. 78:607-610, 1963.
8. Lewis, M. L.: Inner ear complications of stapes surgery. Laryngoscope 71:377-384, 1961.
9. Myers, D., et al.: Stapedectomy failure. Arch. Otolaryng. 76:533-541, 1962.
10. Pratt, L., and Winchester, R.: Polyp of the vestibule. Arch Otolaryng. 75:99-102, 1962.
11. Proud, G.: Personal communication.
12. Rutledge, L. J., Lewis, M. L., and Sanabria, F.: Fatal meningitis related to stapes operation. Arch Otolaryng. 78:637-641, 1963.
13. Schuknecht, H. F.: Sensorineural hearing loss following stapedectomy. Acta Otolaryng. 54:336-348, 1962.
14. Shambaugh, G. E., and Takahara, S.: A clinical and experimental study of the effect of fenestration on the labyrinthine contents. Acta Otolaryng. Suppl. 123, 1955.
15. Williams, H.: The dizzy patient. Trans. Penn. Acad. Ophthal. (May), 1962.
16. Zange and Steurer, quoted by Hohmann: See ref. 6.

OTOSCLEROSIS IN RELATION TO VERTIGO

The question arises of how often dizziness is found with otosclerosis. Rasmussen reported that among 67 patients, 18 (27 per cent) had vertigo prior to operation. He quoted that this figure accorded with Nager's findings. In 6 patients prior to operation, Rasmussen found that postrotatory nystagmus was shortened. In 5 patients, a caloric test was considered abnormal before operation. Felisati reported that he found vestibular disturbance in 30 per cent of his patients, more frequently in women than in men. Stenger reported 5 cases of loss of vestibular function after stapes-plasty even though satisfactory improvement in hearing was achieved. This emphasizes that preoperatively on stapedectomy cases, it would be wise to do a caloric test to make sure that the vestibular function in the unoperated ear is normal. Otherwise, ataxia might inadvertently result in such a case.

Shambaugh advised that the symptoms of vertigo, fullness, or roaring tinnitus preoperatively may indicate a bad prognosis for stapedectomy. In the "Corresponding Letters in Otolaryngology," a case was presented of otosclerosis, with symptoms indicating associated endolymphatic hydrops. The question was asked whether it was wise to do a stapes operation on the ear with hydrops. Some correspondents reported good results with such cases but there was equal division between those against any operation and those for a cautious operation. A "cautious operation" implied minimal opening of the labyrinth. The labyrinth in such a case was considered overly sensitive to surgical manipulation by those advising against any operation.

REFERENCES

1. Corresponding Letters in Otolaryngology 7:142, 1964.
2. Felisati, D.: Subjective vestibular symptomatology in otosclerotic deafness before and after fenestration. Arch. Ital. Otol. 69:26-51, 1958.
3. Rasmussen, H.: Vestibular function prior to and following operation for otosclerosis. Arch. Otolaryng. 49:402-412, 1949.
4. Stenger, H. H.: Isolated loss of vestibular function after stapes plasty. Arch. Ohr. Nas. Kehlkopfheilk. 179:400-408, 1962.

CHAPTER 9

Positional Vertigo and Nystagmus

MARTIN SPECTOR

PERIPHERAL POSITIONAL NYSTAGMUS

Pathology

Experiments in animals by Fernandez and his colleagues have demonstrated that simple cutting of the nerve to one superior semicircular canal, to a horizontal canal, or to the utricle will be followed by positional nystagmus. Electrical stimulation of the utricular nerve never seems to cause nystagmus. Miehlke was able to provoke positional nystagmus in rabbits by inserting a droplet of blood into the perilymphatic space at the upper part of the labyrinth. A fistula in the horizontal semicircular canal may result in positional nystagmus. Positional nystagmus never occurs in seasickness. It has been reported that damage to the utricular macula or atheroma of the utricular artery may cause positional nystagmus. Schuknecht ascribed the condition to occlusion of the anterior vestibular artery.

Lindsay has postulated that positional nystagmus and vertigo results from sudden partial loss of function. A gradual onset of a peripheral lesion was not likely to produce positional nystagmus. After labyrinthectomy, postural nystagmus is never found. Functioning vestibular receptors seem to be necessary for the appearance of positional nystagmus. Harbert reports that positional nystagmus in the first degree position is rotary and that in the third degree position (or direction of the slow component) it is vertical. He ascribes this to the posterior semicircular canal which stimulates the internal rectus eye muscle and the superior oblique eye muscle.

Etiology

Infections of the Ear

Positional vertigo has been reported in association with serous otitis media but it must be rare in this condition. Even in acute suppurative otitis media, positional vertigo is quite uncommon. The incidence is higher in chronic infection of the middle ear and mastoid. In a patient with chronic mastoid infection and/or cholesteatoma complaining of vertigo, positional tests are more often positive than the fistula test. The nystagmus and vertigo is elicited with the affected ear undermost, and it is of the fatigable paroxysmal type.

Trauma

Operations on the Ear. Bergstrom and Ivstam reported that after stapediolysis, positional nystagmus could be elicited in two-thirds of a series of cases by electronystagmography. The positional nystagmus did not begin immediately after operation but took some hours to a day to develop. This delay was ascribed to the development of edema. Practically all these cases cleared within a week. Spector reported 3 cases of prolonged positional vertigo after stapedectomy. In 2 cases, a large piece of the footplate was lost into the vestibule. In a third case, too long a strut was placed. The positional vertigo after stapedectomy was ascribed to trauma to the vestibule, and the types of trauma that seemed to lead to most harm included pressure in the vestibule, suction, foreign material, burring, and a fistula in the membrane over the oval window. Tears into the utricle or saccule are a factor. Positional vertigo was produced during a radical mastoidectomy where the stapes was avulsed even though a graft was immediately laid over the oval window. The positional vertigo lasted 3 months in this case.

Ultrasound Operation. In some cases where ultrasound is applied to the semicircular canals, positional vertigo is produced. This positional nystagmus is of the peripheral type. It occurs with the involved ear undermost. This usually occurs when insufficient ultrasound has been applied. With the application of more ultrasound, or a complete mechanical labyrinthectomy, this reaction disappears. Arslan states that the positional vertigo disappears without treatment after the passage of several months.

Electric shock treatment has caused prolonged positional vertigo.

Head injury will be discussed on page 152.

Altman stated that thrombosis of the internal auditory artery does not induce postural vertigo. Occlusion of the anterior vestibular artery initiates sudden vertigo, which later becomes postural and persists for several months. The caloric response may be depressed or normal. There may be tinnitus.

Probable Vascular Pathology

Lindsay and Hemenway described a symptom complex manifested by a severe attack of vertigo which gradually subsided over a period of several weeks, following which the patients developed positional vertigo of the benign paroxysmal type. This persisted for weeks or years. All were in the fifth, sixth, or seventh decades of life at the time of onset. There was impaired response to the caloric stimulation in the ear positioned undermost during the attack of positional vertigo. Some patients also had tinnitus and hearing loss in the same ear. In one case with studies at autopsy, enlarged vessels were found exerting pressure on Scarpa's ganglion.

Mumps labyrinthitis may cause a prolonged postural vertigo (Altman).

Sudden deafness may be accompanied by postural vertigo.

Benign Paroxysmal Type

In 30 to 50 per cent of all cases seen with positional vertigo, there are no other signs of labyrinthine disease and no definite etiology can be found. The caloric tests, rotatory tests, neurologic examination, and audiologic studies are all normal and there is no spontaneous nystagmus. This group has been labeled the "benign paroxysmal" type.

Some authors have proposed that the condition may be due to coincidental hypertension, arteriosclerosis, drug ingestion, infections, or the hypotensive state. The hypotensive state is described as low blood pressure with frequent headaches and gastrointestinal upsets. The coincidental infections incriminated have included general infections such as tuberculosis or syphilis, and sinusitis or tonsillitis. Vascular occlusion is described as one cause. Minor evidence of aural disease, such as scars or distortions of the tympanic membrane, is considered significant by some authors. The age of greatest incidence is between the years 40 and 60. The cause is actually unknown and the treatment is palliative. Our greatest aid to the patient is to assure him that no serious lesion has been found.

Typical Course

The observer may follow the course of the benign peripheral paroxysmal type of positional nystagmus in stapedectomy in which there has been injury in the vestibule. Initially in these cases—that is, within a day or so—the patient complains that every time he lies on the affected or operated ear, he develops vertigo. The observer, when he places the patient in the critical position, will note a very short latency period; that is, the latency period will not be more than 3 seconds and in some instances the attack seems to come on immediately. Vertigo accompanies the nystagmus and this induces the patient to shut his eyes and arise from the critical position. The nystagmus is rotary to the undermost or to the affected ear. The nystagmus and vertigo lasts about 20 to 30 seconds and will disappear even though the patient remains in the critical position. After the patient sits up, there is often a recurrence of vertigo with nystagmus to the same or the opposite side. Fatigability is very slight at this stage; that is, with repetition of the test, the nystagmus and vertigo are almost as great as at the initial test; the nystagmus and vertigo recur with every test. After a matter of days or weeks, as the condition improves, the latent period lengthens to 2 to 10 seconds, the duration of attacks of nystagmus and vertigo decreases, and the intensity decreases. There is more fatigability; that is, on the second and third consecutive tests, there will be no response elicited. Furthermore, as the condition improves, vertigo does not recur with each test, even after a lapse of a long rest. Toward the termination of the condition, the fatigability is quite marked. Only the most active motion elicits response, and even then it does not occur every time. Fatigue or emotional stress will in many patients increase the frequency of onset. Just before the disappearance of the condition, the positional test may produce no nystagmus and the vertigo, if any, is of short duration. Subsequently, the symptoms will disappear completely.

POSITIONAL VERTIGO DUE TO THE NECK

(See Chapter 17, "Lesions of the Neck and Vertigo," by Bernard Sandler.)

CENTRAL

Experimental Pathology

Allen and Fernandez were able to produce postural nystagmus in cats by ablation of the posterior vermis of the cerebellum. The lesion included the pyramis, uvula, and nodulus of the cerebellum. Postural nystagmus appeared mainly in the supine position and consistently was vertical toward the nose. The nystagmus was fatigable. It was a direction-fixed positional nystagmus toward the lower eyelid. In some animals it was transitory and in others it was persistent. Both types lasted about 10 days. The persistent type changed with time into the transitory. It did not occur in bilaterally labyrinthectomized animals. Positional nystagmus following the removal of the nodulus was temporarily eliminated for about 5 hours by cocaine in the labyrinth and it disappeared permanently following bilateral labyrinthectomy. Bilateral labyrinthectomy followed by removal of the nodulus failed to produce postural nystagmus.

Zlotnikoff placed lead shot in the floor of the fourth ventricle and was able to produce positional nystagmus. In other areas of the posterior fossa he could not elicit positional nystagmus. MacClure felt that in many cases the release of the vestibular centers or vestibulo-ocular reflex from cerebellar inhibitions seemed to be efficient for evoking positional nystagmus, permitting hyperexcitability of the vestibular nuclei. Positional nystagmus may occur when the inhibitory effect of the paleocerebellum is lost. Present evidence indicates that irritation of the vestibular nuclei can cause positional nystagmus. It is evident that supratentorial structures have a more remote inhibiting effect through the cerebellar connections. Change of position may cause positional nystagmus by altering the pressure in the brain stem or by altering the vascular supply.

Central Causes

Multiple Sclerosis. Fromm found that when postural tests were included, a nystagmus was demonstrated in 90 per cent of cases of multiple sclerosis, and of these a positional nystagmus was found in two-thirds. The positional nystagmus was mostly direction-changing but many had a direction-constant type. Multiple sclerosis is the most common cause for the central type of positional nystagmus, according to several observers.

Brain Tumors. Nylen found nystagmus of all types in 346 out of 673 brain tumors—

51 per cent. He reported positional nystagmus of all types present in 69 per cent of his series of subtentorial or posterior fossa tumors. Among all brain tumors with nystagmus, 19.4 per cent displayed spontaneous nystagmus; 52.3 per cent had direction-constant and 28.3 per cent had direction-changing positional nystagmus. He found positional nystagmus in 26 per cent of supratentorial brain tumors, especially in the head-hanging position. Vertical nystagmus which appeared with the head hung back over the table indicated a central, especially supratentorial, lesion. Of the 279 cases who had positional nystagmus, 16.1 per cent had it only on the side, 12.3 per cent had it only in a sagittal position, 30.1 per cent had positional nystagmus in the hanging position, and 41.6 per cent had positional nystagmus in several positions. In the subtentorial, the positional nystagmus occurred in the lateral positions in 23.6 per cent, in several positions in 57.6 per cent, and in the head-hanging position in 4.8 per cent. In the supratentorial, 5.3 per cent had it in the lateral position, 18.4 per cent in several positions, and 66.7 per cent in the head-hanging position. There were 95 cases of acoustic neurinoma. Of these cases, nystagmus, both positional and spontaneous, occurred in 94. Nylen found direction-changing in 28 of the 94, direction-fixed in 37 of 94, and purely spontaneous in 29 without aggravation in any position. Nystagmus was not always aggravated by lying on the side of the tumor. In one case, there occurred a persistent nystagmus on lying on the side away from the tumor. There was no case of pure rotatory nystagmus.

Cawthorne reported a series of patients with positional vertigo as the only evidence of a central metastasis from bronchiogenic carcinoma. They had no other symptoms. The positional nystagmus was direction-changing.

Vascular. An important finding is the high incidence of positional nystagmus in vertebral-basilar artery insufficiency. Hugh Barber reported 72 cases (which included 3 cases of posterior-inferior cerebellar artery thrombosis and 5 other vascular lesions involving the brain stem) where positional nystagmus was demonstrated in 19, an incidence of 26.3 per cent. The ratio of fatigable to nonfatigable positional nystagmus in this group was about 3 to 1. The sign, therefore, represents an important diagnostic feature in ischemic episodes affecting the brain stem. After thrombosis of the posterior-inferior cerebellar artery, prolonged postural nystagmus may follow. Direction-changing nystagmus may occur with vascular disease. Positional nystagmus without dizziness has been reported as fairly frequent in the elderly with intracranial diseases. Hemorrhages, emboli, arteriosclerosis, hypertension, and thrombosis have been reported to cause the central type of positional nystagmus.

A common condition often confused with positional vertigo is dizziness upon first sitting up or arising in the morning. We refer specifically to that vertigo or dizziness which is transient and has no associated nystagmus. This is more common in the elderly but it is not rare in the young adult. It is usually ascribed to inability of the cerebral circulation to adapt, and often this condition is temporary.

Trauma. A direction-changing and irregular type of positional nystagmus may be a sign of post-traumatic disorder. This is thought to indicate damage to the vestibular nuclei. Fischer reported that electric shock may cause positional nystagmus. Microhemorrhages have been reported as the pathologic mechanism.

Drugs. Aschan found barbiturates common in the blood of patients with positional nystagmus. Among 68 cases, with no other sign but positional nystagmus, he found barbiturates in 42. The concentration was above 1 mg. per cent. After imbibing alcohol, patients first get positional nystagmus to one side, and several hours later the nystagmus reverses direction. Chronic alcoholism may be related. Positional nystagmus also has been reported from carbon monoxide, Demerol, morphine, antihistamines, and in animals from quinine and salicylates. Evidence indicates that the modus operandi is central.

Other reported central causes of positional nystagmus include arachnoiditis, encephalitis, brain abscess, Brun's syndrome, and platybasia. Nylen reported a case of encephalitis in which positional nystagmus was the only sign. In platybasia, positional nystagmus particularly occurs in the side positions.

Central-type positional nystagmus is thus likely to be due to (1) neoplasm, often secondary deposits involving the vestibulocerebellar connections, (2) vascular lesions, and (3) disseminated sclerosis.

Edwards reported that demyelination is the most common cause of the central-type positional nystagmus and obstruction of the vertebral arteries is the next most common cause. Further studies should include neurologic and medical examination, air studies, and roentgen study of the chest for primary lung cancer.

Positional Nystagmus in Head Injury

A head injury is an important cause of positional vertigo and nystagmus. In various series of head injuries, positional nystagmus was found in 15 per cent to as high as 43 per cent. Electronystagmography was used to ascertain positional nystagmus in the series with the 43 per cent figure. In Harrison's series of 123 cases of positional nystagmus, 18 were due to head injury. Barber reported that among 165 head-injured patients who complained of dizziness, 24.8 per cent had positional nystagmus. The incidence of positional nystagmus among the head-injured dizzy patients was higher than the incidence of positional nystagmus among the general run of dizzy patients, which was 18.8 per cent in Barber's series. Barber also reported that among the cases of positional nystagmus resulting from head injury, a negligible number had nonfatigable type—that is, only 1 or 2 per cent—whereas the fatigable type constituted a great majority of cases.

Cranial fractures other than those of the temporal bone rarely caused positional nystagmus. Barber reported that only 1 case in 22 cases of extratemporal bone fractures had positional nystagmus. However, in longitudinal fractures of the petrous bone the incidence was 45 per cent, and among transverse fractures of the petrous bone the incidence of positional nystagmus was 10 per cent. Thus, longitudinal fractures of the petrous bone give the highest incidence of positional nystagmus. The more severe the head injury, the higher the incidence and the longer the positional vertigo lasts.

Head injury, theoretically, may cause positional nystagmus and vertigo by injury to either the peripheral labyrinth, to the neck, or to the central mechanisms. Evidence has shown that lesions of the cerebellar vermis, injuries of the fourth ventricle, and the cervical cord also may be responsible for positional nystagmus with a head injury. Positional nystagmus may occur in head injury without any hearing loss. Barber reported that of 16 cases of head injury without fracture but with positional nystagmus, only 50 per cent had hearing loss. The caloric responses seem to give no reliable indications as to the site of the lesion.

Such an injury often is the cause of legal action, and in some instances the patient may be suspected of malingering. Positional nystagmus may be the only sign of organic pathologic change. This may be only definite sign to which the physician may testify in the patient's behalf.

TREATMENT

(See also Chapter 17, "Lesions of the Neck and Vertigo," by Bernard Sandler.)

Those cases associated with neck lesions are more amenable to special treatment, and a cervical collar is often useful. Barber described a patient who had arthritis and positional vertigo. Angiography showed that turning of the head blocked off the vertebral artery. After posterior fusion of C1 and C2, the complaints cleared. Removal of a herniated cervical disc has also been associated with disappearance of severe positional vertigo.

In cases of the benign paroxysmal type, the greatest help seems to be the reassurance that no serious pathology has been found. In the vertigo which occurs when the patient arises to the erect position, ephedrin sulfate, 25 mg. 3 times a day, has been advised. Otherwise, medications are of questionable benefit. Those in use include histamine injections, niacin, Belladenal, Bellergal, and Mesantoin. Most observers feel that the antimotion drugs are not helpful. When the vertigo occurs each morning, a hypnotic or sedative each evening may be found helpful. Balancing exercises and graduated exercises to move the head and eyes are reported to benefit the patient. In cases of positional vertigo with vertebral artery occlusion, anticoagulants have been used. If the vertigo is persistent and incapacitating, then surgical intervention may become necessary. Unilateral labyrinthine ablations have been performed on the ear located undermost in the provocative position, following which positional vertigo could be elicited no longer. Surgical measures in the resistant cases include transcanal labyrinthectomy, ultrasound labyrinthectomy, or vestibular nerve section.

PROGNOSIS

The majority of the benign paroxysmal type clear up in a matter of a few weeks or months. However, recurrence is by no means rare. The usual duration of the benign paroxysmal type is 1 to 9 months. With head injury, the usual duration is 2½ months. If it lasts more than a year after head injury, it may last a long time. I have seen one case with chronic suppurative otitis media with a reliable history for 20 years. Another case associated with a neck lesion had lasted for 8 years. If the peripheral type of positional nystagmus persists for more than 3 months, a complete neurologic examination becomes mandatory.

REFERENCES

1. Barber, H. O.: Positional nystagmus: testing and interpretation. Ann. Otol. 75:838, 1964.
2. Barber, H. O.: Positional nystagmus: especially after head injury. Laryngoscope 74, 1964.
3. Cawthorne, T.: Positional nystagmus. Ann. Otol. 63:481-490, 1954.
4. Hipskind, M. M.: Vertigo. Arch. Otolaryng. 69: 385-389, 1959.
5. Lindsay, J. R.: Postural vertigo and positional nystagmus. Ann. Otol. 60:1134, 1951.
6. Nylen, C. O.: Clinical study of positional nystagmus in brain tumor. Acta Otolaryng. Suppl. 33, 1939.
7. Nylen, C. O.: Otoneurological findings in brain tumors. Acta Otolaryng. Suppl. 33, 1939.
8. Schuknecht, H.: Positional vertigo: clinical and experimental observation. Trans. Acad. Ophthalmol. 66:319-332, 1962.

CHAPTER 10

Miscellaneous Ear Diseases

Vestibular Neuronitis and Acute Toxic Labyrinthitis

Joseph A. Furey

VESTIBULAR NEURONITIS

Vestibular neuronitis, originally described by Dix and Hallpike, characteristically affects the age group of 30 to 50 years. The chief symptom is vertigo, which is usually paroxysmal. There is a conspicuous absence of cochlear signs and symptoms, and dysequilibrium is aggravated by head movements. It is often associated with febrile illness or with evidence of ear, nose, and throat infection. A vast majority of people suffering from this condition showed a direct correlation with coexistent maxillary sinus or tonsillar infection. In many other cases in which infection was discovered, a clear and precise history of an infectious illness at the time of onset of vertigo was elicited. In almost all instances, cochlear function and routine otoscopic examination were normal. An analysis of the labyrinthine response to caloric stimulation in which alternate hot and cold technique was used showed the following: 47 out of 100 had bilateral changes, and 53 had unilateral changes. In the bilateral cases, 7 had complete canal paresis, 25 had severe canal paresis, 7 had moderate canal paresis, and 8 had combined canal paresis and directional preponderance to the same side. In the unilateral cases, 8 had complete canal paresis, 9 had severe canal paresis, 20 had moderate canal paresis, 8 had combined canal paresis with directional preponderance to the opposite side, and 8 had combined canal paresis with directional preponderance to the same side. By explanation: (1) complete canal paresis was defined as no response obtained with irrigation at 20° C. for 1 minute; (2) severe canal paresis was defined as no response obtained with stimuli of normal strength (30° C. or 44° C. for 40 seconds), but response was obtained with water at 20° C. for 1 minute; and (3) moderate canal paresis was reported as obviously reduced responses obtained with stimuli of normal strength. In several of these cases, the abnormal caloric test findings were shown to be the initial and only manifestations of disseminated sclerosis. In most cases, however, there was no evidence of extravestibular nervous disease and an organic lesion of the vestibular nervous pathways at some point up to and including the vestibular nuclei was postulated, and this was termed "vestibular neuronitis." It is felt that the lesion is central to the labyrinth in accordance with the principle that destructive labyrinthine lesions, whatever their pathology, tend to involve the cochlear apparatus. In addition, a high proportion exhibit significant changes in galvanic test responses which are strongly indicative of a lesion central to Scarpa's ganglion.

A significant reduction in galvanic responses was present. This has been borne out not only by the original authors, but by Hatton and the group at Temple University. This reduction of galvanic responses exceeds in degree that which is encountered in cases of Meniere's disease; this observation therefore supports the hypothesis of a central affection of the vestibular neurons.

Vestibular neuronitis is an essentially benign condition which responds well to treatment of focal infection and generally clears up in the course of a few months or years. Palliative medication with antivertiginous medications, such as dimenhydrinate, is helpful. In some instances, it was observed that there was a reestablishment of caloric responses.

ACUTE TOXIC LABYRINTHITIS

Whirling vertigo is the most frequent characteristic of acute toxic labyrinthitis. The onset of symptoms is gradual and reaches a maximum over a period of 24 to 48 hours. At the highest point, vertigo, nausea, and vomiting usually occur. Characteristically, the vertigo disappears within 3 to 6 weeks and a loss of hearing does not occur. Recurrences are infrequent. This syndrome may accompany acute febrile diseases, particularly pneumonia, cholecyctitis, or influenza. It is not unusual that this symptom complex may follow an allergy, extreme fatigue, overindulgence in food or alcohol, or the ingestion of drugs. A great number of drugs, including the thiazides and drugs used in the treatment of hypertension, have been thought to produce acute toxic labyrinthitis. It is true that in many cases the cause cannot be discovered. DeWeese questioned the inclusion of the syndrome under the heading, "Dysfunction of the Internal Ear." It is placed there only because of the severity of vertigo and because the added aggravation from any movement suggests that the end-organ is the probable site of the disturbance. More recently, other men (Furey & Kraus) have suggested reserving the term, "acute toxic labyrinthitis," for a more specific involvement of a toxic or chemical nature. Certainly, in the past, this classification of vestibular dysfunction has fallen heir to many of the symptom pictures which could be termed idiopathic.

Epidemic Vertigo and Anatomic Classification of Vertigo in the Vestibular Tracts

EPIDEMIC VERTIGO

Joseph A. Furey

One of the most interesting of the vestibulopathies is the syndrome of epidemic vertigo, characterized by an acute onset of violent dizziness, with nausea and vomiting, headache and asthenia. The duration may be from several weeks to several months, but recovery is usual. A slight fever frequently accompanies the condition and nystagmus or other vestibular evidence of dysfunction often completes the clinical picture. This condition is epidemic in character and may occur with acute upper respiratory infection or gastroenteritic manifestations. Diagnostically, the caloric test and the audiologic survey are normal. The cerebrospinal fluid analysis is characterized by a slight increase in the number of lymphocytic cells or is normal. It should be noted that epidemic vertigo is often a diagnosis by exclusion, made only after other causes of vertigo have been ruled out. It is imperative to differentiate this condition from labyrinthine hydrops, etc. This can be done best by observing (1) that there is no history of ear affections, (2) that no reduction or fluctuation in hearing or tinnitus is experienced, (3) that the nystagmus presented is of central character, and (4) that the symptoms frequently present a widespread involvement of the central nervous system.

In evaluating the clinical aspects of epidemic vertigo, the most typical feature of an acute episode is dizziness accompanied by nausea and vomiting. Many patients have a local, diffuse, heavy or opprcssive headache.

In about 60 per cent of the cases, lassitude and paresthesia, with a slight fever, were prominent features. About 46 per cent had electroencephalographic dysrhythmias. In only 39 per cent of the cases, was vertigo accompanied by acoustic disturbances, such as hypacusia.

Another author,[1] reporting over 100 cases of epidemic vertigo, described the only objective sign as nystagmus. Caloric tests, which were unspecified, were normal in 41 out of 58 patients. Many of these patients were in excellent health when the initial symptom of vertigo or severe giddiness began. The initial symptom was followed shortly by vomiting and nausea. No ear disease or deafness was present, but transient tinnitus and nystagmus occurred. Oculomotor complications were frequently present, including diplopia and ocular paresis.

The clinical picture of this interesting condition is often divided into two categories: (1) epidemic cases dominated by gastrointestinal manifestations, and (2) epidemic cases dominated by upper respiratory infections, accompanied by a slight fever. Epidemic cases dominated by gastrointestinal manifestations showed a high incidence in mid-January, were more common in the female, and were manifested by the nonneurologic symptoms. There was an incubation period of 1 or 2 days. The most common clinical picture was gastroenteritis with mild vertigo lasting from a few hours to a few days. Concerning epidemic cases dominated by upper respiratory infections and accompanied by slight fever, Pedersen reported that in the autumn of 1953, approximately 50 cases of vertigo of sudden onset occurred within 4 months in a district with a population of only 2000 persons. In another instance, a family epidemic of vertigo (with a complication of encephalitis) was recorded. The family consisted of a 26-year-old mother, two sons aged 5 and 8, and three daughters aged 3, 2, and 1. They all experienced vertigo, nausea, and vomiting within a 24-hour period. Those dominated by upper respiratory infections had an incubation period of 12 to 14 days. These cases were both urban and rural, with no evident relation to water or milk supply or to domestic animals. A large number of diagnostic tests were given these patients, including serologic examinations of the blood and spinal fluid, and in acute cases the feces were examined. Viral studies were done, including poliomyelitis, coxsackie, ECHO, and eastern and western equine type. Bacterial examinations by culture and serologic methods were also performed. All of the tests were negative. It was the general feeling that the most plausible explanation of this condition was a lesion of the second vestibular neuron, including the brain stem, as in vestibular neuronitis. An affection of the brain stem seemed to be most plausible, but since the disease is undoubtedly infectious in nature, it is impossible to exclude the fact that the localization may vary from patient to patient, both in the central and peripheral vestibular system.

In a clinical study of 67 subjects by Leishman, 20 of the subjects showed antral infection, dental sepsis, or attacks of influenza. Cochlear function was tested by pure tone audiometry and normal findings were noted in all subjects. Abnormal responses to vestibular function tests of the Fitzgerald-Hallpike type were obtained in all cases of this series. Many of these cases diagnosed at other institutions as epidemic labyrinthitis were established as vestibular neuronitis on the basis of the vestibular functional tests. In this particular survey the clinical features of the cases accorded closely with the criteria of vestibular neuronitis as defined by Dix and Hallpike.

Furey and Kraus agreed with the similarity of epidemic vertigo, acute toxic labyrinthitis, atypical Meniere's disease and pseudo-Meniere's syndrome, and vestibular neuronitis. Although admitting that these 5 syndromes have more similar than dissimilar characteristics, they tried to point out what they felt were the slight differences. They classified epidemic vertigo as a central vestibulopathy, based on involvement of the brain stem areas and diagnosed by exclusion. In this classification, they felt that the outstanding factor was the epidemic feature. It is quite likely that epidemic vertigo is indeed an encephalitis of viral origin. (See also Chapter 4, the section, "Neurological Examination," by J. U. Toglia.)

REFERENCES

1. Dalsgaard-Nielsen, T.: Further clinical studies on epidemic vertigo, nevraxite vertigineosa. Acta Psychiat. Scand. 28:3-4, 1953.
2. Dix, M. R., and Hallpike, C. S.: The pathology, symptomatology and diagnosis of certain common disorders of the vestibular system. Proc. Roy. Soc. Med. 45:341-354, 1952.
3. Furey, J. A., and Kraus, R. N.: A clinical classification of vertigo. Laryngoscope.
4. Harrison, S. M.: Epidemic vertigo—vestibular neuronitis. Brain 85:613-620, 1962.
5. Leishman, A. W.: Epidemic vertigo with oculomotor complication. Lancet 268:228-230, 1955.
6. Pedersen, E.: Epidemic vertigo: clinical picture, epidemiology and relation to encephalitis. Brain 82:566, 1959.
7. Winther, K.: Vertigo epidemica. Ugeskr. Laeg. 114:1368-1375, 1952.

ANATOMIC CLASSIFICATION OF VERTIGO IN THE VESTIBULAR TRACTS

Joseph A. Furey and Ralph Kraus

I. Peripheral Vestibulopathy.
  1. Vertigo caused by pressure in the external canal.
  2. Vertigo caused by involvement of the middle ear.
  3. Vertigo resulting from end-organ involvement.
  4. Vertigo secondary to involvement of the vestibular labyrinth without cochlear impairment.

II. Central Vestibulopathy.
  1. Vertigo due to involvement of the vestibular nuclei and pathways.
  2. Epidemic vertigo based anatomically on an involvement of the brain stem areas and diagnosed by exclusion.

III. Idiopathic Vestibulopathy.
  1. Postural vertigo.

Eustachian Tube Blockage, Serous Otitis Media, and Intratympanic Neoplasms

Martin Spector

EUSTACHIAN TUBE BLOCKAGE

Eustachian tube blockage is commonly considered a prominent cause for dizziness. The frequency of occlusion of the eustachian tube as a cause for dizziness has, no doubt, been overexaggerated. Formerly, it was common practice to routinely catheterize the eustachian tube of every case of endolymphatic hydrops to relieve the full feeling, and the eustachian catheterization obtained the credit for the passing of an evanescent vertigo attack. Jordan stated that vertigo may result from a sudden eustachian tube blockage, but not from chronic blockage. Shuster stated he never saw a case of vertigo cured by eustachian catheterization. Altman also denied that eustachian tube closure may cause dizziness. Robison indicated that an inflammatory narrowing of the lymph vessels draining the eustachian tube may cause trouble.

Tubal patency may be ascertained by a politzer bag to exert air pressure into the nasal passage, or by the valsalva method, while the examiner either listens for the passage of air into the middle ear or observes the motion of the tympanic membrane. In cases of obstruction of the eustachian tube, the nasopharynx should be examined for pathology.

Many practitioners rely on politzerization for treatment, while others prefer catheterization. The author prefers to try politzerization first; if that fails, eustachian catheterization is used. In obstruction due to the eustachian tube, Williams advised that if the patient is going to benefit, one or two catheterizations are sufficient.

SEROUS OTITIS MEDIA

There are reports in the literature that serous otitis media may cause dizziness. In the author's experience, dizziness has rarely, if ever, been encountered with serous otitis media alone. This opinion is emphasized by the contrast between the great frequency of serous otitis media and the rarity of dizziness with it. It would behoove the examiner to seek some complication or other cause before he assigns the etiology of a case of dizziness to serous otitis media alone.

INTRATYMPANIC NEOPLASMS

Vertigo has been reported to occur with an intratympanic neoplasm in the region of the fenestrae. Most commonly, the lesion is an unsuspected cholesteatoma. A secondary cholesteatoma occasionally will be covered by an almost intact drum without infection. In almost all instances, a crust and annular perforation will indicate that a cholesteatoma exists. On the other hand, a primary cholesteatoma can readily erode bone behind an intact tympanic membrane without any evidence of infection or past history of infection.

Another intratympanic neoplasm which may cause dizziness is a nonchromaffin paraganglionoma. This glomus jugulare tumor, in addition to the vertigo, will present with a pulsating tinnitus. The dusky, discolored appearance of the tympanic membrane will usually denote a mass behind the tympanic membrane. The diagnosis is much easier where a granular, polypoid, easily bleeding mass has already eroded through the tympanic membrane.

CHAPTER 11

Motion Sickness

MARTIN SPECTOR

Motion sickness is a syndrome characterized by nausea and malaise and initiated by movement with acceleration and deceleration. Motion sickness encompasses seasickness, airsickness, and carsickness. The clinical features include malaise, nausea, excessive salivation, cold sweating, and vomiting. The individual becomes quiet, pale, and may, with severe motion sickness, exhibit a facies associated with circulatory collapse. A fall in blood pressure may occur but the pulse exhibits no characteristic change, both fast and slow pulses having been noted. The aftereffects consist of lassitude and mild nausea which may persist for 24 hours. A psychic influence and optic stimuli may contribute to the illness. About 2.4 per cent of the general population are susceptible to undue motion sickness.

It has been shown that removal of the vestibular organs (by labyrinthectomy) or dividing the eighth cranial nerve in dogs and cats immunizes these animals against susceptibility to motion sickness. People whose labyrinths have been destroyed by disease are also immune to motion sickness. It has been shown that extirpation of the nodulus and uvula of the cerebellum in dogs gave immunity. Nausea is reflexly aroused through nerve fibers originating in the labyrinth and connecting to the vagus nuclei. Destruction of the emetic center in the reticular formation of the brain stem rendered dogs immune to motion sickness.

The otolithic apparatus (the utricle and saccule), rather than the semicircular canals, had been incriminated as the site of stimulation. The primary evidence for this was the fact that nystagmus is not found with motion sickness. Johnson has cast doubt that linear motion is of prime importance in causing motion sickness. He stated that weak but prolonged vestibular stimulation may not produce readily detectable nystagmus. He concluded that angular acceleration is a primary stimulus for motion sickness, since he has been able to produce motion sickness under all conditions in which angular accelerations are present and with angular accelerations alone; however, he has been unable to do so with any degree of consistency under conditions in which linear accelerations alone are present.

CORIOLIS REACTION

The coriolis phenomenon has been incriminated as very important in motion sickness. In physical terms, the coriolis phenomenon or effect refers to the linear or tangential velocity produced at the periphery of a rotating sphere. When a sphere rotates, in addition to the angular velocity there is a linear velocity at the periphery. The speed of the linear velocity varies with the radius of the sphere and the angular velocity. The longer the radius of the sphere and/or the faster the angular velocity, the greater the linear velocity or coriolis effect at the periphery. Fernandez wrote in regard to the vestibular coriolis reaction: "The vestibular coriolis reaction appears when a subject exposed to rotation at constant angular velocity tilts his head about an axis perpendicular to the axis of the rotating device. The tilting of the head is associated with strong vestibular disturbances which may include subjective and objective displacements, disorientation, nausea and vomiting, vertigo, and nystagmus. The stimulus arising during the motion of the head is probably due to endolymphatic currents which are induced by bringing one pair of semicircular canals out of the plane of rotation and another pair into it." Guedry and Montague stated: "When a human rider on a rotating structure tilts his head relative to the axis of rotation, he experiences apparent rotation which is uncommonly confusing and which may be accompanied by nausea and vomiting after only a few head movements if the rotating structure has sufficient angular velocity." Johnson stated that any head movement not in the plane of rotation of the vehicle constitutes the most potent labyrinthine stimulus known, at least so far as the semicircular canals are concerned.

The magnitude and direction of the vector representing the coriolis forces depend on several factors, such as the angular velocity and direction of rotation and the rate and direction of the tilting of the head. If a subject is turned constantly in a chair for minutes and then tilts his head forward onto his chest, the vertical semicircular canals will be stimulated. Guedry reported that vertical nystagmus was produced when the head was tilted toward the shoulder during rotation. The vertical nystagmus systematically increased in intensity as the angular velocity of the turntable was increased. Barber reported that Johnson had demonstrated on a model of the labyrinth specific effects on the vertical canals. After steady rotation, tilting the head sagittally influenced the posterior semicircular canals. With a coronal tilt the superior semicircular canals were mostly affected. Arising to the erect position from a tilt elicited a greater response than the original tilt.

Johnson, Fukuda, and others have shown that immobilizing the head of subjects reduced the incidence of motion sickness. They found a correlation between the amount of passive head movement and susceptibility to motion sickness. Experiments on flights confirmed that if the head were fixed to the seat so that it did not move about passively, the subject experienced little motion sickness, whereas if the head was not restrained, most of the subjects were sick. During airplane flights Johnson was able to prevent motion sickness by lying on the floor and by being careful not to move the head.

Guedry and Montague have found that the coriolis stimulation is susceptible to conditioning and habituation.

REFERENCES

1. DeWit, G.: Seasickness—a labyrinthological study. Acta Otolaryng. Suppl. 108:83, 1953.
2. Fernandez, C., and Lindsay, J. R.: The vestibular coriolis reaction. Arch. Otolaryng. 80: 469-472, 1964.
3. Guedry, F. E., Jr., and Montague, E. K.: Quantitative evaluation of vestibular coriolis reaction. Aerospace Med. 32:487-500, 1961.
4. Johnson, W. H.: Some vestibular problems in space flight. Ann. Otol. 70:777-784, 1961.
5. Johnson, W. H., and Taylor, N. B. G.: Some experiments on the relative effectiveness of various types of accelerations on motion sickness. Aerospace Med. 32:205, 1961.
6. Lidvall, H.: Mechanisms of motion sickness as reflected in the vertigo and nystagmus response to repeated caloric stimuli. Acta Otolaryng. 55:527, 1962.
7. McCabe, B. F.: Vestibular suppression in figure skaters. Trans. Amer. Acad. Ophthal. (May), 1960.
8. Schrock, G.: A study of animal reflexes during exposure to subgravity and weightlessness. Aerospace Med. 32:336-340, 1961.
9. Taylor, G. D.: Skin and scuba diving. Laryngoscopy 74:841, 1964.

HABITUATION

Since habituation plays such an important part in motion sickness, habituation and its parameters will be discussed. Habituation refers to a decrease in response after repeated stimulation of the statokinetic labyrinth. Some observers prefer the terms adaptation or suppression to habituation. It is present when an unimportant series of signals is constantly offered to the central nervous system. Adaptation does not change the readiness and alertness of the central nervous system; an unexpected stimulus is perceived quantitatively.

The evidence supports the opinion that

the neuromechanism underlying habituation of vestibular reflexes is a central process. Fatigue of the end-organ does not seem to be a factor. Habituation does not occur in anesthetized animals. Fernandez and Schmidt found that after total ablation of the neocortex and extensive damage to the basal ganglia and diencephalon, animals still exhibited response decline of nystagmus; these authors concluded that these factors were not essential for inducing habituation. The neocortex may be important for retention of the response decline after habituation. Localized or extensive lesions of the midbrain also had no significant effect upon acquisition and retention of the response decline. The phenomenon is apparently located in the vestibular centers, including the vestibular nuclei and reticular formation of both the medulla and pons. It was shown that lesions in the pontine tegmentum (reticular substance of the pons) prevented habituation. Habituation was attributed to changes in the efferent activity to the labyrinths.

Acquisition of habituation signifies the initiation of progressive decrement of nystagmic response after repeated stimulation. The extent may range from a moderate response decline to extinction. Fluur and Mendel found that acquisition of habituation was obtained by repetitive calorization or by repetitive rotation. With consecutive caloric irrigations, both the duration and eye velocity declined. Lidvall showed that the response decline occurred both at minute intervals and at 24-hour or more intervals between caloric stimulations of one ear with water at 30° C. The response decline was more marked in the total number of beats than in the duration of the nystagmus response. He even found some response decline after a 2-week interval between the first and second irrigation. Henriksson, Kohut, and Fernandez performed repeated caloric stimulation on cats and found that the rate of response decline was rapid with initial irrigations and then tended to level off. Most people rapidly develop tolerance to rotation. Hallpike and Hood habituated the human cupula by a revolving chair. They demonstrated habituation by shortening of the duration of nystagmus and shortening of the after-vertigo. Lidvall found no correlation between the degree of neurotic anxiety and the amount of habituation to labyrinthine caloric stimulation. He does mention that many hold the idea that pathological anxiety states are combined with general hyperreactivity.

Whether habituation is attempted in light or darkness does not seem to make much difference. Crampton pointed out that closure of the eyes makes caloric nystagmus response larger in a normal person and smaller in a patient with a central lesion. Spontaneous or positional nystagmus is inhibited by closure of the eyes in cases in which there is a central lesion, but not in cases with a peripheral lesion. Nystagmus inhibited by closure of the eyes may be made apparent by mental arithmetic.

Transfer refers to the possibility that habituation to rotary stimuli in one direction may produce a response decline for rotation in the opposite direction. Lidvall found that the habituation process seems to be specifically linked to the direction of the cupular deflection in the individual labyrinth. In Crampton's studies in cats, habituation to acceleration was not transferred; that is, nystagmus in the untested direction remained undiminished and a directional imbalance was the result. Transfer of habituation occurs in caloric tests, providing the nystagmus is provoked in the same direction as that which was habituated.

The retention of habituation is also important in the study of motion sickness. Henriksson, Kohut, and Fernandez reported that in some cats habituation was retained after 3 weeks of rest, but in some recovery of normal caloric responses occurred after a few days. Also, after several weeks tolerance was lost for rotation. To maintain tolerance, frequent exposure was necessary.

McCabe followed 3 beginners through training for figure skating. At first, they had normal caloric responses. By the end of the season, all had markedly diminished but not completely absent responses to the caloric tests. He reported a figure skater who had attained complete vestibular suppression by physiologic means.

J. J. Groen showed that in newborn infants there was a very slow rate of decline of nystagmus after rotation (20 seconds). As the infant grows, it slows down to a rate of decline of 7 seconds at the age of 3 months.

Most people rapidly develop tolerance to motion sickness. To maintain tolerance, frequent exposure is necessary, because after several weeks tolerance may be lost. Motion sickness occurs much more commonly in children that it does in adults, probably because of the acquisition of tolerance. DeWit found that the threshold for discomfort for rotation was an acceleration of 2.5 degrees per second for average subjects but that it was 4 degrees per second acceleration for seasoned sailors.

Weightlessness

The tolerance for weightlessness has assumed importance for space travel. Johnson stated: "It is the author's impression after having been exposed to about 150 periods of weightlessness of close to 30 seconds each (in an aircraft) that the absence of weight is not capable of producing nausea." Johnson emphasized that marked head movements (nodding and turning) during weightlessness did not cause any nausea or noticeable vertigo. The conclusion that weightlessness is not nauseating seems to have been verified by the reports of the astronauts. When astronauts are rocketed free of the earth's gravitational sphere, it requires at least 8 times the force of gravity, and this might cause small hemorrhages.

Deep-Sea Diving

Taylor stated that 13 of 38 deep-sea divers had noticed a variable degree of dizziness associated with diving. One stated that if he ascended faster than 25 feet per minute, he became dizzy. Ten were prone to seasickness. Three who experienced motion sickness along the bottom of the sea attributed it to positional change due to the movement of water while their eyes were fixed on the bottom as they searched for objects. He advised that a person with dizziness secondary to endolymphatic hydrops or other etiologic factors should not dive.

REFERENCES

1. Crampton, G.: Directional imbalance of vestibular nystagmus in cats following repeated unidirectional angular acceleration. Acta Otolaryng. 55:41-48, 1962.
2. Fernandez, C., and Schmidt, R.: Studies of habituation of vestibular reflexes, effects of caloric stimulation in decorticated cats. Ann. Otol. 71:299-320, 1962.
3. Fernandez, C., and Schmidt, R.: Study of habituation of vestibular reflexes, a revision. Laryngoscope 72:939-953, 1962.
4. Fluur, E., and Mendel, L.: Habituation, efference and vestibular interplay. Acta Otolaryng. 55:136-144, 1962.
5. Groen, J. J.: Postnatal changes in vestibular actions. Acta Otolaryng. 56:390-397, 1963.
6. Henriksson, N. G., Kohut, R., and Fernandez, C.: Studies on habituation of vestibular reflexes, effective repetitive caloric test. Acta Otolaryng. 53:333-348, 1961.
7. Lidvall, H.: Neurotic anxiety and vestibular function as reflected in the vertigo and nystagmus responses to repeated caloric stimuli. Acta Otolaryng. 56:445-455, 1963.
8. Lidvall, H.: Specific and nonspecific traits of habituation nystagmus responses to caloric stimuli. Acta Otolaryng. 50:315-324, 1959.
9. Lidvall, H.: Vertigo and nystagmus responses to caloric stimuli repeated at short and long intervals. Acta Otolaryng. 53:507-518, 1961.
10. McCabe, B. F.: Vestibular suppression in figure skaters. Trans. Acad. Ophthal. (May), 1960.

Part III. Clinical Syndromes of Nonotologic Origin

CHAPTER 12

Neurological and Central Vestibular Syndromes

J. U. TOGLIA

INCIDENCE

Vertigo is a symptom of many neurological diseases but it is more frequently seen in acute vascular diseases of the cerebellum and brainstem; in cysts, tumors, and abscess of the cerebellopontine angle, temporal lobe, and fourth ventricle; and in encephalitis, neurolues, toxic encephalopathy, epilepsy, syringobulbia, and spinocerebellar degenerations.

About 25 per cent of all cases of vertigo have been attributed to diseases of the central nervous system. Lesions in the posterior cranial fossa cause vertigo more frequently than lesions in the anterior and middle cranial fossae.

Macrae[19] reported, in a series of patients with posterior fossa lesions, that vertigo was present in 24 patients with cerebrovascular disease, 16 with multiple sclerosis, 9 with neoplastic diseases, 1 with hydrocephalus, 1 with meningovascular lues, and 1 with olivopontocerebellar degeneration.

Cawthorne[9] found that among 3166 patients afflicted by vertigo, only 367 had diseases of the central nervous system, whereas 2391 had peripheral vestibular diseases and the remaining 358 cases could not be classified. These figures, however, do not accurately represent the frequency of vertigo among neurological patients, because the frequent association of disturbances of consciousness and other neurological signs lead to the neurological diagnosis without necessity for further evaluation of the vertigo.

Most of our neurological textbooks do not elaborate on the subject of vertigo, vestibular testing, and vestibular syndromes. Grinker et al.[13] show some skepticism: "Response to caloric stimulations when there are central lesions are variable and entirely unreliable; one should not depend upon vestibular tests alone for the localization of lesions of the "central nervous system." Wechsler[24] states that enthusiastic claims for the anatomical diagnosis of vestibular lesions in the central nervous system, made for the Barany Tests, are not borne out by clinical experience; he recommends that vestibular tests be carried out in every instance of vestibular lesions in the central nervous system. He also discusses vestibular testing and their results in some detail.

Before proceeding with the discussion about vertigo and central vestibular syndromes, we have outlined in Table 1 the general classifications and some of the clinical features relative to the peripheral vestibular syndromes. These, however, will be discussed in detail elsewhere.

It becomes valuable for clinicians to look at vertigo, nystagmus, and other vestibular disturbances not as separate symptoms, but to group them as specific syndromes. Knowledge of them, with the additional information available from electronystagmography, helps to localize a pathological process in a certain area of the cerebrum, the cerebellum, or the brainstem.

The relations between vertigo and central nervous system lesions were particularly studied by Leidler,[16] who reached the following conclusions:

1. Lesions of vestibular nuclei do not *cause* vertigo in every instance.
2. Lesions close to the vestibular nuclei cause vertigo more frequently than nuclear lesions.
3. Unilateral lesions of vestibular pathways in the brainstem cause intense vertigo.
4. Little or no vertigo is caused by lesions in the brainstem outside the vestibular pathways, including those of the medial longitudinal fasciculus.
5. Lesions in the fourth ventricle and cerebellum do not cause vertigo unless they involve the anterolateral portion of the medulla, the restiform body, and the flocculonodular lobe.
6. Lesions of the middle cerebellar peduncle are not usually associated with vertigo.
7. Lesions of the lateral recess of the fourth ventricle are always associated with vertigo.

Further clinicoanatomical correlations are needed for better evaluation of Leidler's conclusions.

Knowledge of neurological clinical syndromes in which nystagmus is one of the signs helps the anatomical diagnosis of patients with vertigo and other vestibular disturbances. These are grouped according to whether they are related to midbrain, pontine, or bulbar pathology.

Midbrain pathology is suggested by the following syndromes: (1) superior internuclear ophthalmoplegia, and (2) Parinaud's syndrome.

Superior internuclear ophthalmoplegia is characterized by the inability to adduct either eye upon conjugate lateral gaze while nystagmus is present in the abducted eye. Adduction of either eye is present when the patient is tested for convergence. It is therefore not an expression of medial rectus weakness or paralysis of the third nerve.

Parinaud's syndrome is characterized by the loss of upward gaze while the conjugate lateral gaze is normal. It may be associated with vertical nystagmus and dilated fixed pupils. In the above syndromes, vertigo is described as dizzi-

TABLE 1. Retrolabyrinthine Vestibular Syndromes

	Vertigo	Nystagmus	Past Pointing	Romberg	Neuro-vegetative symptoms	Cochlear Symptoms	Vestibula Tests
A. Neuritic Type:							
Cerebrospinal meningitis, mumps, lues, zoster, vestibular neuronitis.	Rotational gradually decreasing.	Horizontal-rotatory.	To side of involved nerve.	To side of involved nerve.	Severe.	Present.	Unilatera or bilate hypoactiv
B. Radicular Type:							
Pontocerebellar angle tumors, pontocerebellar arachnoiditis.	Rotational positional paroxysmal with fewer crises.	Variable horizontal-rotatory or purely horizontal, bilateral or positional.	To either side.	To either side.	Present or absent.	Present or absent.	Unilatera hypoactiv absent.
C. Nuclear Type:							
Viral, vascular toxic, vasomotor vestibular neuronitis.	Violent rotational crisis, short duration or positional.	Purely rotatory during crisis or positional.	To either side.	To either side.	Present or absent.	Absent.	Contrala loss of rotatory nystagmu

ness or imbalance, rather than rotatory hallucination of the environment or of the subject.

Pontine pathology is suggested by the following syndromes: (1) inferior internuclear ophthalmoplegia, and (2) Raymond-Cestan's syndrome.

Inferior internuclear ophthalmoplegia is characterized by the inability to abduct either eye upon conjugate lateral gaze while the opposite eye has normal adduction.

This syndrome is not due to paralysis of the lateral rectus or of the sixth nerve, as demonstrated by the presence of abduction of either eye upon caloric stimulation of the labyrinths.

Raymond-Cestan's syndrome is characterized by tetraplegia, anesthesia and bilateral horizontal nystagmus. In the above syndromes, true vertigo may be present if the pathology extends to the nuclear and paranuclear vestibular areas.

Bulbopontine pathology is suggested by the following syndromes: (1) Babinski-Nageotte's syndrome, and (2) Wallenberg's syndrome.

The Babinski-Nageotte's syndrome is characterized by the following neurological findings: true vertigo, horizontal-rotatory nystagmus directed toward the side of the lesion, ipsilateral paralysis of the tongue, pharynx, and larynx, ipsilateral loss of taste on the posterior third of the tongue, ipsilateral Horner's syndrome, ipsilateral ataxia of the extremities, contralateral hemiplegia, crossed anesthesia, and analgesia.

The Wallenberg's syndrome resembles Babinski-Nageotte without hemiplegia.

The central vestibular syndromes have been grouped in classifications based on combined anatomical and clinical grounds or on experimental data. We are following a classification which combines those of Arslan and Aubry (Table 2).

When the patient complains of vertigo, imbalance, and other symptoms of neurological nature without tinnitus and deafness, we may pose a diagnosis of central vestibular syndrome and attempt first to distinguish infratentorial from supratentorial pathology.

The vertigo in infratentorial lesions is more objective and may be paroxysmal as labyrinthine vertigo, increased by head motion and by opening the eyes. Nausea and vomiting are not infrequent, but they are seldom severe as in patients with disease of the labyrinth. The nystagmus may be unilateral or bilateral and may be present on looking straight forward. The type of nystagmus may be horizontal, vertical, rotatory, pendular, multiple, retractorious, or alternating. The vestibular tests are unilaterally or bilaterally hypoactive and may show directional preponderance.

TABLE 2.
Classification of the Central Vestibular Syndromes

I. *Infratentorial Vestibular Syndromes*
   - A. Localized vestibular brainstem syndromes
     - 1. Bulbar syndromes
       - a. Inferior bulbar syndromes
       - b. Superior or bulbo pontine syndromes
     - 2. Pontine syndromes
     - 3. Mesencephalic syndromes
   - B. Diffuse brainstem vestibular syndromes
   - C. Cerebellar and extrinsic brainstem vestibular syndromes

II. *Supratentorial Vestibular Syndromes*
   - A. Optostriate vestibular syndromes
   - B. Cortical vestibular syndromes

The vertigo in supratentorial lesions is not rotatory; it is less intense and more like instability of the equilibrium. Rotatory vertigo has been recorded more frequently with temporal lobe pathology than with pathology of the occipital, parietal, central, and frontal lobes. Spiegel[23] was able to isolate vestibular responses in the occipital lobes, computing electroencephalographic vestibular responses discriminated from other cerebral electrical activities. The nystagmus in a supratentorial lesion is not constant and only of first degree and small amplitude. The vestibular tests may be normal or may show bilateral hyperactivity, directional preponderance, or absence of the fast phase of the nystagmus. Hypoactive response has been recorded bilaterally following epileptic seizures. Once a level is established of an infratentorial or of a supratentorial lesion, it may be possible to attempt further localization of the pathology by studying vestibular symptoms and specific vestibular syndromes, as outlined in Tables 3 and 4.

INFRATENTORIAL VESTIBULAR SYNDROMES

These syndromes may be related to localized or diffuse pathology in the brainstem, to extrinsic brainstem lesions, and to cerebellar lesions.

Localized Brainstem Vestibular Syndromes

These syndromes may be subdivided into (1) bulbar syndromes, (2) pontine syndromes, and (3) mesencephalic syndromes.

Bulbar Syndromes

These syndromes include the lower or inferior bulbar syndrome and the superior or bulbopontine syndromes.

The Inferior Bulbar Syndrome. This syndrome is related to pathology of the medulla at the entry or below the level at which the auditory nerve enters the brainstem. The primary symptoms include (1) vertigo, paroxysmal or continuous, increased by head motion and opening the eyes, (2) spontaneous rotatory nystagmus directed toward the side of the lesion (clockwise with left side lesion; anticlockwise with right side lesion), (3) poor equilibrium, (4) ataxic gait and past pointing, (5) absence of tinnitus and deafness. The caloric tests may show no responses or absence of rotatory nystagmus in the III head position of Brunning. In the most caudal form, nystagmus may be absent and the vestibular tests normal. This syndrome, defined as vestibulospinal or Deiterospinal, is more commonly encountered with platybasia. Other inferior bulbar syndromes are caused by vascular insufficiency of the vertebral arteries (Wallenberg's syndrome) and to inflammatory diseases, multiple sclerosis, neoplasms, or syringobulbia. Vertebrobasilar insufficiency, Wallenberg's syndrome, and syringobulbia will be discussed in this section, whereas multiple sclerosis and encephalitis will be discussed with the diffuse forms of brainstem pathology. Neoplasms will be discussed elsewhere in this volume.

Vertebrobasilar insufficiency is the most common cause of vertigo in neurological practice. The mechanism varies from intrinsic

TABLE 3. Bulbar Vestibular Syndromes (Aubry et al.)

	Inferior Bulbovestibular Syndrome		Superior Bulbovestibular Syndrome	
	Syringo-bulbia	Wallenberg Syndrome	Neoplasm	Vascular Lesions
Total Number of Cases	30	9	23	16
Nystagmus	30	6	19	13
Horizontal	3	—	7	3
Horizontal-Rotatory	—	1	—	3
Rotatory	24	4	2	4
Vertical	2	—	—	1
Multiple	1	1	10	2
Deviation of the Index				
Present	7 (unilateral)	3	6 (unilateral)	5 (unilateral)
Vestibular Tests				
Abnormal	30	7	23	14
Deafness	2	2	9	1
Pharyingolaryngeal Signs	20	4	—	—

vascular disease (atherosclerosis, arteritis) to congenital vascular anomalies or to mechanical vascular obstruction secondary to cervical arthritis, spondylosis, or trauma. Often more than one mechanism is involved so that a patient with a congenital anomaly or with cervical spondylosis may be symptomless for years until an atheromatous process obstructs either the vessel directly involved or other vessels in the circle of Willis, which have been up to now sufficient to supply collateral circulation.

The congenital anomalies are a difficult diagnostic problem unless arteriography is used. In a series of 2000 angiograms,[11] asymmetry of the vertebral arteries with regard to size was found not only in the intracranial portion, but also in their extracranial course. The left cervical vertebral artery was larger than the right in 45.2 per cent of the cases, the right more than the left in 20.7 per cent, and they were approximately equal in 34.1 per cent. In 8 per cent of the cases the left vertebral artery originated directly from the aortic arch, emphasizing the need for complete angiographic studies whenever possible before making a definite diagnosis and most of all before any vascular surgery is considered.

The mechanical obstructions of vertebral arteries have been studied angiographically and anatomically. Hyperextension of the neck and extreme rotation of the head may compress the vertebral arteries at the atlantoaxial joint or in the intervertebral foramina. The relation between vertigo and cervical pathology (spondylosis, trauma, traction) will be discussed elsewhere in this volume.

Whatever the mechanism, vertebrobasilar insufficiency may cause vertigo because of insufficiency either to the vestibular nuclei or to the peripheral labyrinth via the internal auditory artery. In both instances the vertigo is severe, paroxysmal, or continuous; with insufficiency to the vestibular nuclei, deafness and tinnitus are more likely to be absent, whereas with insufficiency to the end-organ they are almost always present. Sooner or later, other neurological symptoms develop: visual disturbances, drop attacks, somatic sensory changes of face and extremities, dysarthria, dysphagia, ataxia, and paresis of the extremities.

Wallenberg's Syndrome. Insufficiency of

TABLE 4. Pontomesencephalic Vestibular Syndromes (Aubry et al.)

	Pontine	Mesencephalic	Diffuse Brainstem
Total Number of Cases	Degenerative 76 Neoplasms 10 Vascular 9	Neoplasm 9 Vascular 16	Multiple Sclerosis 296
Nystagmus	49	20	168
Horizontal	27	3	47
Horizontal-Rotatory	1	1	7
Rotatory	2	1	8
Vertical	1	8	11
Multiple	18	4	77
Pendular	—	2	6
Deviation of the Index			
Present	20	—	46 (21 unilateral)
Vestibular Tests			
Abnormal	80	19	242
Deafness	8	5	3

blood supply to the lateral medullary areas below the entry of the acoustic nerve is responsible for this syndrome, also defined as the posterior inferior cerebellar artery syndrome. The symptoms and signs have been already described. We emphasize that vertigo may be as severe as labyrinthine vertigo. The nystagmus may be unilateral and directed to the opposite side, or it may be bilateral, horizontal, or rotatory. Caloric responses may be absent or unilaterally hypoactive, or they may show directional preponderance or no rotatory nystagmus with the patient in position #3 of Brunning.

Electronystagmographic studies of Wallenberg's syndrome may show changes of the vestibular function as the disease evolves. If vertebrobasilar insufficiency is suspected, blood pressure and pulses should be taken in both arms, bruits listened for in the carotid and supraclavicular spaces, temporal and retinal arteries examined for tortuosity, and the head rotated and the neck hyperextended in order to elicit vertigo and/or nystagmus. Additional studies include cervical spine x-rays (AP, lateral, and oblique views), electrocardiogram, electroencephalogram, ophthalmodynamometry; occasionally, when spondylosis or cervical arthritis is suspected, cerebrospinal fluid examination with manometrics, electromyography of the upper extremities, and myogram may be indicated. When the case warrants, complete cervicocerebral angiography will be performed. In treating vertebrobasilar artery insufficiency, each case should be considered separately.

Syringobulbia signifies presence of cavities in the medulla oblongata. Paroxysmal vertigo may be the first symptom of syringobulbia, followed by disturbances of equilibrium and positional nystagmus. However, vertigo may be continuous or absent altogether. Spontaneous rotatory nystagmus is very frequent (80 per cent in a series by Aubry). Its intensity and degree vary but they are not altered by changing head position.

Jonesco and Sisesti[15] reported that with unilateral syringobulbia, the fast phase of the nystagmus is to the same side; with bilateral lesions, greatest pathology is at the side toward which the rotatory nystagmus is directed. Syringobulbia causes pharyngeal and laryngeal, but no auditory, symptoms. Abnormalities of caloric tests include absence of rotatory nystagmus and directional preponderance.

The clinical diagnosis of syringobulbia is very difficult unless this is in association with syringomyelia, in which case the diagnosis is established by the typical sensory dissociation (absence of pain and temperature with preservation of touch), a large cervical spinal canal, and abnormal myelography. In syringobulbia respiratory difficulties endanger the patient's life. The treatment is conservative management of the patient, as opposed to the neurosurgical treatment of syringomyelia.

The Superior Bulbovestibular syndrome. This syndrome is determined by pathology of the vestibular nuclei in the bulbopontine areas. The vertigo may be violent, paroxysmal or positional. Aubry analyzed 16 cases of vascular etiology and 23 cases of neoplastic etiology. His vestibular findings are summarized in Table 4. These show that spontaneous nystagmus is frequent and mostly horizontal or multiple. The direction of the nystagmus is to the normal side. The vestibular signs are more often bilateral than unilateral. The index deviation is present in one-third of the cases and more evident in the homolateral arm. The patients have a tendency to fall to the side of the lesion. The caloric responses may be absent or hypoactive homolaterally or bilaterally. Other signs include frequent homolateral or bilateral deafness (more so with neoplastic lesions).

Pontine Syndromes

Vascular insufficiency of the basilar artery, neoplastic lesions (usually gliomas), tuberculoma, gumma, heredodegenerative diseases including olivopontocerebellar atrophy, Friedreich's ataxia—all and many others are responsible for pontine symptomatology.

Vertigo is usually not severe or may be absent. Spontaneous nystagmus is observed in 50 per cent of the cases (Table 4), and is horizontal or multiple. It is more common with heredodegenerative diseases than with vascular and neoplastic diseases. Deafness is recorded in 20 per cent of the cases. Abnormal caloric tests, recorded in 80 per cent of the cases, include absence of rotatory nystagmus, absence of the fast phase, and bilateral inexcitability. Disturbance of the horizontal conjugate motility of the eyes is frequently seen. Other neurological signs include weakness of the extremities, Bell's palsy, deafness, crossed analgesia and anesthesia (one side of the face, the opposite side of the body, and the opposite extremities), loss of the corneal reflex, masticatory difficulties, and disturbances of consciousness.

As to the etiology, we limit our attention to the hereditary ataxias, mainly the Friedreich's and the olivopontocerebellar deegnerations, since these two have been usually associated with vertigo and vestibular disturbances.

Friedreich's ataxia is due to pathology of the spinal cord and of the brainstem, including the vestibular nuclei, and of the cerebellar cortex. The disease begins with ataxia of the legs in the first two decades of life and ends with heart failure in about 20 years. Symptoms include staccato, explosive speech, loss of proprioceptive sensations, absent tendon reflexes, often a positive Babinski, optic atrophy in 9 per cent of the cases, and nystagmus. Other features include pes cavus, kyphoscoliosis, and electrocardiographic abnormalities. We are primarily concerned with the vertigo and vestibular disturbances. Attacks of vertigo were originally reported by Friedreich himself. They usually appear early in the course of the disease and may be troublesome for a time, but they are rarely permanent. Nystagmus is present in more than 50 per cent of the cases; it may be bilateral and horizontal but with no rotatory component. Rarely, the nystagmus is vertical or alternating. Objective signs of vestibular dysfunction have been seldom investigated, but caloric responses may be absent. Deafness may be occasionally present.

Olivopontocerebellar atrophy is due to pathology of the central portion of the pons with degeneration of the pontine nuclei, pathology of the olivary nuclei, cerebellar hemispheres, substantia nigra, and basal ganglia. The onset of this disease, which is not heredofamiliar in most instances, is late in middle life and is characterized by cerebellar signs, extrapyramidal signs, and rigidity more than tremor. Although Aubry described several cases with vestibular disturbances, the majority of patients have no vertigo or nystagmus. Further attention from a vestibular point of view is needed. The diagnosis of hereditary ataxia is only of clinical importance. There is no treatment other than supportive.

Mesencephalic Syndromes

Almost all pathologic processes mentioned in the discussion of bulbar and pontine syndromes may be found in the mesencephalon. The following diseases are specifically related to this area: lethargic encephalitis of *V. Economo*, polioencephalitis hemorrhagica superior (Wernicke's syndrome), and pinealoma.

Lethargic Encephalitis of V. Economo. This encephalitis is probably caused by a virus. The pathology involves the periaqueductal gray matter, the ocular motor nuclei, and the substantia nigra; the pons and the medulla are less involved. The disease has occurred in epidemics, although it may occur sporadically. The epidemics occur more frequently in winter. Patients of all ages and of either sex are equally involved. The transmission of this disease from one subject to another is not clear. The incubation period varies from 9 to 21 days. The onset is most frequently announced by fever, upper respiratory infection, headache, and vertigo. The clinical picture is polymorphous. The most constant symptoms are hypersomnia, reversed sleep pattern, delirium and other mental symptoms, ophthalmoplegia, and disturbances of the pupillary reflexes and of the convergence.

Vertigo is a very frequent complaint. Examination of the spinal fluid reveals presence of 20-100 lymphocytes and some elevation of the proteins. The disease lasts from weeks to months; full recovery may occur, although death occurs in 25 per cent of the cases and sequelae in 35 per cent. The most common sequelae are Parkinson and psychiatric disorders. Vestibular studies are lacking, with the exception of those done in patients with postencephalitic Parkinson's disease. In these cases caloric responses show dissociated patterns and monocular and/or perverted nystagmus.

Polioencephalitis Hemorrhagica Superior. This condition is more frequent in alcoholics but has been demonstrated in patients with carcinoma of the gastrointestinal tract, pernicious anemia, and nutritional deficiencies. The pathology involves mainly the periventricular gray matter, the mammillary bodies, the ocular nuclei, the vestibular nuclei, the thalamus, and the hypothalamus. The clinical picture varies from case to case but invariably shows cloudiness of the consciousness, ophthalmoplegia, ataxia, and often peripheral neuropathy and myelopathy. The duration varies from days to weeks. Recovery is often dramatic following high doses of thiamine chloride, nicotinamide, and other vitamins of the B group. Mortality has been as high as 15-20 per cent. Evaluation of vertigo and caloric tests in these cases are rather difficult because of disturbances of consciousness, drowsiness, delirium, and ophthalmoplegia.

Pinealoma. This entity is discussed by neurosurgeons, but is mentioned here for its specific relation to the mesencephalon. The mesencephalic syndromes are characterized by the following findings: impairment of the vertical gaze (upward more commonly than downward), vertical nystagmus, and loss of the pupillary light reflex. Vertigo is described as instability of the surrounding objects (oscillopia). Vestibular findings were elicited by Aubry. The spontaneous nystagmus may be vertical, multiple, monocular, pendular, or retractorius. The disturbance of balance and gait is not severe. Deafness is relatively frequent because of pathology of the inferior nuclei. Caloric responses may be hyperactive bilaterally or show perverted nystagmus. With the patient in Brunning's position #3, they may fail to produce rotatory nystagmus. Deviation of the index may involve only one arm and is often to the side of the slow phase of the nystagmus.

Diffuse Brainstem Vestibular Syndromes

The brainstem may be diffusely affected by a wide variety of diseases, among which are multiple sclerosis, encephalitis, vascular lesions, neoplasms, degeneration and demyelinization associated with malignancies, alcoholism, malnutrition and vitamin B deficiency, sarcoidosis, Behçet's disease, porphyria, and hemoglobinopathies. The evaluation of vestibular dysfunction is rather difficult because of the diffuse character of the lesions, although a large-scale vestibular investigation has not been done, with the exception of multiple sclerosis, herein reviewed.

Multiple Sclerosis

The incidence of vertigo and vestibular symptoms in patients with multiple sclerosis varies from one report to another. Charcot wrote that vertigo represents the onset of multiple sclerosis in 75 per cent of the cases; Alpers[1] reported 10 per cent. Williams and Corbin[25] found that among 50 consecutive cases of multiple sclerosis, only 2 had episodic vertigo, 4 dizziness (not vertigo), and 5 vertigo or dizziness on change of position. Macrae[19] found that among 84 patients with posterior fossa lesions complaining of vertigo, 16 had multiple sclerosis. The history of transient symptoms — such as visual blurring, scotomas, unilateral, blindness, diplopia, tumor and ataxia, paresthesias, paresis, and bladder disturbances—makes it possible in many instances to establish this diagnosis. The presence of white blood cells, increased gamma globulin, and abnormal colloidal gold in the cerebrospinal fluid determines the stage of activity of this disease. No treatment is available other than supportive and psychological ones.

Barre[4] described two clinical forms of multiple sclerosis with relation to vestibular findings: (1) The acute vestibular form was characterized by severe vertigo and gait disturbance, horizontal, vertical, or rotatory nystagmus, and normal caloric responses or hypoactive responses in the presence of marked nausea and vomiting. (2) The second form was characterized by less vertigo and gait disturbance, rhythmic nystagmus of first degree and small amplitude, and hyperactive caloric response.

Aubry analyzed 296 cases of multiple sclerosis and his vestibular findings are summarized in Table 4. Vestibular symptoms were present in 76 per cent and spontaneous nystagmus in 70 per cent, being multiple in 45 per cent of the cases. Hyperactive caloric responses were noted in 23 per cent of the cases and loss of the rotatory nystagmus in 27 per cent. One of the characteristic features of multiple sclerosis is the occurrence of transient acute vestibular symptoms in the absence of cochlear signs. Arslan[2] reported that in multiple sclerosis (and in gliomas as well) the nystagmus may be of a pendular type. This pendular nystagmus should be distinguished from the congenital fixation nystagmus by the anamnesis and by studying the interference between pendular nystagmus and the nystagmus induced by caloric and optokinetic stimulations. The acquired central pendular nystagmus is not abolished by caloric and optokinetic stimulations.

Cerebellar and Extrinsic Brainstem Vestibular Syndromes

Cerebellar lesions and lesions adjacent to the brainstem cause vertigo and vestibular symptoms rather frequently, because of their proximity to vestibular pathways. The extrinsic brainstem lesions include cerebellopontine angle tumors, aneurysms, and cystic arachnoiditis. The cerebellar lesions include neoplasm, hemangioendothelioma, abscess, tuberculoma, ataxia-telangiectasia, and degeneration associated with malignancies, lymphoma, dilantin intoxication, alcoholism, and vitamin B deficiency.

Discussion about vertigo relative to cerebellopontine angle lesions and cerebellar vascular and neoplastic diseases will be noted elsewhere in this volume. Vertigo is not a relevant symptom in the slow developing cerebellar degenerations, from whatever etiology, although nystagmus and loss of balance may be as disturbing as the cerebellar ataxia.

SUPRATENTORIAL SYNDROMES

The functional relation of the vestibular system to basal ganglia and cerebral cortex is not corroborated as yet by anatomical and experimental data. This group includes diseases of the basal ganglia and of the cerebral cortex.

Optostriate Vestibular Syndromes

Vertigo and other vestibular symptoms are not severe or more usually absent in basal ganglia diseases. Vestibular tests are normal unless the pathology extends to the brainstem. Caloric responses have been reported absent in 55 per cent of choreas during their acute stage.[3]

Cortical Vestibular Syndromes

Although anatomical connections between the vestibular brainstem pathways and the cerebral cortex are not well established, the functional relation of the vestibular system to the cerebral cortex has been physiologically and clinically demonstrated. In this group we include discussions on encephalitis and epilepsy. The relation of vertigo to neoplasm of the cerebral hemispheres and to other intracranial space-taking lesions will be discussed elsewhere.

Encephalitis

Barre and Reys[5] described epidemics characterized by vertigo and vestibular signs with or without neurological abnormalities. There was a suggestion of encephalitis, although supporting data relative to cerebrospinal fluid examination were not available. Herbert,[14] however, reported a large series of upper respiratory infections followed by vertigo and attributed to encephalitis because of increased white cells and proteins in the cerebral spinal fluid. Dalsgaard-Nielsen[10] reported 21 cases of epidemic vertigo attributed to encephalitis because electroencephalographic abnormalities were present in 46 per cent of the cases and neurological signs in 24 per cent. In one of the epidemics reported in Denmark by Pedersen,[21] vertigo occurred in epidemiological association with encephalitis; although he attributed these cases to pathology of the brainstem (in spite of the presence of normal caloric tests), he mentioned the possibility that these were cases of cortical encephalitis. In a series of 152 consecutive cases of encephalitis Pedersen found vertigo to be conspicuous in 43 patients, although 22 of these cases had other neurological signs indicating brainstem involvement.

Epilepsy

In the discussion of vertigo with relation to epilepsy we must first distinguish vertigo as a seizure per se from the vestibulogenic epilepsy which is characterized by grand mal seizures following either an attack of Meniere's syndrome or caloric stimulation. Vestibulogenic epilepsy is one of the various forms of "reflex epilepsy." Vertigo as a seizure is attributed to the heterogeneous group of temporal lobe epilepsy.[20] The question of whether or not every patient who loses consciousness during a vertiginous attack is epileptic remains a controversial matter. Some authors[6] feel that consciousness may be lost in cases of labyrinthine ictus, whereas others[9] would ascribe these cases to epilepsy. The presence of electroencephalographic abnormalities during a vertiginous attack without nystagmus, whether consciousness is lost or not, should establish a diagnosis of temporal lobe epilepsy. At the other end, absence of such electrographic abnormalities in patients who lose consciousness during a vertiginous attack and have no nystagmus cannot necessarily rule out epilepsy. In such cases, activation techniques may be helpful, such as hyperventilation, hypoglycemia, metrazol, and barbiturates. If these induce vertigo and EEG abnormalities without nystagmus, vertigo may be defined as cortical or temporal lobe seizures. If, at the other end, activation by means of caloric test induce vertigo (followed or not by grand mal seizures) and nystagmus, these represent cases of vestibulogenic epilepsy, originating in the brainstem reticular system as a result of labyrinthine discharge. The frequency of vertigo in epilepsy varies from one report to another. Gowers wrote in 1907[12]: "Vertigo occupies a large province in the borderland of epilepsy, perhaps the largest (18 per cent)." Lennox[17] found among 750 epileptic patients that 126 had dizziness as aura (16.8 per cent) and that dizziness represented 12.5 per cent of all types of aura. Penfield[22] found it 9 times out of 259, 8 of which had lesions in the posterior temporal lobe gyrus. When vertigo occurs in children, the first diagnosis suspected is epilepsy rather than vestibular disorder. However, Bridge[7] reported that only 10 out of 742 epileptic children had vertigo. Lerique et al.[18] reported that out of 52 young children affected by paroxysmal vertigo, which disappeared by the age of 5, only 2 had grand mal seizures and the majority revealed no clinical or electrographic evidence of epilepsy. Therefore, other causes for sudden vertigo in children should include Meniere's syndrome, hypoglycenic states, tetany, increased intracranial pressure, and migraine equivalents.

REFERENCES

1. Alpers, B. J.: Vertigo and Dizziness. New York, Grune and Stratton, 1956.
2. Arslan, M., and Sala, O.: Fisiopatologia e clinica delle vie Vestibolari centrali. Soc. Coop. Tipogr. Padova. 1956.
3. Aubry, M., and Pialoux, P.: Maladies de L'Oreille Interne et Oto-Neurologie. Paris, Masson et Cie, 1957.
4. Barre, J. A.: Sur la description et le diagnostic

de la sclerose en plaque; ses phases vestibulo-oculaire, vestibulo-pyramidale et vestibulo-pyramido-cerebelleuse. Sem. op. Paris 24:462-466, 1948.

5. Barre, J. A., and Reys, L.: L'Encephalite epidemique a Strasbourg; sa forme labyrinthique. Bull. Med. Paris 35:256-361, 1921.
6. Boudin, G., et al.: Vertiges et pertes de connaissance. Rev. Neurol. 101:742-750, 1959.
7. Bridge, E. M.: Epilepsy and Convulsive Disorders in Children. New York, McGraw-Hill Book Co., 1944.
8. Buckley, R. E.: Vertiginous temporal lobe seizures stimulated by functional hyperinsulinism. J.A.M.A. 186:204-205, 1963.
9. Cawthorne, T.: Vertigo, president's address. Proc. Roy. Soc. Med. 52:529-536, 1959.
10. Dalsgaard-Nielsen, T.: Further clinical studies on epidemic vertigo, "nevraxite vertigineuse." Acta Psychiat. Neurol. Scand. 28: 263-269, 1953.
11. Fields, W. S., and Alford, B. R.: Neurological Aspects of Auditory and Vestibular Disorders. Springfield, Ill., Charles C Thomas, Publisher, 1964.
12. Gowers, W. R.: Epilepsy and Other Chronic Convulsive Diseases: Their Causes, Symptoms and Treatment. New York, Dover Publications, Inc., 1964.
13. Grinker, R. R., and Bucy, P.: Neurology, 5th Ed. Springfield, Ill., Charles C Thomas, Publisher, 1960.
14. Herberts, G.: Post-infectious meningo-encephalitis as an etiologic factor in certain cases of vertigo. Acta Otolaryng. Stock. Suppl. 118:109-113, 1954.
15. Jonesco-Sisesti, N.: La Syringobulbie. Paris, Masson et Cie, 1932.
16. Leidler, R.: Wie Weit Kann man aus der vestibularuntersuchung auf art und sitz einer Hirner Kran Kung Schliessen. Pract. Otolaryng. 2:152-190, 1939.
17. Lennox, L. G.: Epilepsy and Related Disorders. Boston, Little, Brown & Co., 1960.
18. Lerique, A., et al.: Une manifestation paroxystique propre aux jeunes enfants: les crises vertigineuses. Rev. Neurol. 105:214-217, 1961.
19. Macrae, D.: The neurologic aspects of vertigo, analysis of 400 cases. Calif. Med. 92:4: 255-259, 1960.
20. Nielsen, J. M.: Tornado epilepsy simulating Meniere's syndrome. Neurology 9:294-296, 1959.
22. Penfield, W., and Kristiansen, E.: Epileptic seizure pallans; study of localizing value of initial phenomena in focal cortical seizures. Springfield, Ill., Charles C Thomas, 1951.
23. Spiegel, E. A.: Personal communication.
24. Wechsler, I. S.: Clinical Neurology. Philadelphia, W. B. Saunders Co., 1963.
25. Williams, H. L., and Corbin, K. B.: The differential diagnosis of vertigo. Trans. Amer. Otol. Soc. 46:275-299, 1958.

CHAPTER 13

Neurosurgical Aspects of Vertigo

LYCURGUS M. DAVEY

Vertigo as a symptom of disorders having neurosurgical importance plays only an ancillary role in the diagnosis of such conditions, since the vertiginous episodes are usually overshadowed by symptoms of greater neurological prominence. It is these rather than the characteristics of the vertigo itself that lead to a diagnosis. When vertigo is of peripheral origin, it is apt to be violent and unmistakably clear to the patient, while, as the cause of the vertigo becomes more centrally located, the vertiginous complaints are less clearly definable and are often described as dizziness of the type classified as "nonsystemized dizziness" by DeWeese.[35] Thus, true vertigo does have some localizing value, whereas dizziness does not. This general statement may serve as an introduction to the orderly presentation of those neurosurgical problems in which vertigo may appear, in the hope that a view in perspective will clarify some of the perplexities of the situation. No claim is made to any neat formula for the complex problem of vertigo.

Lesions of the posterior fossa manifest vertigo in about 50 per cent of cases. This is especially true of cerebellar tumors, and, in fact, early concepts regarding the function of the cerebellar hemispheres were confused with those of the vestibular system.[73] It would seem clearest, then, in the evaluation of vertigo as a neurosurgical symptom to start with lesions of the posterior fossa.

LESIONS OF THE VIII CRANIAL NERVE

General Characteristics

In general, lesions of the VIII cranial nerve will give symptoms varying according to the manner in which the nerve becomes involved. Thus, irritative lesions, such as infections and metastatic implants, will cause recurrent episodes of vertigo, milder but not unlike those of peripheral origin; lesions that involve the internal auditory artery may produce a syndrome indistinguishable from Meniere's syndrome; slowly expanding lesions may yield only vague signs of dizziness as in the case of most acoustic neurinomas.

Vascular

Anomalous vessels crossing the VIII nerve have been reported to produce Meniere's syndrome. In Dandy's series of VIII nerve section for relief of Meniere's disease, such vessels gave rise to no symptoms that would identify the true nature of the pathology until disclosed by the surgical approach to the nerve.[54] Thiébaut et al.[91] believe that the occurrence of vertiginous crises in association with anomalous vessels and the relief of these symptoms by sectioning the VIII nerve lends support to the vasomotor theory in Meniere's disease. Further support of this theory may be adduced from the encouraging results obtained by Golding-Wood[52] in his treatment of Meniere's disease, especially the bilateral type, by sympathectomy. Bilateral Meniere's disease may also be treated by differential section of the VIII nerve according to the technique of McKenzie.[72] In this era of microscopic surgery, this procedure has been pushed into the background, but its successes are not to be ignored as attested by the recent review of Dandy's cases.[54]

Metastatic

Metastatic tumors may seed on the VIII

cranial nerve. Since their growth is apt to be rapid and is usually associated with tissue reaction, symptoms arise abruptly and follow a rapid course. Vertigo in this situation is prominent. One such case from the Yale-New Haven Hospital was diagnosed by appropriate neuro-otological studies, and a metastatic melanoma from the eye measuring only 5 x 6 mm. in size was removed from the VIII nerve at surgery.[29] Meningeal carcinomatosis, often from the lung[63] or breast,[10] may occur in the region of the cerebellopontine angle and invade the VIII nerve, with vertigo as one of its prominent symptoms.

Traumatic

Trauma of the VIII cranial nerve, usually due to a fracture of the petrous apex, frequently involves the VII and often the VI cranial nerves. Thus, vertigo is associated with hearing loss, ipsilateral facial paralysis, and often palsy of the lateral rectus muscle. House[58] has described a case of persistent vertigo following head trauma which was successfully treated by partial section of the vestibular nerve through a middle fossa approach. As noted at the time of surgery, the vertigo resulted from an unrecognized fracture at the petrous apex extending in a thin line through the superior semicircular canal.

LESIONS OF THE CEREBELLOPONTINE ANGLE

Classification

Many lesions have been described in the cerebellopontine angle. Evans and Courville[43] have offered a classification of these new growths, amplifying an earlier classification by Henschen. This is repeated here to emphasize the numerous possibilities that exist in the differential diagnosis of the most important of the lesions in this area — namely, acoustic neurinoma.

a. Primary Tumors: (1) tumors arising from the adjacent nerves, particularly the acoustic: neurinomas; (2) tumors arising from the dura mater: meningiomas; (3) tumors arising from the soft membranes (pia-arachnoid): cholesteatomas; (4) the adjacent brain structures, especially the flocculus of the cerebellum, the lateral recess, and the choroid plexus; (5) tumors arising from the petrous portion of the temporal bone (including the bone itself and labyrinth).

b. Secondary and Metastatic Tumors.

c. Cysts of the Cerebellopontine Angle .

d. Infectious Granulomas: (1) tuberculomas; (2) gummas; (3) torula.[67]

To this classification should be added a group of cases of recent interest:

e. Vascular Lesions: (1) aneurysms of the vertebral artery and its branches simulating brain tumor; (2) arteriovenous anomalies.

Acoustic Neurinoma

Incidence

Of this wide variety of lesions, acoustic neurinoma is the most important. In a series of 6000 consecutive autopsies, 100 cases of intracranial tumor were found.[43] Of this number, five (5 per cent) were located in the cerebellopontine angle and three (3 per cent) were acoustic neurinomas. This low figure for angle tumors in this series only indicates that many such cases recover and leave the hospital, which is not true for the patients with the malignant gliomas. Among Cushing's series of 2023 verified intracranial tumors,[23] 176 proved to be acoustic neurinomas (8.7 per cent). In the series reported by Borck and Tönnis,[11] there were 217 (32.2 per cent) acoustic neurinomas among a group of 671 tumors of the posterior fossa. Thus, it is apparent that this tumor is the most common benign lesion of the posterior fossa.

Symptoms—General Comments

Although the tumor is one of the VIII nerve, it is usually considered in relation to the cerebellopontine angle rather than to this nerve alone because it grows sufficiently before diagnosis to compress contiguous structures. This situation may be corrected in another generation or so as the increasing use of currently available diagnostic measures permits the diagnosis of acoustic neurinomas while they are still classifiable as lesions of the VIII nerve alone.

Early Symptoms

Its early symptoms are usually vestibular and cochlear but either may precede the other. In Cushing's first reported series, 25 of 30 cases had inaugural auditory symptoms.[22] Associated signs of involvement of the VII, VI, and V cranial nerves and the cerebellum are usually late. Symptoms may rarely simulate a peripheral labyrinthine disorder—e.g., Meniere's disease.[2] In such instances, it is probably their involvement of the auditory artery instead of their origin from the vestibular nerve which is responsible for those cases mistaken for Meniere's disease.

Symptom of Vertigo

Vertigo has not been as prominent a symptom as one might suppose. When it does occur, it is transitory and more frequently described as a vague dizziness, aggravated by standing and moving and relieved by lying down. This may be explained by the slow expansion of the tumor, which allows time for the vestibular nuclei to compensate for the disturbance.

Incidence of Vertigo

As an initial symptom, vertigo occurred in 6 per cent (3 of 50 cases) studied from Cushing's series,[50] in 18 per cent (29 of 157) of the cases studied by Edwards and Patterson,[42] in 5 per cent (2 of 42) of cases studied by Givre,[51] and in 6.5 per cent (8 of 122) of cases studied by Pool and Pava.[75] As a late symptom, it occurred in 36 per cent of Cushing's cases,[50] 49 per cent of the cases studied by Dix and Hallpike,[36] 42 per cent of those of the Edwards and Patterson series,[42] and 58 per cent of those of Pool and Pava.[75] Although 66 of 157 cases (42 per cent) examined by Edwards and Patterson had complaints of vestibular symptoms, only 36 cases had true vertigo. The other 30 were found to have "giddiness" without movement and, in many instances, a marked loss of balance. With minor reservations, these authors felt that since this giddiness occurred in circumstances similar to those which were associated with vertigo in other patients, it too was of vestibular origin. Dix and Hallpike[36] go so far as to say: ". . . the early vestibular symptoms of VIII nerve tumors take the form of a sense of imbalance and unsteadiness of gait, and this was complained of in 73 per cent of our 70 cases." From a review of the literature and personal experience with patients, the statokinetic disturbances of vestibular function cannot be overemphasized. These symptoms usually appear earlier than vertigo and are not, as often supposed, of cerebellar origin.

Paroxysmal Vertigo

When vertigo occurs in paroxysmal and severe form and is an initial symptom, it may easily simulate the vertigo of Meniere's disease.[2] Although this occurrence has been reported, it is rather the exception. Four of the 6 cases of small tumors of the VIII nerve found at autopsy by Hardy and Crowe[56] were seen to originate from its vestibular portion. When one considers this finding, it is surprising that vertigo is not a more common or early symptom of acoustic neurinoma. The studies cited, however, attest that it is not.

Early Appreciation of Vertigo in Diagnosis of Acoustic Neurinoma

Edwards and Patterson[42] pointed out many years ago that the vertigo occurring with acoustic neurinomas is usually mild and is commonly a "giddiness" which is passed as unimportant (just as is the early and minimal hearing loss, the importance of which is missed in adults) by both the patient and physician. These complaints are usually attributed to some lesser aural disorder. Unless evidence of these symptoms is carefully sought at the time of the anamnesis and unless the presence of acoustic neurinoma is suspected, the actual diagnosis, as Cushing[22] pointed out, may be missed. Often the patient is not referred to a neurosurgeon until the symptoms become more persistent and perhaps even disabling. It is strongly urged that either they be encouraged to return for adequate follow-up or that they be referred for further work-up in this early stage of the disease. Now that the otologists have developed a translabyrinthine approach to tumors of the VIII nerve, early diagnosis is essential to the application of this operation.

Diagnosis

Cardinal diagnostic symptoms of acoustic neurinoma are deafness, cerebellar incoordination, and dizziness. In the examination of the patient, the presence of nystagmus, hearing loss, diminished or absent corneal or facial sensation, cerebellar signs, and papilledema leave little room for doubt about the diagnosis of acoustic neurinoma. Two early signs of facial nerve involvement may prove extremely helpful: (1) loss or diminution of sensation over the skin of the posterior portion of the external auditory canal, and (2) loss or disturbance of taste over the anterior two-thirds of the tongue on the suspected side. Deafness unassociated with these symptoms and signs is unlikely to be due to an acoustic tumor. In the last few years it has been possible to reduce these cardinal symptoms to hearing loss and dizziness when appropriately investigated with auditory, vestibular, and radiological studies.

Laboratory Studies

Since details of these various tests may be found elsewhere in this volume, it is sufficient to list simply the following examining procedures: A full battery of audiological studies; a careful test of vestibular function, preferably the bicaloric test of Hallpike and Cawthorne;[27] where available, radiological evaluation of the petrous ridges by plesiotomography,[65] which can show sections of only 1 mm. thickness; and Pantopaque radiography[7,83] of the cerebellopontine angle with its capacity to outline neatly even small lesions pouching out of the internal acoustic meatus. Lumbar puncture is an unwise procedure in a patient with papilledema or other signs of increased intracranial pressure. Although some dispute this position on lumbar puncture, it should be emphasized that the fear is not that the procedure always carries a serious risk, but that when disaster strikes, the results can be devastating. In those cases in which the results of lumbar puncture have been reported, the spinal fluid protein is apt to be greatly elevated in acoustic neurinomas, whereas in other lesions it is apt to be normal or only slightly elevated. One typical study should suffice to illustrate this point. D'Errico[34] reported that in 6 cases of acoustic neurinoma, spinal fluid protein ranged from a low of 50 mg. per cent to 725 mg. per cent, with an average of 231 mg. per cent. In contrast, among 9 meningiomas, the lowest spinal fluid protein value was 5 mg. per cent, the highest 65 mg. per cent, and the average 35 mg. per cent.

Treatment

With a strongly suspicious attitude toward the cardinal symptoms of hearing loss and dizziness, House[59] has been able to diagnose and treat an impressive number of small tumors. Results appear far more favorable when the tumor is discovered in its smallest possible state. The case of the metastatic tumor cited above, which measured as little as 5 x 6 mm., indicates a worthy goal in early diagnosis.

Critique on Translabyrinthine Approach. Treatment of these tumors deserves special mention because the new translabyrinthine technique of House[60] is an exciting advance in management of these lesions. His approach is particularly suited to the preservation of the facial nerve and to the removal of those lesions within the porus acousticus so small as not to be evident through the posterior fossa. From the viewpoint of a neurosurgeon, the chief criticism that might be leveled at this procedure would be against its use in the removal of the larger acoustic neurinomas or other large angle growths in which adequate access to sources of major hemorrhage and visualization of surrounding neural structures may be limited. In such instances, the strictures imposed by the translabyrinthine exposure would amount basically to poor surgical technique.

Posterior Fossa Approach. The best operative method for the larger tumors is through the posterior fossa. Although it may necessitate the sacrifice of a cap of cerebellum, the wide angle of visualization which this provides makes identification and the handling of important veins, arteries, and cranial nerves easier. Uncapping the cerebellum avoids retraction on this structure and its attendant risk of tearing a tentorial vein which is difficult to reach. Moreover, the cerebellar deficit incurred leaves the patient with no disability of practical importance.

Preservation and Reconstruction of the Facial Nerve. Wherever feasible, the lateral portion of the tumor is uncovered early in the dissection and the facial nerve identified at the internal auditory meatus. Preservation of the facial nerve is not always possible when it is thinly attenuated and stretched out over the capsule. If a proximal segment of the facial nerve can be preserved, it should be identified with a suture and a secondary facial anastomosis should be performed.[37-39] Dott first carried out successfully an extrapetrous graft to a facial nerve which had become detached at the porus during complete removal of an acoustic neurinoma. Drake,[38] without knowledge of Dott's work, had occasion to perform a similar extrapetrous autogenous graft with a 2-inch length of lateral femoral cutaneous nerve. Subsequently, Drake[39] described a direct anastomosis of the facial nerve at the internal auditory meatus which he had done in 1959. Just prior to the publication of this last technique, an occasion was presented to us in July 1963 to perform, with 7-0 silk sutures on a swedged needle, an intracranial direct reanastomosis of the severed ends of the VII and VIII nerves during the removal of a huge pearly tumor. The patient died 4 months later without evidence of recovery of facial function. This case is cited to emphasize the feasibility of the technique. The use of a special needle holder as recommended by Dott[37] and the aid of magnifying glasses as suggested by Drake[40] should put this procedure within the competence of all neurosurgeons.

Total vs. Intracapsular Enucleation. Total removal is preferred to intracapsular enucleation. Dandy[26] was able to reduce his mortality from 11 per cent in his first 46 cases to 3 per cent in the next 36 cases reported in which this method was employed. Since not all neurosurgeons have that late master's skill or volume of experience, there are times when an intracapsular resection might be the more prudent choice. In particular, should the capsule be strongly adherent to the brainstem or too intimately related to the anterior cerebellar artery, to separate the tumor from these structures is to court disaster.

Unroofing Internal Auditory Meatus. Before terminating the procedure, the internal auditory meatus should be unroofed and the poral portion of the tumor removed from the auditory nerve to eliminate an important source of recurrence of tumor growth. This may be done with an osteotome or a fine punch. Drake[40] has used a small dental burr and magnification with a loupe and "the posterior wall of the meatus can be removed easily and safely to expose the nubbin of tumor within and its origin from the acoustic nerve." He has used this technique to expose and preserve the facial nerve as well.

Decompression of the Arch of the Atlas. Finally, in those cases with increased intracranial pressure, the arch of the atlas may be removed and the bony suboccipital decompression enlarged. The dangers of postoperative edema are thereby lessened, an important advantage of this method in the difficult cases.

Differential Diagnosis

In other tumors of the cerebellopontine angle, vertigo is seen even less frequently. In the early Cushing's series,[22] the tumors which were mistaken for acoustic neurinoma included a meningioma of the posterior fossa, papilloma of the choroid plexus of the fourth ventricle, ependymal glioma, and a pontile glioma extending into the right recess in such a way that, when exposed from behind, it could be easily mistaken for an acoustic tumor. Revilla[79] reported vertigo in 4 of 13 meningiomas and 2 of 13 cholesteatomas (pearly tumors). This symptom was not present with astrocytoma, astroblastoma, medulloblastoma, or ependymoma. Pool and Pava[75] include in the differential diagnosis also tumors of the petrous portion of the temporal bone, such as meningiomas, osteosarcomas, myelosarcomas, and epitheliomas of the middle and inner ear. In such lesions, vertigo is usually quite secondary and the diagnosis is made by the more primarily associated neurologic disturbances.

Cysts of the Cerebellopontine Angle

Of the lesser lesions, glomus tumors, arachnoiditis, and arachnoidal cysts of undetermined etiology have been described as causes of vertigo.[92] Chronic arachnoiditis frequently affects the vestibular function, but overt vestibular symptoms are rare.[62] Evans and Courville[43] describe arachnoidal cysts as a chronic process following middle ear infection with resulting arachnoiditis. They describe the meninges as becoming thickened, whitish, and opaque and producing adhesions which trap fluid. The fluctuation of the clinical symptoms is attributed to rupture and subsequent refilling of these inclusions.

Infectious Granulomas

In this era of antibiotics, improved public health measures, and generally better living, it is purely an encyclopedic gesture to mention tuberculomas and gummas of the cerebellopontine angle as causes of vertigo.[43,57] Apparently, torulosis may give rise to a similar lesion.[67] Even in India, where tuberculomas of the brain are not uncommon, those of the cerebellopontine angle are.

Vascular Lesions

Large aneurysms of the vertebral artery were accompanied by dizziness in 54 per cent and nystagmus in 62 per cent of cases studied.[31] In an analysis of the complaint of dizziness, no clear differentiation was made between the terms dizziness and vertigo. The commonest error of diagnosis in such cases was to operate upon them in the mistaken impression that they harbored an acoustic neurinoma. With increasing use of angiography, such errors may be minimized.[64] Moreover, with the ability to recognize these aneurysms preoperatively, their surgical management may be well planned in advance and even handled successfully.[1] Similar experiences have been described with arteriovenous malformations in the posterior fossa.[74] Holmes[57] indicated that the pressure of an arteriosclerotic vessel or arteriosclerotic aneurysm on the VIII nerve was "not an infrequent cause" of vertigo. "In these cases, there is usually a sensation of rotation of self from the healthy side towards the side of the lesion and external objects toward the opposite side, but this is not such a definite rule as Grainger Stewart and I suggested many years ago."[57] Another characteristic of such lesions is that the vertigo persists long after the hearing is gone, a point which differentiates such lesions from peripheral aural diseases.

LESIONS OF THE FORAMEN MAGNUM

Development Anomalies—Including Platybasia

Developmental anomalies such as the Arnold-Chiari and the Dandy-Walker syndromes may have concomitant vestibular disturbances.[71,86] The associated nystagmus is coarse, spontaneous, and often vertical. Platybasia, or primary basilar impression, stemming from bony anomalies of occipital development is frequently accompanied by vertigo. Basilar impression secondary to Paget's disease and to such less common causes as osteoporosis, rickets, and osseous dysplasias is less often associated with neurologic disturbances, including vertigo. Vertigo as a presenting symptom in basilar impression is unusual. It occurred in but one of the cases reported by Garcin and Economos[48] in their exhaustive monograph on this subject and in only one of 10 cases reported by Taylor and Chakravorty.[90] Actually, the clinical picture associated with basilar impression is overshadowed by more prominent neurologic symptoms. These symptoms have been divided into four categories: those due to (1) spinal cord compression, (2) cerebellar compression, (3) fourth ventricular obstruction, and (4) secondary syringomyelia. Taylor and Chakravorty[90] have added two new symptom complexes: sudden attacks of altered consciousness without neurologic signs, and a syndrome of vertebrobasilar insufficiency or infarction beginning with hemiparesis. In the light of increasing interest in disturbances of the vertebral circulation (which will be discussed more fully later in this chapter), the authors reexamined the etiology of this condition and stressed the vascular disturbances caused by this anatomical abnormality of basilar invagination. Surgical decompression of the area of the foramen magnum and upper cervical spine has been helpful in arresting and, in some instances, relieving the preoperative symptoms.

Tumors—Including Aneurysms

Among other lesions of the foramen magnum, Symonds and Meadows[88] reviewed 7 cases and only one, an aneurysm of the right vertebral artery, showed any associated signs of vertigo. Several reports of posterior fossa meningiomas were reviewed[16,24,70,81] and among those at the foramen magnum, no instance of vertigo as a symptom was mentioned.

LESIONS OF THE CEREBELLUM AND FOURTH VENTRICLE

Incidence of Vertigo

"Vertigo is one of the most constant symptoms of extracerebellar and intracerebellar tumors, and it is specially frequent in the former." So stated Stewart and Holmes[87] in 1904. Although a review of their cases demonstrated many more seriously ill than one might expect today, their contention is still tenable. For example, in a series of 480 cases of cerebellar tumors analyzed by Borck and Tönnis,[11] 43 per cent demonstrated dizziness; in Grant's series comprising 158 verified cases, 44 per cent had this complaint.[53] Among hemangioblastomas, this percentage rises to as much as 68 per cent among the solid tumors with cysts in the 48 cases studied by Cramer and Kimsey.[19] In the overall group, vertigo occurred in 53 per cent of their cases and in 57 per cent of the 46 cases of Borck and Tönnis.[11]

Localizing Value of Vertigo

In both extracerebellar and intracerebellar tumors, according to Stewart and Holmes,[87] objective vertigo or the sense of displacement of external objects in front of the patient is directed toward the side opposite the lesion; that is, in a left-sided tumor apparent movement of objects is from left to right. Unfortunately, this often-repeated dictum is neither so helpful nor so simple a matter, for much depends upon whether the lesion is destructive or irritative; whether it compresses the inferior cerebellar peduncle, where the cerebellovestibular connections course; whether the lesion compresses the vestibular nuclei in the floor of the fourth ventricle; or whether the lesion is bilateral. In this last instance, for example, a medulloblastoma will often be associated with cerebellar nystagmus, but when the tumor has affected both sides the nystagmus will disappear as the effect upon the paired vestibular nuclei becomes equal. Hence, the direction of vertigo or nystagmus (and by translation the movement of objects in front of the patient) can be helpful only when considered with other findings. Borck and Tönnis[11] state that the direction of nystagmus was not helpful in the localization of lesions in their 480 cases of infratentorial tumors. Apparently, Holmes[57] at a later time came to the same conclusion regarding the direction of vertigo.

Vertigo in Specific Tumors of the Cerebellum

In a study of medulloblastomas, vertigo was one of the symptoms in 34 of 116 of Tönnis' cases, or 27 per cent, whereas nystagmus was present in 64 per cent of 22 cases described by Cuneo and Rand.[20] Since this tumor is found commonly in children, it seems improbable that accurate appraisals of the symptom of vertigo will be made. With astrocytomas, the incidence of dizziness was 40 per cent and for ependymomas it was 50 per cent.[11] Meningiomas on the convexities of the cerebellum may be associated with vertigo but their slow growth can scarcely endow them with characteristic signs or symptoms.[16,24,70,81] Among the less frequent lesions of this area demonstrating vertigo are included metastatic lesions, abscesses, arteriovenous angiomas, tuberculomas, sarcomas, arachnoid cysts, and gummas.[11]

Cerebellar Abscess

A special word about cerebellar abscess is in order at this point. In spite of its great infrequence in this era of antibiotics, its recognition is essential to avert the catastrophic consequences of this disease. It commonly occurs, according to Aubry and Pialoux,[6] with a retrolabyrinthine osteitis, especially at the level of the posterior semicircular canal. In turn, this results in a localized area of pachymeningitis, first externally, then internally. A fistulous communication may appear, but it is not essential to the propagation of the infection to the cerebellum. This occurs by means of a septic retrograde thrombophlebitis of the pial veins, or a perivasculitis or endarteritis of the pial vessels. A cerebellar abscess must be suspected after the aural infection has cleared if there persists or reappears vertigo or a marked nystagmus, which usually changes in direction with positional tests. This suggests its central origin. In time, the abscess will be accompanied by homolateral cerebellar signs. Naturally, as it increases in size or cerebellar edema progresses in response to the inflammatory process, signs of increased intracranial pressure and papilledema will ensue. Intractable occipital headache is common. General symptoms, such as low-grade fever, malaise, and increase of polymorphonuclear white cells in the peripheral blood count may be seen. Among diagnostic studies, the persistence of an abnormal cellular response in the cerebrospinal fluid, despite evidence of resolution of the external focus of infection, should alert one to the possibility of cerebellar abscess.

Total excision of the abscess is ideal treatment, but often the pressure of circumstances may necessitate marsupialization as the wiser choice. Adequate antibiotic coverage is essential. Sensitivity studies on the purulent contents of the abscess will prove rewarding. Since one reason for the formation of cerebellar abscesses is inadequate antibiotic therapy of the external lesion, it may be found that the causative organism is resistant to antibiotics that seemed previously effective.

Vertigo with Lesions in and near the Fourth Ventricle

Vertigo as an early symptom has been found with angiomas, meningiomas, cerebellar cysts, ependymomas, and choroid plexus papillomas. It would appear that the larger lesions, the vascular anomalies, and those lesions extending into or occupying the fourth ventricle are more likely to manifest the symptom of vertigo. Thus, among tumors of the fourth ventricle, such as choroid plexus papillomas, cysticercus, ependymomas, and other gliomas, it is not surprising to find that they are commonly ushered in by vertigo.

Bruns' Syndrome

Special reference should be made to a syndrome, originally described by Bruns[13] in 1902, consisting of episodic attacks of great vertigo, violent headaches, and vomiting with changes in head posture in a man having cysticercus of the fourth ventricle. Freedom from symptoms between attacks is characteristic. A third characteristic was added by Alpers and Yaskin[3]: a constant anterior flexion of the head usually in the midline but at times with lateral flexion and rotation. These same authors have observed the Bruns' syndrome with a cerebellar astrocytoma, varied lesions of the fourth ventricle, and with lesions of the third and even lateral ventricles.

LESIONS OF THE BRAINSTEM

Characteristics of Vertigo

Vertigo having its origin in peripheral causes tends to be paroxysmal; but that produced by lesions in the brainstem is more continuous, with durations of hours or days at a time, and with increase in severity by movement. Postural vertigo of central origin usually persists so long as the critical position is maintained, while that of peripheral origin is fatiguable.

Incidence of Vertigo

Tumors of the brainstem were studied by Barnett and Hyland,[8] who found vertigo as an early or initial symptom in 8 of 33 cases; however, in the series of Bray et al.[12] and Bucy and Kiplinger,[14] dizziness is not listed as a prominent symptom even though involvement of the VIII cranial nerve occurred in 7 of 48 cases in the former and 31 of 100 cases in the latter series. Bucy and Kiplinger[14] state that tumors of the pons are frequently associated either at the onset or later with nausea, vomiting, and dizziness. Nystagmus has a more specific position in the analysis of these cases with a 36 per cent incidence in Bucy and Kiplinger's cases and a 26 per cent incidence of horizontal and 14 per cent of vertical nystagmus in the series of Bray and associates.[12]

Among the vascular lesions of the brainstem, hematomas of the pons may act as space-occupying lesions, the initial evidence of which may be sudden vertigo. The incidence of dizziness in basilar aneurysms is 24 per cent as compared to 50 per cent in basilar insufficiency. In contrast, the figures for nystagmus are 25 per cent and 12 per cent respectively.[30]

Trauma to the Brainstem and Post-Traumatic Dizziness and Vertigo

Trauma to the brainstem as a cause af post-traumatic vertigo and dizziness has been studied by Friedman, Brenner and Denny-Brown.[47] Since initial signs in a significant number of their cases pointed to damage to the brainstem, they were led to believe that "there was remarkably little evidence that post-traumatic dizziness is related to damage to the vestibular end-organ." However, in the absence of associated neurologic signs, the evidence is stronger for the more likely locus of pathology to be in the peripheral organ, most probably in the utricle.[28] This will be discussed more fully later, as it is more pertinent to the general object of head injury and the syndrome of labyrinthine concussion.

Syringobulbia

Aubry and Pialoux[6] have published on the neuro-otological studies in 30 cases of syringobulbia. In this condition many varied forms of nystagmus may be seen. Positional nystagmus induced in one of our cases of syringobulbia showed a dissociation in which the frequency of the nystagmic beat of one eye was twice that of the other.

Diagnosis of Brainstem Tumors

Diagnosis of brainstem tumors is generally easy because of the multiple cranial nerve palsies which progress to such complete paralysis as to indicate destruction of nuclei. These tumors occur mostly in children, approximately 87 per cent in patients under the age of 20. Early diagnosis is frequently possible. For example, in one of our cases, a 6-year-old white girl presented with weakness of the lateral rectus muscle of the right eye and a left Babinski response. Despite the paucity of findings, a diagnosis of pontine glioma was made, much to the consternation of the disbelieving parents. Other advice was sought, and the diagnosis was confirmed by air studies. In reviewing these cases, vertigo, though a symptom of pontine lesions, is not apparently an important consideration. In the differential diagnosis, one need bear in mind that such tumors are uncommon in adults. Before making a diagnosis of pontine glioma in a patient over the age of 20 years, the possibility of a lesion external to the pons compressing that structure should be excluded first. Among such possibilities are included acoustic neurinoma, meningioma, pearly tumors (cholesteatomas), and aneurysms.

Treatment of Brainstem Lesions

Treatment, despite early diagnosis, is hardly ever surgical, since manipulation in this area will cause medullary paralysis and death will ensue within a few hours. Dandy[26] did report successful evacuation of an encapsulated intrapontine hematoma but, as he stated: "The number of encapsulated removable tumors within the brainstem must be exceedingly few." Bray and co-workers[12] have reported clinical remission in 24 of their 37 patients treated with radiotherapy. With higher doses, up to 4000 r in 28 days, these authors felt that there resulted "a remission of symptoms and signs in a greater percentage of patients." No cures were affected, and it was questionable whether there was any increase in survival time.

SUPRATENTORIAL LESIONS

Lesions in and near the Third Ventricle

Tumors of the third ventricle may produce dizziness but only rarely has vertigo been specifically reported and associated with these lesions. In a review of the literature, Dandy[25] reported 31 cases of colloid cysts of the third ventricle and added 5 cases of his own. Of the cases in which the symptom of dizziness was considered, there were 9 instances in which this was one of the symptoms. Among these 9 cases, there was one case in which the first symptom was attacks of vertigo, and another case in which the first symptom consisted of headaches and dizziness. Of Dandy's cases,[25] 2 showed dizziness and 3 did not. In addition, he reported on 16 other types of tumors in this site that he felt were removable and added 16 of his own cases. Among the histological types of tumors mentioned, there were included pearly tumor, meningioma, ependymoma, dermoid, epidermoid, and encapsulated solid sarcomas. Only 3 of the reported cases mentioned dizziness as a symptom. Among Dandy's 16 cases,[25] one had an onset with headaches and dizziness. His cases included 7 ependymal gliomas, among which dizziness occurred in 5 of the 6 cases in which this symptom was mentioned. Among 3 cases of cysts of the cavum Vergae and septum pellucidum, only one was accompanied by the symptom of dizziness.

Zimmerman and German[93] reported 2 cases of colloid cysts, one of which demonstrated dizzy spells. However, in their examination of 28 cases from the literature (including those reviewed earlier by Dandy[25]), they noted only 4 cases of vertigo. Vertigo and dizziness, therefore, may be symptoms of growths in this area, but they are scarcely of diagnostic importance. In pinealomas, dizziness is seen but rarely. In the study of Freeman et al,[46] dizziness was present in only 3 (9 per cent) of their cases of pinealoma, and absent in all 7 cases of Barnett and Hyland.[8]

Hydrocephalus

Arrested hydrocephalus in adults may give rise to a vestibular syndrome.[69] The following case is illustrative of the problem and its eventual treatment.

Case 1. M.E. Arrested hydrocephalus presenting with vertigo. Ultimately treated with a ventriculoatrial Holter valve shunt with symptomatic improvement.

A 38-year-old white married female was first seen on November 8, 1956, for evaluation of dizziness. This had been present since childhood when she noted that she could not do somersaults because of dizziness. On November

4, 1956, she had noted gradual onset of subjective vertigo, and upon moving she became aware of objective vertigo with objects spinning in a counterclockwise direction. This trouble prevented her getting out of bed, and even at rest she had considerable nausea but no vomiting. There was no hearing loss, tinnitus, numbness of the face, or awkwardness in the use of her hands. Slight unsteadiness and a tendency to veer to the left had been noted over the preceding 5 years. Long-standing bifrontal headaches and aching in the back of the neck were present. There was no history of birth injury or postnatal difficulty. She had done well in school until she became interested more in boys than studies, and she finished with a B average in high school.

On examination, she performed rapidly alternating movements a little awkwardly with the right hand. Slight ataxia was noted on the finger-to-nose test on the right. Mild swaying on Romberg test and awkwardness on the right heel-to-shin test was seen. She was admitted to the Yale-New Haven Hospital (45-38-88) from March 3 to 9, 1957, where diagnostic studies were done. X-rays of the skull showed increased digital markings with posterior displacement of the calcified pineal shadow, thinning of the posterior clinoids and enlargement of the sella turcica (19 x 11 mm.). The electroencephalogram was diffusely abnormal with a suggestive left frontal focus. A pneumoencephalogram demonstrated a severe grade of hydrocephalus involving all four ventricles but no evidence of tumor or obstruction. Spinal fluid protein was 25 mg. per cent.

She showed slight improvement and was not seen again until March 1962, when she complained of bifrontal headaches following a fall one month earlier. There was now marked unsteadiness of gait but no other changes on examination. She had given up her job as a bookkeeper in 1960. Her next visit was on June 13, 1963, and she indicated that in November 1962, she was driving, swerved to avoid a dog in the road, and hit a utility pole. On May 28, 1963, she had fallen in her bedroom and sustained a laceration of the right occipital area. Following this, she had become aware of diplopia and blurring of vision. On examination, no ocular palsies could be demonstrated.

She was readmitted to the Yale-New Haven Hospital from August 11 to 31, 1963. The pneumoencephalogram now demonstrated an obstruction at the foramen magnum. Spinal fluid protein was still only 25 mg. per cent. A vertebral angiogram was performed, and it demonstrated normal left vertebral and basilar arterial supply, but no reflux into the right vertebral was achieved. Discussion of the case led to a decision to offer the patient a ventriculoatrial shunt using a Holter valve rather than a posterior fossa exploration. This shunt was effected on August 27, 1963, and the patient felt sufficiently improved to be discharged on her fourth postoperative day. When last seen on July 9, 1964, she still complained of some unsteadiness of gait but blurring of vision and diplopia appeared only when fatigued.

Lesions of the Temporal Lobes

Tumors of the posterior temporal lobe may cause vestibular disturbance with caloric directional preponderance to the side of the lesion.[15] Similar involvement of the angular and supramarginal gyri produces well-marked directional preponderance of optokinetic responses but only slight directional preponderance of caloric responses.[15] Such alterations of caloric and optokinetic responses may be seen with porencephalic cysts, cortical scars, hematomas, and abscesses.[4] Otogenic temporal lobe abscess may still be seen occasionally.[80]

Lesions of the Frontal Lobes

Dizziness has been described in frontal tumors by Freeman and associates.[46] They indicated that 4 cases, 6 per cent of their frontal tumors, had dizziness as a symptom; and in 3 of these a horizontal nystagmus was reported. In frontal lesions it is presumed that the symptom of dizziness is caused by increased intracranial pressure being transmitted to the labyrinthine circulation which is connected to the subarachnoid pathways through the ductus and saccus endolymphaticus.

Lesions of the Occipital Lobes

In World War I casualties who suffered gunshot wounds of the occipital lobes,

Holmes[57] observed vertigo in those patients "who were subject to epileptiform seizures in which visual phenomena were prominent symptoms." He described a clonic jerking of the head and eyes toward the field in which the visual phenomena were referred. To this, he ascribed the immediate cause of the vertigo. The vertigo was not always associated with convulsive manifestations. It is clear that he did not imply a cortical center for vertigo but rather affirmed that the vertigo was the by-product of the spasmodic movements of the head and eyes which movements could also "be excited from frontal, temporal, and parietal lobes and irritating lesions involving these (might) in the same manner give rise to vertigo."[57]

HEAD INJURY AND THE SYNDROME OF LABYRINTHINE CONCUSSION

Psychogenic vs. Organic Dizziness Following Head Injury

The complaint of dizziness frequently seen in the postconcussion syndrome is seldom of vestibular origin. Neuro-otologic studies in such cases have uniformly given negative results. On the other hand, when a history of true vertigo is elicited, especially in the period immediately after injury, it is probable that an organic basis exists for the complaint of dizziness. The onset of such vertigo occurs immediately or very soon after the trauma to the head and is aggravated by change of position. Ordinarily, it follows a self-limiting course. In such cases, the commonest cause of vertigo is a concomitant concussion of the labyrinth.[28] The following case is illustrative of the syndrome of labyrinthine concussion.

Case 2. B.L. Syndrome of labyrinthine concussion. A 28-year-old white male truck driver was admitted to the Yale-New Haven Hospital (43-19-17) on July 29, 1955, after a boulder being loaded on his truck hit the cab of the truck and the patient's head was struck forcibly. He was rendered unconscious for only a few seconds. When he regained consciousness, he could not remove his hands from the steering wheel. He was transferred promptly to the hospital where x-rays of the cervical spine revealed no fracture or dislocation. The skull was intact. After the radiological examination had been completed, the patient turned his head to the right and experienced objective vertigo. Upon his return to the emergency room, this positional vertigo recurred violently and was accompanied by nausea and vomiting.

Examination was essentially normal except for markedly positive positional tests, with nystagmus being induced in every position of the head, but greatest with the head turned to the right, in which position nausea and vomiting ensued. No hearing loss to whispered voice was noted. Within 2 days he had become sufficiently comfortable to withstand caloric tests, which were done on August 1, 1955. They demonstrated a marked directional preponderance of induced nystagmus to the right. (At 30°C., the left ear showed duration of nystagmus to be 150 seconds; right ear = 85 seconds; at 44°C., left ear = 98 seconds; right ear = 136 seconds). Positional tests induced nystagmus but only mild vertigo. At the time of his discharge from the hospital on August 4, 1955, he experienced only mild transient vertigo on sudden quick movements of the head.

When seen on August 10, 1955, he still complained of mild vertigo with sudden turns. By August 27, 1955, he complained only of mild dizziness but not vertigo. He returned to his job as a truck driver on August 29, 1955. When seen on September 17, 1955, the dizziness had cleared except for mild episodes when going over bumps in his truck, but by the following week, September 24, he was free of all complaints. Caloric tests done on August 17, 1955, were completely normal, with following durations of nystagmus: at 30°C. left ear = 87 seconds and right ear = 94 seconds; at 44°C., left ear = 99 seconds and right ear = 99 seconds.

Summary of Syndrome of Labyrinthine Concussion

This case demonstrates the three characteristic phases of labyrinthine concussion: the acute phase lasting about 48 hours, the recovery phase lasting about 2 weeks, and the convalescent phase which may persist for several months, although it cleared within 2 months in this case. The chronic phase was not seen with this patient. This is the syndrome of labyrinthine concussion.

EXTRACRANIAL CAUSES OF VERTIGO—VASCULAR AND CERVICAL

Sensitivity of Carotid Sinus

A vertiginous syndrome, often violent, may be the only symptom of hyperexcitability of the carotid sinus, according to Aubert.[5] Irritation of the sinus by enlarged lymph nodes may also produce this condition. Symptoms may be altered by turning the head. Since there is no direct connection between the arterial supply to the labyrinth and the carotid system, there is postulated an interference with the anterior petrovestibular parasympathetic plexus, which produces vasodilatation. Aubert[5] further states that injections of procaine around the carotid sinus have provided symptomatic relief.

Carotid Arterial Insufficiency

Carotid arterial insufficiency may produce symptoms of vertigo in those instances in which important collaterals from the carotid circulation supply the base of the brain.[44] The importance of these collaterals may be related either to anomalies of the circle of Willis or to insufficiency of the vertebral arteries. Relief of such vertebrobasilar symptoms by carotid endarterectomy has been reported.[61]

Vertebral Artery Insufficiency in Posterior Fossa Syndromes

With increasing use of angiography, the importance of the vertebral circulation is being discovered in a variety of clinical syndromes, such as basilar impression, the Barré-Liéou syndrome, and neck injuries. The importance of lesions in the vertebral artery was underscored in a recent study of Wallenberg's lateral medullary syndrome by Currier et al.[21] Previously regarded as the result of thrombosis of the posterior-inferior cerebellar artery, it has now been identified by these investigators with vertebral artery thrombosis. Since their own 39 cases were without anatomical verification, they reviewed 38 additional cases from the literature and found that in 32 of these, "there was no primary thrombosis of the posterior-inferior cerebellar artery but rather involvement of the vertebral artery." Although the symptoms are variable, vertigo is common and nystagmus is reported in 36 of 39 cases.

Intermittent Vertebral Artery Compression—Powers' Syndrome

Intermittent vertebral artery compression, described by Powers, Drislane, and Nevins,[76] constitutes a more readily understood cause of vertiginous crises. The syndrome as described by these authors consists of episodic vertigo, syncope, tinnitus, and deafness without evidence of arteriosclerosis. It is differentiated from arteriosclerotic disease of the vertebral arteries in that periods of freedom from symptoms alternate with almost explosive onset of true vertigo. The onset of vertigo is unpredictable but is often associated with rotation or extension of the neck or with emotional tension. The afflicted may show a central type of hearing loss and tinnitus, which may persist after the vertigo ceases. Headache is common and is usually of the tension type, but unilateral and extending from the parieto-occipital to the supraorbital area. Accompanying gastrointestinal symptoms include nausea, vomiting, and occasionally explosive diarrhea. Visual disturbances are manifested by inability to maintain visual concentration for any period of time and hallucinations of flashing lights or horizontal lines. Finally, paresthesia of the upper extremity with vasospastic signs point to the region of the subclavian artery as the source of pathology. Findings in these cases included a positive scalenus tension test, vertigo with the Adson maneuver, and a supraclavicular bruit in one-third of the patients. Accordingly, the treatment was directed toward relieving the compression of the vertebral artery as it arose from the subclavian. This was accomplished by sectioning the scalenus anticus muscle, ligating the thyrocervical trunk when it arose in common with the vertebral artery, and stripping the periarterial sympathetics of the vertebral artery. Results obtained were highly satisfactory, according to the report of the authors.

Subclavian Steal Syndrome

The subclavian steal syndrome can give rise to true vertigo. This interesting syndrome was so named by an editorialist[41] reviewing an article by Reivich and associates,[78] who described the ability of the vertebral arteries to serve as a collateral pathway in occlusion of the subclavian artery. As often occurs with important medical observations, there appeared a little earlier, but almost simultaneously, in Italy an article by Contorini[17] describing this same series of clinical events. Its discovery was made possible by the increasing interest and use of cerebral angiography. The pathological anatomy of this disease consists of occlusion of the subclavian artery proximal to the origin of the vertebral artery. The collateral pathway is up one vertebral pathway and down the other to the involved subclavian. The anastomatic shunt is at the point where the vertebrals join to form the basilar artery. The pathophysiology is equally simple. With increased circulatory demand by activity of the arm on the side of the occluded subclavian artery, there is a greater shunting of blood from the vertebral on the sound side to that of the involved side. This results in a relative ischemia of the brainstem, and vertigo ensues as one of the earliest symptoms. The degree of ischemia will be determined by the demands made upon the shunt and even more so upon the anatomical integrity of the carotid arteries and the adequacy of the anteroposterior communications of the circle of Willis. Thus, the condition may be asymptomatic when the collateral supply from the carotid arteries can compensate for the flow lost through the "subclavian steal." The diagnosis may be suspected when there is a disparity between the blood pressure obtained in the two arms. In a typical case, the blood pressure in one arm may be 100/70, whereas in the other arm it may be 200/80. The brachial and radial pulses will be weak in the involved arm, and a bruit may be heard over the subclavian artery at the medial edge of the scalenus anticus muscle or over the mastoid process. Definite diagnosis will be made by angiography, which should demonstrate contrast medium passing up one vertebral artery and flowing down its opposite number into the subclavian artery. The basilar artery may not be visualized because of this shunt. Treatment will necessitate subclavian endarterectomy and probably patch grafting.

Injuries of the Cervical Spine

Cervical spine injuries may have a causal relation to vestibular symptoms.[18,32,85] In a series of 10 cases with cervical root avulsion, 8 had vestibular symptoms which were more marked with involvement of the lower cervical segments, especially when a Horner's syndrome was present.[33]

Cervical Vertigo and its Mechanisms

Ryan and Cope[82] use the term cervical vertigo to describe a condition accompanying neck injuries or diseases. They reported 5 cases and these were classified in three categories—vertigo due to (1) cervical spondylosis, (2) treatment with neck traction, and (3) trauma, i.e., specific neck and head injuries. In their opinion, the most likely cause is interference of tonic reflexes rather than occlusions of the vertebral artery or disease or damage to the cervical sympathetic system. In a later article,[18] they maintained this position and demonstrated that a positional nystagmus with vertigo similar to that occurring in otolith disease may result from the conditions cited above. It was also their opinion that in the differential diagnosis of cervical vertigo, pain and stiffness of the neck are invariable in the conditions described by them.

In a contrary view, Fields[44] maintained that compression of the vertebral artery resulting in vertigo can be assigned to the following etiological categories: (1) hyperextension and extreme rotation of the head and neck, (2) cervical spondylosis, and (3) cervical trauma and cervical manipulation. Tatlow and Bammer[89] described 3 cases showing neurological signs and symptoms related to turning of the head. All 3 had vertigo. They demonstrated that the vertebral artery can be markedly narrowed by turning of the neck as shown by injections of the artery in a cadaver. Fields[44] demonstrated the same phenomenon in one of his patients. With regard to cervical spondylosis, Fields felt that symptoms would not ensue unless the patient had either atherosclerosis or a vascular anomaly of the collateral channels in addition to cervical spondylosis. The suggestion that removal of the offending osteoarthritic spurs should be beneficial in relieving vertigo and other symptoms has been advanced by Fields[44] and others.[55,84]

Serious Complications of Cervical Trauma—Including Manipulation

Several articles have appeared on the relationship of cervical trauma and cervical manipulation to vascular accidents of the brainstem.[89] Death as a result of cervical manipulation has been documented.[45,77] Increasing interest in the role of cervical trauma in vascular accidents related to the vessels in the neck, both carotids and vertebrals, has arisen as a result of the increasing use of angiography, but it still seems speculative to apply the mechanisms demonstrated in these specific cases to an interpretation of similar symptoms in less well-documented clinical problems. Continued interest in the role of the vertebral arteries in vestibular syndromes should prove rewarding.

REFERENCES

1. Abbott, K. H., Hubbell, D. V., and Vogel, P. J.: The surgical treatment of vertebral aneurysms. Bull. Los Angeles Neurol. Soc. 26: 79-85, 1961.
2. Alpers, B. J., and Forster, F. M.: Atypical clinical features of acoustic nerve tumors. J. Nerv. Ment. Dis. 108:271-284, 1948.
3. Alpers, B. J., and Yaskin, H. E.: The Bruns syndrome. J. Nerv. Ment. Dis. 100:115-134, 1944.
4. Andersen, H. C., Jepsen, O., and Kristiansen, F.: The occurrence of directional preponderance in some intracranial disorders; a study of the Fitzgerald-Hallpike caloric test. Acta Otolaryng. Suppl. 118:19-31, 1954.
5. Aubert, M.: Vertiges et Surdités d'Origine Vasculaire. Paris, Masson et Cie, 1958.
6. Aubry, M., and Pialoux, P.: Maladies de l'Oreille Interne et Otoneurologie. Paris, Masson et Cie, 1957.
7. Baker, H. L.: Myelographic examination of the posterior fossa with positive contrast medium. Radiology 81:791-801, 1963.
8. Barnett, H. J., and Hyland, H. H.: Tumors involving the brain-stem. A study of 90 cases arising in the brain-stem, fourth ventricle, and pineal tissue. Quart. J. Med. 21:265-284, 1952.
9. Barré, J.: As quoted in Laskiewicz.
10. Bauer, E.: Tumorzellen im Liquor cerebrospinalis (meningitis carcinomatosa). Z. Laryng. Rhinol. 43:191-195, 1943.
11. Borck, W. F., and Tönnis, W.: Zur Differentialdiagnose infratentorieller Geschwülste. Fortschr. Neurol. Psychiat. 4:125-166, 1955.
12. Bray, P. F., Carter, S., and Taveras, J. M.: Brain-stem tumors in children. Neurology 8:1-7, 1958.
13. Bruns: As quoted in Alpers and Yaskin.
14. Bucy, P. C., and Kiplinger, J. E.: Tumors of the brain-stem with special reference to ocular manifestations. Arch. Opthal. (Chicago) 62:541-554, 1959.
15. Carmichael, E. A., Dix, M. R., and Hallpike, C. S.: Lesions of the cerebral hemispheres and their effects upon optokinetic and caloric nystagmus. Brain 77:345-372, 1954.
16. Castellano, F., and Ruggiero, G.: Meningiomas of the posterior fossa. Acta Radiol. Suppl. 104:1-177, 1953.
17. Contorini, L.: Il circolo collaterale vertebro-vertebrale nella obliterazione dell'arteria succlavia alla sue origine. Minerva Chir. 15:268-271, 1960.
18. Cope, S., and Ryan, G. M. S.: Cervical and otolith vertigo. J. Laryng. 73:113-120, 1959.
19. Cramer, F., and Kimsey, W.: The cerebellar hemangioblastomas. Review of 53 cases with special reference to cerebellar cysts and the association of polycythemia. Arch. Neurol. Psychiat. (Chicago) 67:237-252, 1952.

20. Cuneo, H. M., and Rand, C. W.: Brain Tumors of Childhood. Springfield, Ill., Charles C Thomas, 1952.
21. Currier, R. D., Giles, C. L. and Dejong, R. N.: Some comments on Wallenberg's lateral medullary syndrome. Neurology 11: 778-791, 1961.
22. Cushing, H.: Tumors of the Nervus Acusticus. Philadelphia, W. B. Saunders Co., 1917.
23. Cushing, H.: Intracranial Tumors. Springfield, Ill., Charles C Thomas, 1932.
24. Cushing, H.: Meningiomas. Springfield, Ill., Charles C Thomas, 1938.
25. Dandy, W. E.: Benign Tumors in the Third Ventricle of the Brain: Diagnosis and Treatment. Springfield, Ill., Charles C Thomas, 1933.
26. Dandy, W. E.: Lewis' practice of surgery. *In:* The Brain. Hagerstown, Md., W. F. Prior Co., 1963.
27. Davey, L. M.: Evaluation of bicaloric test of vestibular function. U.S. Naval Med. Res. Lab. Report No. 411, Vol. 22, 18pp., 1963.
28. Davey, L. M.: Labyrinthine trauma in head injury. Conn. Med. 29:250-255, 1965.
29. Davey, L. M.: Neuro-otological studies in neurosurgical diagnoses. (In preparation.)
30. Davey, L. M., and German, W. J.: The vestibular system and its disorders. Ann. Rev. Med. 13:431-446, 1962.
31. Davey, L. M., and German, W. J.: Aneurysms of the posterior cerebral circulation simulating brain tumors. (In preparation.)
32. Decker, H.: Disorders of equilibrium in the cervical syndrome. HNO 8:328-332, 1960.
33. Decker, H., Rohr, H., and Unterharnscheidt, F.: The influence of traumatic cervical root avulsion on the auditory and labyrinth apparatus. HNO. 7:365-372, 1959.
34. D'Errico, A.: Meningiomas of the cerebellar fossa. J. Neurosurg. 7:227-232, 1950.
35. DeWeese, D. D.: Dizziness: An Evaluation and Classification. Springfield, Ill., Charles C Thomas, 1954.
36. Dix, M. R., and Hallpike, C. S.: Discussion of acoustic neuroma. Proc. Roy. Soc. Med. 51:889-897, 1958.
37. Dott, N. M.: Facial paralysis—restitution by extra-petrous nerve graft. Proc. Roy. Soc. Med. 51:900-902, 1958.
38. Drake, C. G.: Acoustic neuroma. Repair of facial nerve with autogenous graft. J. Neurosurg. 17:836-842, 1960.
39. Drake, C. G.: Intracranial facial nerve reconstruction. Arch Otolaryng. 78:456-460, 1963.
40. Drake, C. G.: Personal communications.
41. Editorial: New vascular syndrome—"The Subclavian Steal." New Eng. J. Med. 265:912-913, 1961.
42. Edwards, C. H., and Patterson, J. H.: A review of the symptoms and signs of acoustic neurofibromata. Brain. 74:144-190, 1951.
43. Evans, N., and Courville, C. B.: The nervus acousticus. Pathologic conditions involving the eighth nerve and the cerebellopontine angle. Laryngoscope 42:432-455, 1932.
44. Fields, W. S., and Weibel, J.: Effects of vascular disorders on the vestibular system. *In:* Neurological Aspects of Auditory and Vestibular Disorders. Springfield, Ill., Charles C Thomas, 1964, pp. 305-340.
45. Ford, F. R., and Clark, D.: Thrombosis of the basilar artery with softenings in cerebellum and brain stem due to manipulation of the neck; report of 2 cases with one postmortem examination. Reasons are given to prove that damage to vertebral arteries is responsible. Bull. Hopkins Hosp. 98:37-42, 1956.
46. Freeman, D. G., Petrohelos, M. A., and Henderson, J. W.: Neurologic symptoms and signs in 347 cases of verified brain tumor. Neurology 3:437-452, 1953.
47. Friedman, A. P., Brenner, C., and Denny-Brown, D.: Post-traumatic vertigo and dizziness. J. Neurosurg. 2:36-46, 1945.
48. Garcin, R., and Oeconomos, D.: Les Aspects Neurologiques des Malformations Congénitales de la Charnière Cranio-Rachidienne. Paris, Masson & Cie., 1953.
49. Gelb, H., and Arnold, G. E.: Syndromes of the head and neck of dental origin: I. Pain caused by mandibular dysfunction. J. Dent. Med. 14:201-212, 1959.
50. German, W. J.: Acoustic neurinomas: a follow-up. Clin. Neurosurg. 7:21-39, 1961.
51. Givre, A.: Clinical-statistical studies of tumors of the cerebellopontine angle. Arch. Neurochir. 2:97-108, 1945.
52. Golding-Wood, P. H.: Observations on sympathectomy in the treatment of Meniere's disease. J. Laryng. 74:951-970, 1960.
53. Grant, F. C., Webster, J. E., and Weinberger, L. M.: Unusual symptomatology with tumors of the cerebellum based on 158 verified cases. Amer. J. Med. Sci. 202:313-329, 1941.
54. Green, R. E.: Surgical treatment of vertigo with follow-up on Walter Dandy's cases: neurologic aspects. Clin. Neurosurg. 6:141-152, 1959.
55. Hardin, C. A., Williamson, W. P., and Steegman, A.: Vertebral artery insufficiency produced by cervical osteoarthritic spurs. Neurology 7:331-340, 1957.

56. Hardy, M., and Crowe, S. J.: Early asymptomatic acoustic tumor. Report of 6 cases. Arch. Surg. 32:292-301, 1936.

57. Holmes, G.: Vertigo from the neurological standpoint. Proc. Roy. Soc. Med. 17:6-10, 1924.

58. House, W. F.: Vestibular nerve section and its effect on hearing. *In:* Neurological Aspects of Auditory and Vestibular Disorders. Springfield, Ill., Charles C Thomas, 1964, pp. 94-103.

59. House, W. F. (Ed.): Monograph. Transtemporal Bone Microsurgical Removal of Acoustic Neuromas. Arch. Otolaryng. 80:597-756, 1964.

60. House, W. F.: Evolution of transtemporal bone removal of acoustic tumors. Arch. Otolaryng. 80:731-742, 1964.

61. Humphries, A. W.: Relief of vertebrobasilar symptoms by carotid endarterectomy. Surgery 57:48-52, 1965.

62. Jatho, K.: Die Arachnitis des Kleinhirnbrückenwinkels und ihre audiologische Diagnostik. Z. Laryng. Rhinol. 34:156-170, 1955.

63. Knowles, J. H., and Smith, L. H., Jr.: Extrapulmonary manifestations of bronchogenic carcinoma. New Eng. J. Med. 262:505-510, 1960.

64. Krayenbühl, H., and Yasargil, M. G.: Die vaskularen Erkrankungen im Gebiet der Arteria vertebralis und Arteria basialis. Stuttgart, Georg Thieme Verlag, 1957.

65. Lapayowker, M. S., Carter, B. L., and McGann, M. J.: The use of plesiosectional tomography in the diagnosis of eighth nerve tumors. Amer. J. Roentgen. 88:1187-1193, 1962.

66. Laskiewicz, A.: Cervical spondylosis and the ear. Acta Otolaryng. 51:403-411, 1960.

67. Levy, I., and O'Leary, J. L.: Incidence of vertigo in neurological conditions. Ann. Otol. 56:557-575, 1947.

68. Liéou: As quoted in Laskiewicz.

69. Macrae, D.: The neurologic aspects of vertigo. Calif. Med. 92:255-259, 1960.

70. Markham, J. W., Fager, C. A., Horrax, G., and Poppen, J. L.: Meningiomas of the posterior fossa. Arch. Neurol. Psychiat. (Chicago) 74:163-170, 1955.

71. Mayoux, R.: Quelques Notions Nouvelles sur le Vertige. Methodes d'Exploration de l'Appareil Vestibulaire. Paris, Masson & Cie, 1953.

72. McKenzie, K. G.: Intracranial divisions of the vestibular portion of the auditory nerve for Meniere's disease. Canad. Med. Ass. J. 34:369-381, 1936.

73. Miller-Guerra: Le Syndrome Cérébelleux et le Syndrome Vestibulaire. Paris, Masson & Cie, 1954.

74. Olivercrona, H., and Ladenheim, J.: Congenital arteriovenous aneurysms of the carotid and vertebral arterial systems. Stuttgart, Springer Verlag, 1957.

75. Pool, J. L., and Pava, A. A.: The Early Diagnosis and Treatment of Acoustic Nerve Tumors. Springfield, Ill., Charles C Thomas, 1957.

76. Powers, S. R., Drislane, T. M., and Nevins, S.: Intermittent vertebral artery compression: a new syndrome. Surgery 49:257-264, 1961.

77. Pratt-Thomas, H. R., Berger, K. E.: Cerebellar and spinal injuries after chiropractic manipulation. J.A.M.A. 133:600-603, 1947.

78. Reivich, M., Holling, H. E., Roberts, B., and Toole, J. F. Reversal of blood flow through the vertebral artery and its effect on cerebral circulation. New Eng. J. Med. 265: 878-885, 1961.

79. Revilla, A. G.: Differential diagnosis of tumors at the cerebellopontile recess. Bull. Hopkins Hosp. 83:187-212, 1948.

80. Ruggles, R. L., and Cassady, C.: Otitic temporal lobe abscesses. Laryngoscope 75:1259-1267, 1965.

81. Russell, J. R., and Bucy, P. C.: Meningiomas of the posterior fossa. Surg. Gynec. Obst. 96: 183-192, 1953.

82. Ryan, G. M. S., and Cope, S.: Cervical vertigo. Lancet 2:1355-1358, 1955.

83. Shafron, M.: Pantopaque examination of the cerebellopontine angle. Radiology 85:921-925, 1965.

84. Sheehan, S., Bauer, R. B., and Meyer, J. S.: Vertebral artery compression in cervical spondylosis. Neurology 10:968-986, 1960.

85. Spector, M.: Positional vertigo due to neck lesions. Med. Times, April 1962.

86. Spillane, J. D.: Developmental anomalies in the region of the foramen magnum. *In:* Modern Trends in Neurology, 2nd Series. New York, Paul B. Hoeber, Inc., 1957, pp. 240-258.

87. Stewart, T. G., and Holmes, G.: Symptomatology of cerebellar tumors: a study of 40 cases. Brain 27:522-591, 1904.

88. Symonds, C. P., and Meadows, S. P.: Compression of the spinal cord in the neighborhood of the foramen magnum. Brain 60:52-84, 1937.

89. Tatlow, W. F. T., and Bammer, H. G.: Syndrome

of vertebral artery compression. Neurology 7:331-340, 1957.

90. Taylor, A. R., and Chakravorty, B. C.: Clinical syndromes associated with basilar impression. Arch. Neurol. 10:475-484, 1964.

91. Thiébaut, F., Rohmer, F., Greiner, G. F., and Mengus, M.: Vertiges et surdité gauche; malformation vasculaire; guérison aprés section du VIII. Rev. Otoneurolog. 28:115-118, 1956.

92. Torok, N.: Review of neuro-otology pathogenesis of neuro-otological diseases. Amer. J. Med. Sci. 246:496-513, 1963.

93. Zimmerman, H. M., and German, W. J.: Colloid tumors of the third ventricle. Arch. Neurol. Psychiat. 30:309-325, 1933.

CHAPTER 14

Ocular Causes of Vertigo

OWEN BELMONT

If by vertigo one means a sense of rotation, then there is no truly ocular vertigo. Ocular vertigo is rather an unsteadiness or disorientation caused by a conflict in the data gathered by the eyes, the labyrinths, and the proprioceptive receptors. Most commonly, ocular vertigo is caused by a recent paralysis of an extraocular muscle. Milder forms of ocular vertigo are seen in patients made uncomfortable by spectacles, great heights, or travel.

PARALYSIS OF AN EXTRAOCULAR MUSCLE

The most common extraocular muscle palsy is that of the lateral rectus. For example, following a blow on the head, a man can no longer abduct his right eye. He complains of the classic symptoms of lateral rectus palsy: diplopia (in this case, worse on looking to the right), confusion (superimposition of dissimilar images), vertigo, and past pointing when fixing with the paretic eye.

The severity of these symptoms varies with the age of the patient. Infants and young children suffer less than those over the age of 6. Visual maturity occurs at 5 to 7. After this, suppression of one eye becomes increasingly difficult, so that a 3-year-old may complain of diplopia for only a few days after the onset of a paralytic squint, while a 20-year-old may complain of diplopia for years.

When a patient with paralysis of the right lateral rectus muscle looks to the right, the image falls on the fovea of the left eye and nasal to the fovea of the right eye. The further he turns his eyes to the right, the greater the separation of the images. As he turns his head to the right, the images approach each other and fuse. To minimize this variable diplopia he may turn his head to the right, so that his eyes remain turned left when viewing an object straight ahead.

In paresis of the right lateral rectus muscle, diplopia will be greater and more annoying if the patient fixes with the paretic (right) eye than if he fixes with the nonparetic (left) eye. In order to fix an object straight ahead, when fixing with the right eye, abnormally strong nervous impulses are sent to the paretic right lateral rectus muscle, and equally strong impulses are sent to the yoke muscle, the left medial rectus. On the other hand, if the nonparetic (left) eye is fixing, a normal impulse is sent to the left lateral rectus muscle and to its yoke muscle, the right medial rectus. For this reason, the amount of esotropia will be greater with the paretic eye fixing than with the nonparetic eye fixing.

When a vertically acting muscle, such as the superior oblique, is paralyzed, in addition to the vertical separation of the retinal images a torsional displacement of the images adds to the patient's discomfort. In an effort to minimize the separation of the retinal images, the patient may adopt a torticollis. Children are usually more successful than adults in finding a position that will minimize diplopia. An adult may not show a head tilt, but will suffer more from nausea, diplopia, and faulty orientation in space.

When vertigo is caused by paralysis of an extraocular muscle, the cause is usually obvious. The ocular etiology is easily verified; if both eyes are closed, relief is quick. Occlusion of the paretic eye eliminates the diplopia, vertigo, and past pointing. Occlusion of the sound eye eliminates the diplopia but not the vertigo and past pointing.

Past Pointing in Paralysis of an Extraocular Muscle

In the instance of a patient with a paresis of the right lateral rectus muscle, when he attempts to fix an object to the right with his right eye and then points to the object, he will past point. That is, he will point out the object as though it were farther to the right. In the past it has been suggested that because increased innervation was required to abduct the right eye, the individual concluded that the object was farther right than it was; so he past pointed. This explanation has now been rejected. It is now believed that the reason for past pointing is that the abduction of the eye is not strong enough to center the image directly on the fovea. Instead, it is focused slightly nasal to the fovea. Since the retinal elements nasal to the fovea have a temporal directional value, the object is seen as more temporal than it actually is. The larger the test objects used, the greater the past pointing, since retinal elements stimulated are apt to be located further away from the fovea on its nasal side.[2]

DISTURBED ORIENTATION IN SPACE FROM SPECTACLE LENSES

Vertigo and disturbed orientation from spectacles present no diagnostic problem, since the symptoms are relieved by removing the offending glasses. Nevertheless, the subject deserves some attention. Spectacles may disturb an individual's orientation in space through overcorrection of his error, prismatic effects, meridional magnification, and aniseikonia (inequality in size of retinal images).

Overcorrection. A patient overcorrected for myopia or hyperopia frequently complains of giddiness or confusion. This is associated with intermittent blurring and clearing of the retinal images. In most instances the cause is obvious and the patient sees to it that the lenses are replaced by a suitable pair.

Prismatic Effects. When the shape of a spectacle frame is changed, the height of the optical centers may be different from that in the previous spectacles. A hyperope who looks through his lenses decentered up, or a myope who looks through his lenses decentered down, will complain of feeling as if he were on stilts. This results from a base-up prismatic effect. Since images are displaced toward the apex of a prism, the floor is displaced down, and the patient feels 10 feet tall.

On the other hand, if a myope looks through his lenses decentered up, or a hyperope through his lenses decentered down, he feels as if he is standing in a hole. Or, he may complain that the glasses magnify. We tend to judge the size of objects by their height. The illusion is created by a base-down prismatic effect, which displaces images up. The remedy is to correct the adjustment of the frame, raising or lowering it as indicated, or to revert to a frame identical to the previous one. If nothing is done, the patient may adapt to the new lenses in many instances.

Meridional Magnification. Astigmatic corrections, made by cylindrical lenses, cause a small but definite change in image size which is not the same in all meridians. Convex cylindrical lenses magnify at right angles to their axes. Concave cylindrical lenses minify at right angles to their axes. When strong cylindrical lenses are prescribed at oblique axes, there is a tilting of the vertical and horizontal meridians when the patient looks through them. The patient may feel that the sidewalk is tilted, and buildings may seem about to fall. This sensation may disappear after wearing the glasses several weeks, or it may persist for years. In those who remain uncomfortable, the power of the cylindrical lens may be reduced, and the equivalent of the reduction substituted as a spherical lens.

Aniseikonia. In a binocular individual with good depth perception, after correction of the refractive error by spectacle lenses, a difference in the size of retinal images in the two eyes may occur, usually when the refractive error is radically different in the two eyes. This causes faulty orientation in space and may result in a sensation described by the patient as giddiness or dizziness.

Meridional magnification in binocular individuals is a form of aniseikonia, although meridional magnification can cause distortions in a monocular individual, while aniseikonia by definition is always a binocular phenomenon. Patients suffering from aniseikonia likewise complain that the floor is slanted and buildings seem about to topple; they may also make errors in judgments requiring accurate depth perception. One patient said that when driving with her glasses on, an approaching car would at first seem a block away and then would suddenly appear close before her. When the retinal images were equalized by use of contact lenses, she felt much more sure of herself in driving.

In most people, the confusion and disorientation that occurs on first wearing a pair of glasses that create unequal retinal images will disappear in a few days to a few weeks. Such patients have learned to suppress their binocular clues to depth perception in favor of monocular clues, the clues born of experience. These have been listed by Adler[2] as interposition of one object before another, customary size of objects, color and haziness of objects, convergence of lines to the vanishing point, and shadows. However, in unfamiliar surroundings, as in a forest, this suppression may suddenly fail and the disturbed orientation in space reappear. Failure to suppress stereoscopic depth perception is more apt to occur when fatigued. In any case, the conflict between monocular and binocular clues may cause tension and a vague malaise.

The disturbing effects of aniseikonia may be minimized by several stratagems:

1. *Substituting overall aniseikonia for meridional aniseikonia.* This is done by using equivalent spherical lenses for part or all of strong cylindric lenses. Clinically, overall aniseikonia is better tolerated than meridional aniseikonia.

2. *Undercorrection of one eye.* This helps in two ways. First, by using a weaker lens to undercorrect the poorer eye, the magnifying effect of the lens is smaller and the disparity in image size is decreased. Second, approximately equal visual acuity is one of the prerequisites for binocular vision, and since only a binocular individual can suffer from aniseikonia, the patient is given relief by thus converting him into a monocular individual.

3. *Contact lenses.* Because they are much closer to the eyes, contact lenses cause less magnification or minification of the retinal image. When substituted for spectacle lenses, they will cause formation of retinal images less disparate in size.

4. *Size, or iseikonic lenses.* By altering the shape and thickness of spectacle lenses, their effect on retinal image size can be changed while keeping their dioptric power constant. Since corneal contact lenses have become popular, they have been used for many patients who formerly might have been given thick and unsightly size lenses.

OCULAR VERTIGO CAUSED BY HEIGHTS

Adler[1] has pointed out that although fear of falling plays a part, vertigo caused by heights is chiefly ocular in origin. The person who looks down from a cliff or a tall building is upset by the transfer of the vanishing point from the horizon to a point below him. The lower part of his body is also seen as he looks down to the vanishing point, and this adds to his confusion. The same individual who cannot bear to look down to the street from a 30-story building will be able to look out the window of an aircraft at 30,000 feet without fear. Now there is no structure below him that vanishes to a point below. If the aircraft descends and passes low over a skyscraper, the ocular vertigo may reappear.

Ocular Vertigo in Blind Flying. A pilot who is flying blind through fog may develop vertigo because of conflicting data gathered by his eyes and his labyrinths.[1] Since the horizon is invisible, his visual sensations are used to orient himself within the plane only. The labyrinth meanwhile registers changes in orientation to the horizon, and the conflict between the ocular and labyrinthine data may cause confusion and dizziness. The much-touted sensation arising from the seat of the pants is of little help. The pilot who is untrained in instrument flying and cut off from a view of the horizon will go into a tight spiral dive to the left (the "graveyard spiral") within 12 seconds. "You can't depend on your normal senses to control an airplane when you are shut off from the ground or from the horizon. You will get a strong sensation that you are climbing, when actually you are flying straight and level, so you shove the wheel to get the nose down and all of a sudden you are in a dive."[5]

OCULAR VERTIGO IN TRAVEL

Certain individuals may complain of headache, nausea, and even vertigo when riding in a train or automobile. Looking out the side window, the eyes reflexly fix passing objects, follow them out of sight, then return to fix on new objects. The result is optokinetic nystagmus. In susceptible individuals this activity is poorly tolerated, resulting in the so-called panoramic headache.

This type of car sickness occurs more frequently and more severely in patients with vertical oculomotor imbalance. It is therefore important to try to correct vertical phorias by incorporating appropriate vertical prisms into the spectacle prescription. Often this gives relief. If this fails, the simplest remedy for those suffering from panoramic headache is to refrain from looking out side windows. Such patients may often read a book on a vibrating, bouncing train with impunity so long as they remember not to look out the window.

Physiologic Basis for Optokinetic Nystagmus. Adler[2] has stated:

> In man, the most important source of reflex tonus comes from the visual impulses themselves. The importance of this source of tonus increases as one ascends the scale of animal life, and at the same time the effectiveness of the vestibular and neck reflexes diminishes in the same proportion. Thus, we find in the lower vertebrates, such as the rabbit or guinea pig, that the tonic reflexes of the neck and otolith apparatus are extremely effective in determining the position of the eyes in their orbits. It is at the same time difficult to demonstrate any change in position of the eyes of this animal with changing patterns in the animal's visual field. In man, however, the neck reflexes are relatively ineffective, and the eyes show no deviations in response to turning the head on the neck, provided of course that the head is turned slowly to avoid stimulation of the semicircular canals. On the other hand, changes in the visual fields, even when of slight attention value, can be shown to produce marked changes in the ocular muscle tonus.

When, as occurs in a person looking out a train window or observing an optokinetic drum, a series of moving objects attract the attention, the following movements of the eyes and the recovery movements when the object passes out of sight cause a rhythmic oscillation of the eyes called optokinetic nystagmus. The amplitude of this nystagmus depends on the interest aroused by the passing objects. Thus, people or houses will excite a nystagmus of greater amplitude than telegraph poles or trees. Optokinetic nystagmus may be considered an adaptation to movement of the environment, while labyrinthine nystagmus is an adaptation to movement of the head.

Clinical Methods for Eliciting Optokinetic Nystagmus. The most powerful method for eliciting optokinetic nystagmus is to seat the patient in the center of a huge drum, the inner surface of which is painted with vertical stripes. When the drum is rotated about the patient, it is almost impossible for a normal individual to suppress optokinetic nystagmus. For practical reasons, the usual device for eliciting optokinetic nystagmus is a drum about 30 cm. high by 25 cm. in diameter. The surface has black and white vertical stripes, 1.5 cm. wide. The drum is rotated about its vertical axis, taking 1 to 2 seconds for a complete revolution.[3]

The optokinetic drum may be used to help differentiate between spontaneous vestibular nystagmus and fixation nystagmus.

> If a patient shows spontaneous nystagmus, and it is doubtful whether it is a fixation nystagmus from infancy or a vestibular nystagmus, the optokinetic drum is rotated in front of the patient. If the drum is rotated to the right,

nystagmus to the left (and vice versa) should appear, or rather should be superimposed on the pre-existent spontaneous nystagmus. If, e.g., in a case of spontaneous vestibular nystagmus to the left, the drum is rotated to the right, the left nystagmus becomes stronger, as it is the sum of the spontaneous vestibular and the newly elicited optokinetic nystagmus; whereas, on turning the drum to the left, the spontaneous left nystagmus becomes weaker or is even changed to a right nystagmus.

In contrast, in spontaneous fixation nystagmus the appearance of the spontaneous nystagmus either remains unchanged in spite of the turning of the drum, or irregular jerks *in* the direction of the drum movement are superimposed (inversion of the O.N.).[3]

Optokinetic Nystagmus and Topical Neuro-ophthalmologic Diagnosis. J. Lawton Smith has written a valuable monograph on optokinetic nystagmus and its use in topical neuro-ophthalmologic diagnosis.[5] Smith quotes numerous case histories to support Cords' hypothesis.

Cords proposed the most reasonable explanation thus far provided to explain the interrelationship between homonymous hemianopias and optokinetic disturbances. He reasoned that the most logical site for a single lesion to simultaneously produce a hemianopia and an optokinetic abnormality was where the corticopetal and corticofugal visual fibers lie in apposition. This is in the area of the internal and external sagittal strata as they pass around the posterior and lateral aspects of the lateral ventricles, and involves the middle and posterior one third of the optic radiations. Involvement here is seen clinically with deep *parietal* lobe lesions. According to this reasoning, therefore, lesions involving the optic tracts, lateral geniculate body, temporal lobe and occipital lobe may produce full hemianopias, but normal optokinetic responses (a negative O.N. sign) would be expected in such instances. On the other hand, with parietal lobe lesions, hemianopias would be seen with asymetric horizontal optokinetic responses (positive O.N. sign).[5]

Smith points out that diminished or absent optokinetic responses may occur in normal individuals who are inattentive, or in those who have been taking barbiturates, tranquilizers, sedatives, narcotics, dilantin, etc. Barbiturates may cause drug nystagmus to appear, while simultaneously suppressing optokinetic nystagmus. Such drug nystagmus is not seen when the patient looks straight ahead, but may occur in extreme lateral gaze (end position nystagmus) and also as a vertical nystagmus in upward gaze.

Smith also describes the use of optokinetic nystagmus to differentiate the vertical nystagmus of brainstem lesions and drug nystagmus: "One must be quite cautious in making any neurologic interpretations of the optokinetic responses found in patients with brainstem lesions. Lateralization of the lesion is particularly fraught with difficulty."[5] Nevertheless, he points out numerous applications of the optokinetic response in lesions of the brainstem. For instance, in parkinsonism there may be an optokinetic response to up-targets but not down-targets, or vice versa. See-saw nystagmus may not be suppressed with cold caloric stimulation or by rotation, yet it may be suppressed by the optokinetic drum. See-saw nystagmus, Smith states, is always associated with a lesion involving the chiasm and causing bitemporal hemianopia.

Smith emphasizes that one must differentiate cerebral from brainstem lesions when interpreting optokinetic responses. In patients complaining of perioral paresthesias, diplopia, or vertigo, one suspects basilar rather than carotid arterial involvement.

BASIC EYE EXAMINATION IN VERTIGO

One need not be an ophthalmologist to examine the eyes as part of an evaluation of a patient with vertigo.

History. The patient can be asked whether he has noted any visual symptoms in association with his dizziness. Diplopia, visual field defects, apparent movement of the environment, distress on looking out of a car window, and recent changes of glasses are all valuable leads. Is the vertigo relieved by occlusion of one eye, or both eyes? If it is not relieved by closing one eye, it is not caused by extraocular muscle palsy; if it is not relieved by closing both eyes, it is not ocular in origin.

Visual Acuity. Patients are sometimes blind in one eye without knowing it. A visual acuity with and without glasses takes little time and may surprise both doctor and patient.

Ocular Rotations. Watch for fine fixation nystagmus, slower pendular nystagmus, or vestibular nystagmus. Look for end-position nystagmus, as well as paresis of one of the oculorotary muscles.

Pupils. Check for equality, regularity, response to light and accommodation, direct and consensual response.

Fundus. The most common error made by the nonophthalmologist in fundus examination is false economy in the choice of an ophthalmoscope. This is usually a battered veteran of medical school days which would be difficult for even an expert to use. The less experienced the examiner, the more important it is that he use a good ophthalmoscope. This need not be expensive. The writer's personal preference is the Keeler Practitioner with the large battery handle. This sells for $65.00 and has a macula attachment which enables one to visualize the fundus through a small pupil.

Every ophthalmoscope should be kept in a dust-proof case when not in use, because the clarity and brightness of the fundus view is soon dimmed by accretions of dust and grease. Even so, the head should be mailed back to the factory every few years for cleaning and reconditioning. This is inexpensive.

If a mydriatic is necessary, 1 per cent Paredrine may be used. After the examination, this should be neutralized by a drop of one-half per cent pilocarpine to minimize the hazard of acute narrow-angle glaucoma. No mydriatic should be used if a patient has glaucoma. Because the fundus is magnified 16 times when viewed with the direct ophthalmoscope, one often picks up a very fine fixation nystagmus that was missed on external examination.

The examiner should familiarize himself with the appearance of the normal nerve head, so that he can detect papilledema, optic atrophy, or excavation of the nerve head. The degree to which long-standing hypertension has caused sclerosis of the arteriolar walls and arteriovenous nicking can be observed. Abnormalities of the retinal vessels are usually matched by similar changes elsewhere in the central nervous system. The same may be true of retinal hemorrhages and exudates.

Confrontation Fields. The examiner confronts the patient and occludes his own left eye while the patient occludes his own right eye. The test object, preferably a 3 to 5 mm. white ball on a wand, is brought in from the periphery at different meridians. The patient signals his first glimpse of the test object as the examiner compares the patient's visual field with his own. This is then repeated for the other eye. If a visual field defect is suspected, it should be confirmed by perimetry.

SUMMARY

As perhaps the most important avenue of sensory data gathered by the central nervous system, the eyes should be evaluated as part of any study of a patient with vertigo. Ocular vertigo is a sense of unsteadiness and confusion rather than rotation.

Ocular vertigo can be associated with paralysis of an extraocular muscle, faulty spectacles, great heights, and travel.

Optokinetic nystagmus may be elicited clinically as an aid in topical neuro-ophthalmologic diagnosis.

A brief ophthalmic survey should be part of every evaluation of a patient complaining of vertigo.

REFERENCES

1. Adler, F. H.: Ocular vertigo. Trans. Amer. Acad. Ophthal. 46:27, 1942.
2. Adler, F. H.: Physiology of the Eye, 3rd ed. St. Louis, C. V. Mosby Co., 1965.
3. Kestenbaum, A.: Clinical Methods of Neuro-Ophthalmological Examination. New York, Grune and Stratton, 1961.
4. Smith, F. K.: Week-End Pilot. New York, Random House, 1957.
5. Smith, J. L.: Optokinetic Nystagmus. Springfield, Ill., Charles C Thomas, 1963.

CHAPTER 15

Odontogenic Dizziness and Related Symptoms

DAVID J. GOODFRIEND

Dizziness and related auditory, vagal, and ocular symptoms may be predisposed and caused by traumatic malrelationships of the temporomandibular joints as the result of abnormalities of the masticatory system. The temporomandibular joints are situated in a critical part of the head in close anatomical relations with the auditory and vestibular conduction systems. The fossa of the temporomandibular joint is in the temporal bone, separated from the pars tympani by the petrotympanic or glacerian fissure. This fissure is an opening between the middle ear or tympanic cavity and the temporomandibular joint. It is traversed by the anterior tympanic artery, the chorda tympani nerve, and the malleus-mandibular ligament. The malleus-mandibular ligament extends from the anterior process of the malleus to the capsule and meniscus of the temporomandibular joint, as illustrated by Figure 1.

The nerve and blood supply of the external auditory meatus, the tympanic membrane, the tensor tympani and tensor veli palatini muscles, and the temporomandibular joint are provided by branches of the auriculotemporal segment of the fifth cranial nerve and by branches of the internal maxillary artery. The

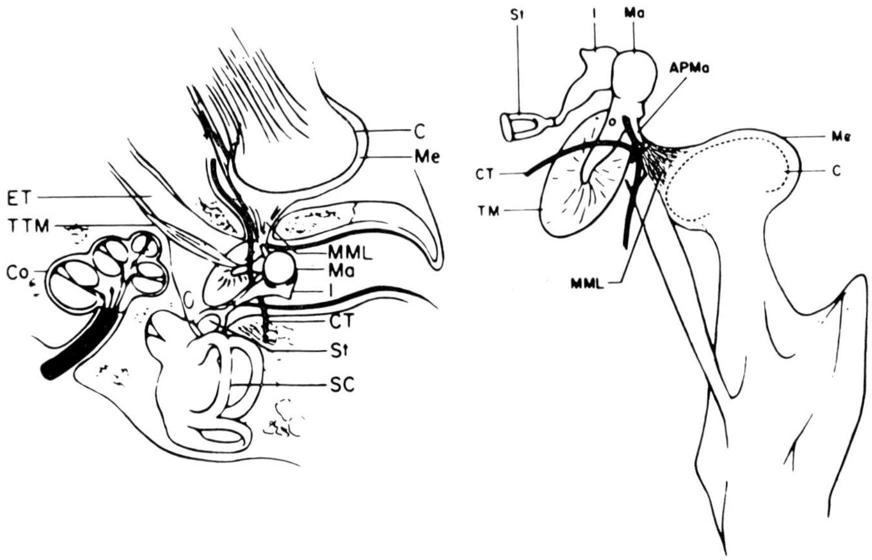

FIG. 1 (left). Anatomical interrelationships of the auditory and vestibular systems with the temporomandibular joint viewed from above, showing anterior malleolar ligament (MML) and chorda tympani (CT) traversing the petrotympanic fissure (an opening from the middle ear to the fossa of the temporomandibular joint).

FIG. 1 (right). Middle ear and temporomandibular joint region viewed from behind, showing ligament (MML) extending from the anterior process of the malleus (APMa) to the meniscus (Me) and capsule of the temporomandibular joint condyle (C).

nerves and blood vessels which supply the meatus, drum, middle ear, and the temporomandibular joint pass behind the joint condyle to enter the ear and joint. The veins that drain these parts and the labyrinth traverse the temporomandibular joint region to enter the pterygoid venous plexus, as illustrated by Figure 2.

The significance of these close anatomical and neurovascular interrelationships in considering auditory and vestibular symptoms is shown by the fact that the temporomandibular joint condyle moves backward and upward with the closing of the jaws. The backward-upward movement of the condyle stops with the contact of the teeth. If the contact of the teeth permits the jaws to overclose, the temporomandibular joints overclose and the overclosed joint condyle is in traumatic malrelations with the organs of the auditory and vestibular conduction systems and their neurovascular supply.

Normal adequate contact of the teeth or dental occlusion locates the closed condyle in the center of the joint fossa about 5 mm. anterior and lateral to the external auditory meatus, the anterior attachment of the tympanic membrane, the petrotympanic fissure, the tympanic cavity, and the bony part of the eustachian tube, as shown by Figure 3. The space between the posterior and medial border of the joint condyle is occupied by a cone of the parotid gland and loose connective tissue. It is traversed by the nerves and vessels that supply the joint and adjacent parts of the ear, and by the malleus-mandibular ligament and the chorda tympani nerve. The interarticular fibrocartilagenous meniscus of the temporomandibular joint surrounds the condyle and acts as a protective shock absorber to the adjacent organs of the ear. The meniscus also moves backward and upward with the closing of the jaw, and since the malleus and tympanic membrane are attached to the meniscus by the malleus-mandibular ligament, they also move with movements of the temporomandibular joint.

Dental occlusal abnormalities—such as attrition, breakdown, loss and irregularities of the bite-supporting teeth, and inadequate fillings, crowns, bridges, and dentures which permit the jaw and temporomandibular joint to overclose—result in traumatic malrelations of the closed condyle with the adjacent organs of the ear and their neurovascular supplies. This may result in contact of the condyle

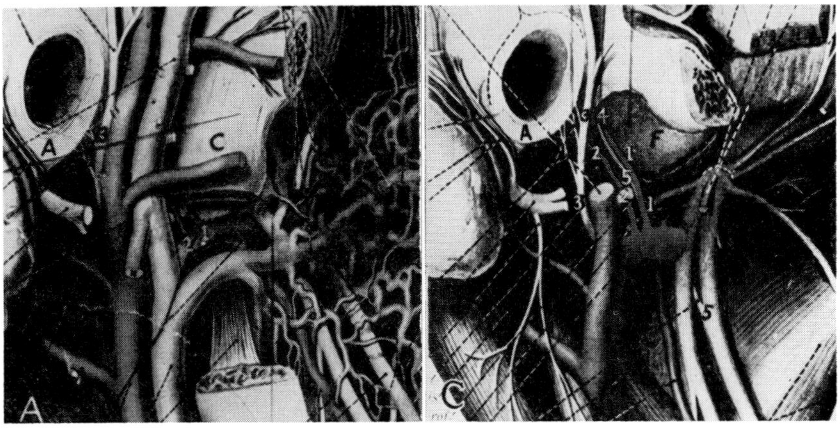

FIG. 2 (left). Nerves and blood vessels that supply the auditory and vestibular systems and the temporomandibular joint. A shows auditory meatus (A), anterior tympanic artery (1), deep auricular artery (2), auriculo-temporal nerve (3), and pterygoid venus plexus (P).

FIG. 2 (right). Shows anterior tympanic artery (1) and chorda tympani (5) passing behind condyle (C) to traverse the Petrotympanic fissure (4) on the posterior border of the temporomandibular joint fossa (F).

with, or penetration of, the meatus, petrotympanic fissure, tympanic cavity, and eustachian tube. These malrelations displace the nerves and blood vessels that normally pass behind the condyle and traverse the petrotympanic fissure. The posterior-superior displacement of the closed condyle and the resultant abnormal intra-articular pressure results in displacement and degeneration of the meniscus, which decreases its shock-absorber role and results in tensional disorder of the movements of the malleus-mandibular ligament. The traumatic factors result in roughening and resorption of the surfaces of the condyle, the fossa, and the bony partitions that are normally between the joint and the meatus, middle ear, and eustachian tube. The abnormal relations and resultant irritation, injury, degeneration, and deformity of the meatus, drum, petrotympanic fissure, middle ear, and Eustachian

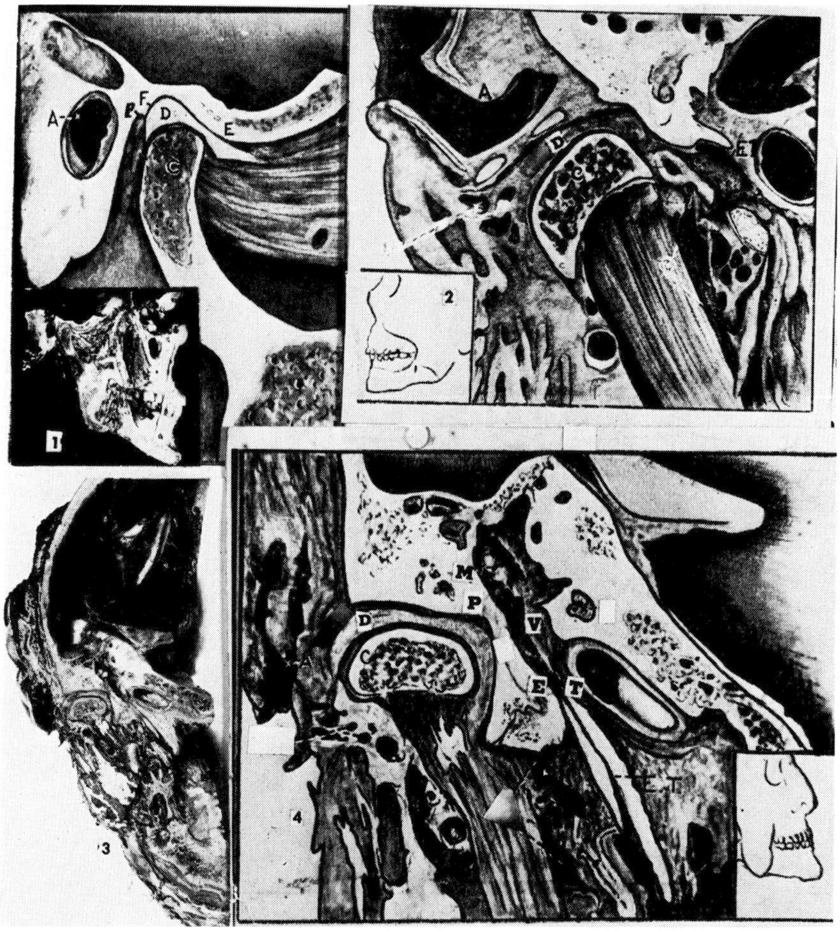

FIG. 3. Dissections of auditory-temporomandibular joint regions associated with normal dental occlusions. The figure shows (1) lateral section with condyle (C) in center of fossa (F) in contact with inferior surface of meniscus (D), the thick portion of which protects the petrotympanic fissure (P) and the space between the condyle and the ear (A); (2) transverse section with rounded, smooth surface of condyle (C) situated anterior to auditory meatus (A), anterior attachment of drum (D), separated therefrom by extension of parotid gland and loose connective tissue; (3) transverse oblique section illustrated by drawing 4 showing normal, oval condyle (C) situated anterolateral to petrotympanic fissure (P), middle ear (M), tympanic cavity (V), and bony eustachian tube (ET).

tube, and the displacement and irritation of their nerve and blood supply, which are caused by dental occlusal and temporomandibular joint malrelations and trauma (as shown by Figures 4, 5, 11 and 13), may be assumed to be pathognomonic of dizziness and related auditory, vagal, and ocular symptoms.

PATHOGENIC HYPOTHESES

Many hypotheses of the mechanism of action of the role of dental occlusal-temporomandibular joint abnormalities in the etiology of dizziness and related symptoms have been offered, including those of Goodfriend,[1] Costen,[2] Cawthorne,[3] and Myrhaug.[4]

Cawthorne reported the study of 1523 cases

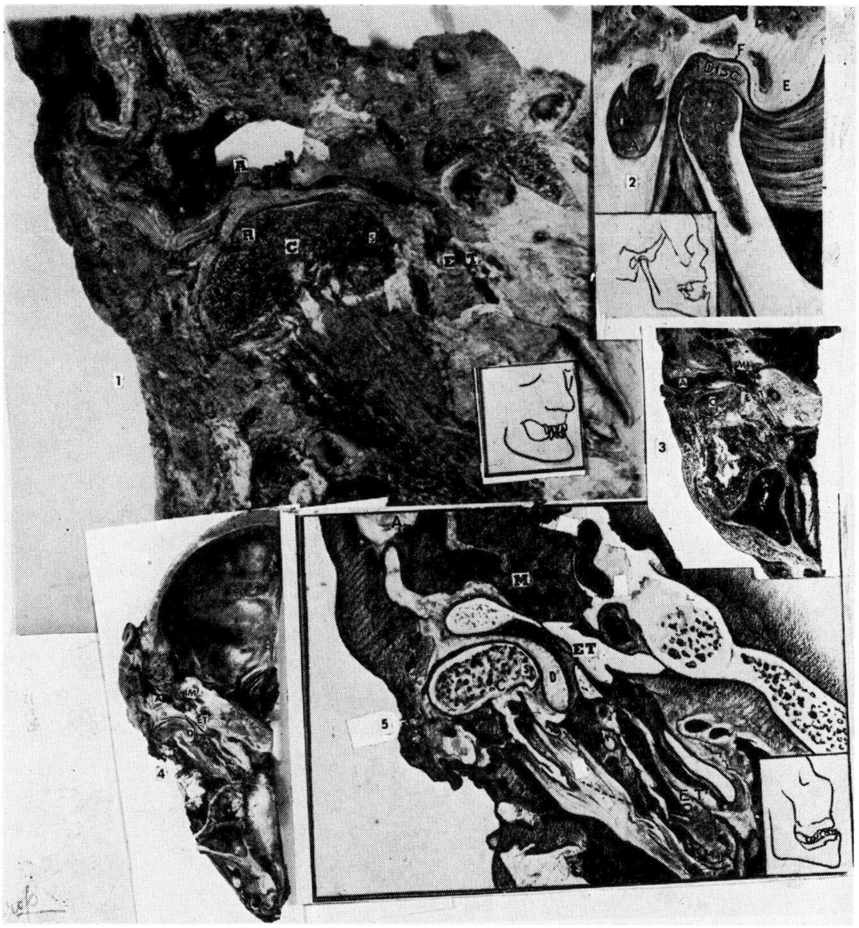

FIG. 4. Dissections of auditory-temporomandibular joint regions associated with abnormal dental occlusions. (1) Transverse section showing malrelations and malformations of condyle (C) that have displaced the tissues, nerves, and vessels that normally are situated between the condyle and auditory meatus (A) which the condyle has penetrated. The spur (S) on the medial surface of the condyle is in relation to the distorted lateral wall of the eustachian tube (E.T.). (2) Lateral section showing posterior displacement of condyle (C) with erosion of its superoposterior surface and the floor of the joint fossa (F), and traumatic irregularity of the articular surface (F-E). (3) Transverse-oblique section showing posterior-medial displaced condyle in contact with anterior attachment of drum and middle ear (M) and lateral wall of eustachian tube (ET). (4) Transverse-oblique section illustrated by drawing of 5, showing posterior displaced condyle (C) with medial spur (S) in relation to anterior displaced meniscus (D) and anterolateral wall of middle ear (M) and eustachian tube (ET).

of dizziness and related symptoms. He attributed the cause to the difference of the conduction of impulses by one ear as compared with the other. He found that the severity of vertigo attacks was directly influenced by the degree of difference and the suddenness of its occurrence. Myrhaug attributed the pathogenesis to contraction of the tensor tympani and tensor veli palatini muscles which he observed to contract during otologic surgery with the clenching of the jaws. His study of 1391 cases of dental occlusal defects showed that 378 (30 per cent) had dizziness and related symptoms. He described typical changes of the tympanic membrane as the result of spastic contraction of the masticatory and tensor muscles. He said that the light reflex is lost and the blood supply reduced. The tympanic membrane becomes thinner, transparent, and atrophic. Later, a sickle-shaped, grey-white precipitate, called the arcus lipoides myringes, is formed peripherally in the pars tensa.

Clinical findings support Cawthorne's hypothesis that dental anomalies which result in overclosure of the jaw and temporomandibular joint occur unilaterally and displace one condyle posteriorly and the other medially. Although both may be traumatic to the conduction systems, the resultant interference with transmission of impulses would differ from one ear to the other. Malocclusions of deciduous and permanent dentitions usually do not cause dizziness and related symptoms, because they occur gradually with tooth eruption. They are potential etiologic factors that are exacerbated by the breakdown and loss of bite supporting teeth to become frequent causes of vestibular symptoms. Long-standing dental occlusal and temporomandibular joint abnormalities become causes of symptoms as the result of external trauma and traction, and factors which increase vestibular sensitivity. Costen's hypothesis of the cause of vertigo includes disorders of vestibular impulses by irritation of the chorda tympani nerve. Dissections of Figure 4, and roentgenograms of Figures 11, 13, and 15, show that dental occlusal anomalies displace temporomandibular joint condyles into contact with the petrotympanic fissure and thereby irritate the chorda tympani nerve.

Myrhaug's hypothesis is supported by the clinical findings of Schwartz[5] and of Perry,[6] who showed that masticatory muscular spasms are concomitant with dental occlusal anom-

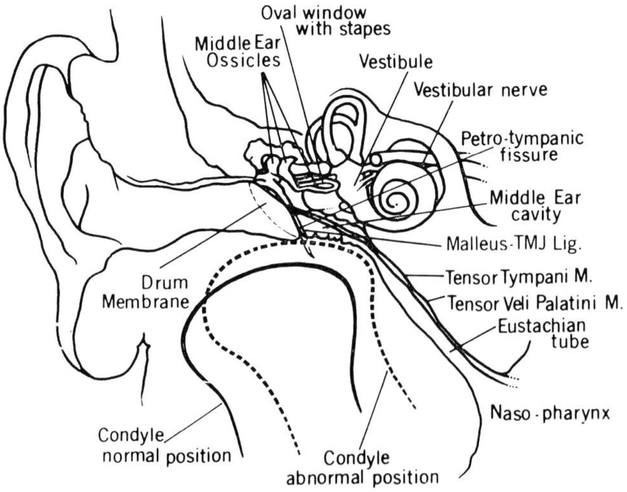

FIG. 5. Sketch showing the normal and abnormal relationships of the temporomandibular joint condyle with the auditory meatus, tympanic membrane, petrotympanic fissure, middle ear, and eustachian tube that are associated with normal and abnormal dental occlusions.

alies and relax as the result of dental corrective treatment.

The most significant validation of the pathogenic role of dental occlusal and temporomandibular joint abnormalities is correlation of the diagnosis of the dental occlusal cause and the effectiveness of dental corrective treatment in the relief of dizziness and related auditory, vagal, and ocular symptoms.

DIAGNOSIS

Diagnosis of dental occlusal and temporomandibular joint causes of dizziness and related symptoms includes (1) case history, (2) palpation of joint movements, (3) examination of the teeth and bite, and (4) roentgenography of the joint and ears.

In taking the case history, it is difficult for the physician to elicit dental complaints and experiences and for the dentist to secure history of auditory and vestibular symptoms. There are usually no subjective dental symptoms and no dental dysfunctions. Patients can eat and talk and have no pain in their teeth. There may be past or present joint symptoms —including noisy, traumatic, painful, limited, and excessive joint movements—but since patients do not associate these with the etiology of vertigo, they have to be elicited.

Case histories may correlate the onset of vertigo with dental treatments—such as the the removal, reconstruction, and replacement of teeth—or with traumatic and overclosed new dentures, or old dentures that have been worn for too many years. Traumatic oral surgery, the use of a mouth gag, head and neck injuries, and traction may also be pathogenic factors. Patients frequently associate the triggering of vertigo attacks with eating; they attribute the attack to food allergy rather than to the trauma of dental occlusal and temporomandibular joint anomalies. Vertigo attacks frequently occur upon awakening and could be caused by clenching and bruxing teeth during sleep.

The joints are palpated by placing the fifth fingers in the auditory meatuses and the finger tips in front of the traguses during jaw movements (Fig. 6). Joint trauma may be felt as crepitic, traumatic, and displacing condyle movements. Traumatic condyle movements may be heard by placing the stethoscope over the meatus and tragus.

Facial measurements compare the distance from the base of the nasal septum to the point of the chin, with that from the pupil point to the corner of the lips. These are about the same if the dental occlusion is normal, as shown by Figure 6B. Overclosed dental occlusions diminish the distance from the nasal septum to the chin (Fig. 6A) and result in temporomandibular joint trauma.

Examination of the teeth may show loss and breakdown of molar and bicuspid teeth. The bite may be interlocked and traumatic as the result of inadequate support of posterior teeth and a deep overbite of anterior teeth. Occlusions which prevent lateral gliding contacts of the posterior teeth and irregularities of the plane of the biting surfaces are likely to be pathogenic (Fig. 7) and also, old dentures and bridges which permit the jaws to overclose (see Fig. 16).

Roentgenography of the temporomandibular joint and ear is presently a limited procedure which should be as routine in otology and dentistry as is roentgenography of the teeth. Diagnostic procedures include lateral oblique and vertex oblique roentgenograms which traverse the ear and joint, as shown by Figure 8. The lateral views are made by directing the central x-ray beam through the joint and ear from the opposite side at an angle of 20 degrees above the horizon on the vertical plane and 90 degrees to the cassette held in contact with the meatus and temporomandibular joint, as shown by Figures 9A and 9B.

These views are taken with the teeth occluded as in swallowing, and with a cork held between the posterior teeth at a wide opening of the jaw. Diagnosis is based upon the normal location of the occluded condyle in the lower center or forepart of the fossa and the opened condyle below the crest of the articular eminence, as shown by Figure

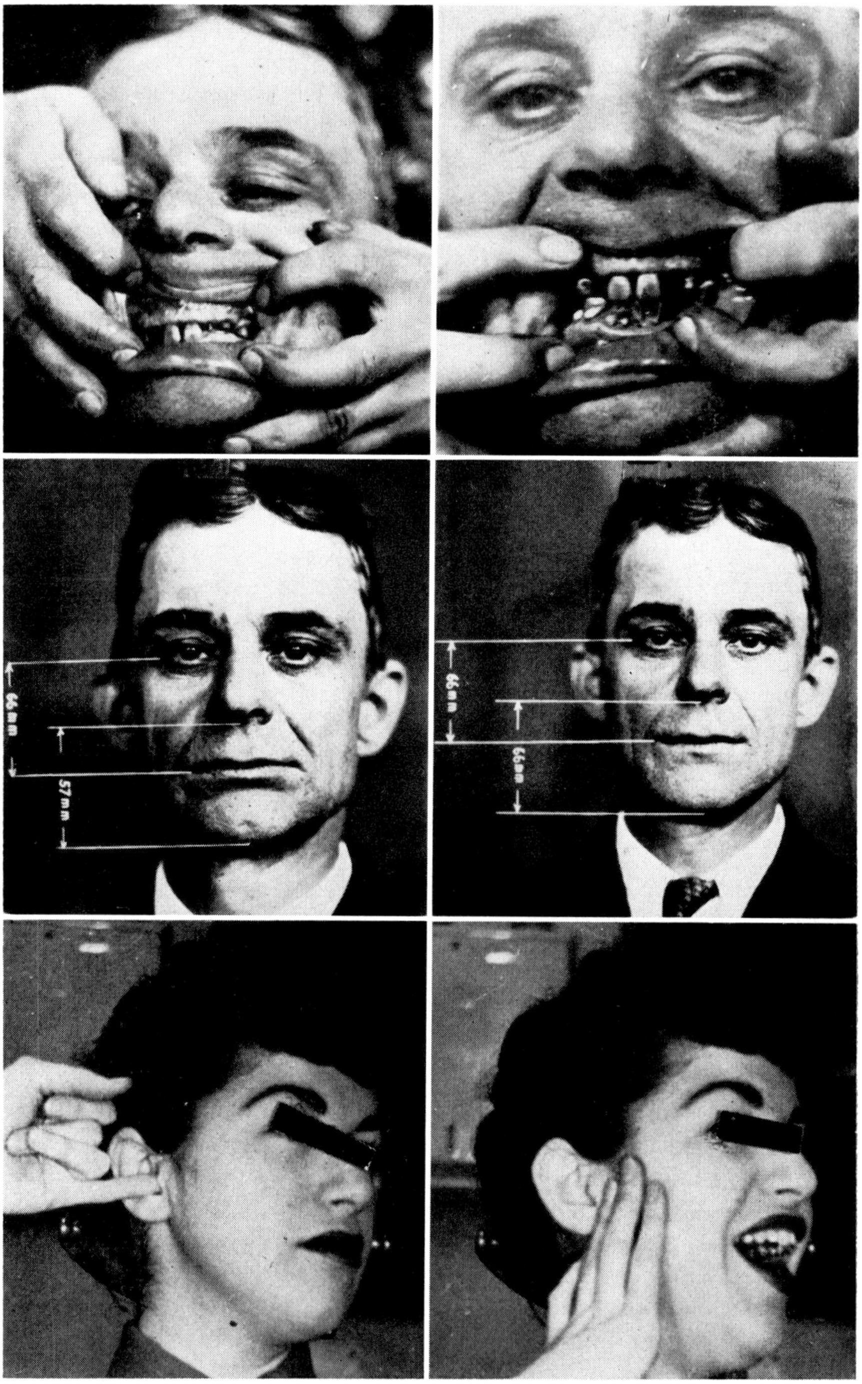

Fig. 6. Procedures for diagnosis of dental occlusal-temporomandibular joint cause of dizziness and related symptoms. *A* shows overclosed attritioned dental occlusion that diminished nose-to-chin dimension 9 mm. as compared with that from the pupil to the corner of the lips. *B* shows corrected maxillomandibular relations that equalized the aforementioned dimensions. *C* shows method of palpating joint with jaw movements by placing fifth finger in meatus and finger tips on front of the tragus.

10. Abnormalities show the condyle in the posterior and superior part of the fossa, close to or in contact with the anterior bony wall of the meatus, as shown by Figure 11A. The diagnosis of abnormal roentgenograms is aided by reference to the dental occlusal cause by means of clinical and model studies (Fig. 7). The findings may be checked by repeating the roentgenograms with bite-blocks or occlusion rims which correct the mandibular overclosure. The latter roentgenograms which show the condyle in normal relations guide the extent of dental corrective treatment. Repetition of these studies after dental treatment check its adequacy in establishing optimum environment of the adjacent auditory organs, as shown by Figure 11B.

Vertex roentgenograms of the temporomandibular joint and ear are made with the head tilted back to locate the gonial angle of the mandible above the tragus of the ear in the horizontal plane. The central x-ray beam is directed in a zero horizontal degree through the region medial to the tragus from the submaxillary region of the side of the joint and ear to be studied as illustrated by Figures 9C and 9D. These studies are made with the teeth occluded, as in swallowing, and with corrective occlusal rims. They show the long axis outline of the condyle of the joint and the meatus, middle ear, petrotympanic fissure, and eustachian tube. Diagnosis is based upon the normal, which shows the condyle as a smooth-surfaced oval with rounded posterior and medial surfaces that are situated about 5 mm. anterior and lateral to these parts of the auditory conduction system, as illustrated by Figure 12.

Vertex roentgenograms of the temporomandibular joint and ear lesions that are

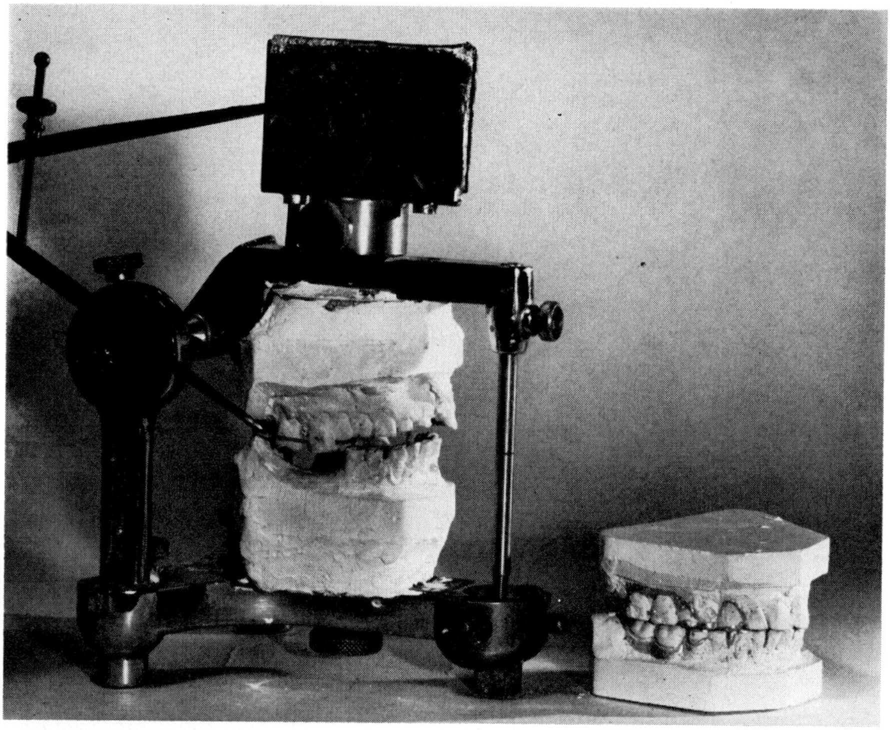

Fig. 7. Severely attritioned, overclosed, dental occlusion with irregular occlusal surfaces involving extruded molars and loss of bite-supporting teeth. The articulated cases have been adjusted to establish corrected maxillomandibular relations. The calipers indicate the location and form of harmonious occlusal surfaces which are incorporated in the dental treatment shown by the accompanying casts of the completed case.

caused by abnormal dental occlusions, which are illustrated by Figure 13, show malrelations and deformities of the joint condyles and adjacent structures. These include diminished space between or contact of the posterior and medial surfaces of the condyle and the anterior wall of the meatus, the anterior attachment of the tympanic membrane, the anterior orifice of the petrotympanic fissure, and the anterolateral wall of the tympanic cavity and eustachian tube. The condyle may have a flat or concave posterior surface and a spur on its medial surface. Diagnostic interpretation of these roentgenograms of joint abnormality in relation to pathogenesis is based upon the pathological anatomy shown by Figure 4, which was caused by abnormal dental occlusion.

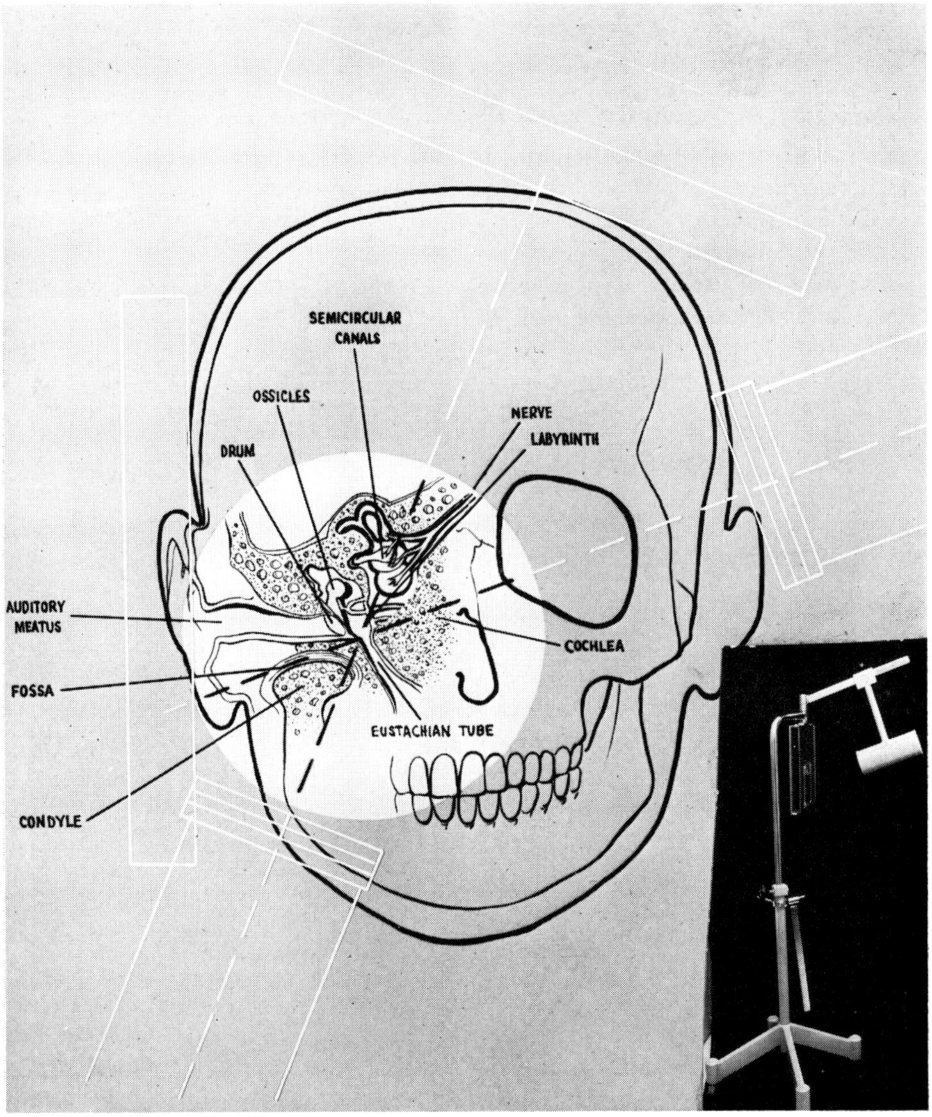

FIG 8. Sketch showing the location of the cassette and film, and the direction of the central x-ray beam for lateral-oblique and vertex-oblique roentgenograms of the temporomandibular joint and ear regions. The spot-focusing instrument provides for these angulations as illustrated by Figures 9-13.

CLINICAL FINDINGS

Clinical findings are based upon a 10-year research at the University of Pennsylvania in cooperation with George M. Coates and others,[7] a 12-year study of vertigo cases in cooperation with Herbert T. Kelly,[8] and 40 years of treatment of temporomandibular joint lesions in private practice.[9]

Vestibular and auditory, vagal and ocular symptoms attributable to dental occlusal and temporomandibular joint abnormalities may have been preceded by symptoms localized to the joint and mandible. These consist of traumatic joint and mandibular movements that may be felt by palpation as crepitus or knocking, and heard audibly or with the stethoscope. The mandible may deviate from the center line in opening and closing, or its movement may be limited or excessive. Patients frequently accept these symptoms as normal or adjust to them. The symptoms occasionally disappear or become more bearable, only to be followed by the more serious symptoms for which patients seek medical treatment.

Dizziness and related symptoms that are attributable to dental occlusal anomalies and temporomandibular joint trauma and displacement are similar to those attributable to other causes, except lesions of the central nervous system. The dizziness of central vertigo is likely to be continuous, of progressing severity, and associated with increased cranial pressure and paralysis of muscles supplied by the facial cranial nerve. The dizziness that is caused by temporomandibular joint trauma is usually, although not necessarily, paroxysmal and severe. Patients may be well between attacks of dizziness, or they may complain of light-headedness, wooziness, and staggering or lateral walking. They are frequently afraid and uncertain of heights, steps, and platforms, and susceptible to motion sickness.

Auditory symptoms include tinnitus, aerotitis media and eustachian tube blocking, inability to discern the source of sound and the nuances of language, and varying degrees of acute and progressive deafness. Ocular symptoms include disorders of focusing, disorders of ocular musculature, and halos and hallu-

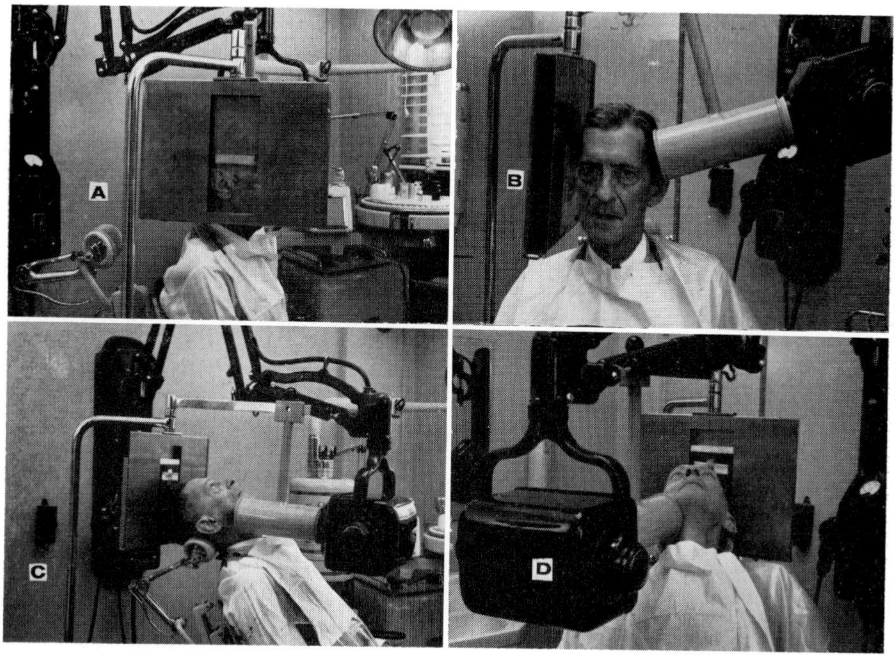

FIG. 9. Application of spot-focusing instrument for lateral (A and B) and vertex (C and D) roentgenograms of the temporomandibular joint and ear regions.

cination. Vagal symptoms include pallor, sweating, nausea, and vomiting. These symptoms may be accompanied by blackout, syncope and loss of consciousness, and loss of sphincter control. Pain of the termini of the trigeminal nerve involving the supraorbital, infraorbital, mental, auriculotemporal, and occipital regions is a frequent concomitant with the auditory, vestibular, and vagal symptoms of temporomandibular joint trauma and displacement.

This broad spectrum of symptoms may occur in part or in total. There is no syndrome in the sense of a definite combination, that differentiates the dental and temporomandibular cause, and no absence of symptoms which eliminates its possibility. Experience with thoroughly documented cases from the clinics of the University of Pennsylvania,[7] and the Kelly-Goodfriend study,[8] shows that these cases are not diagnosed by otological studies, that neuro-otological studies usually show labyrinthitis with nystagmus following caloric testing, etc. Many cases in which dental correction of the temporomandibular joint malrelationships relieved the vestibular symptoms had previously been suspected to be caused by cholecystitis, gastrointestinal disor-

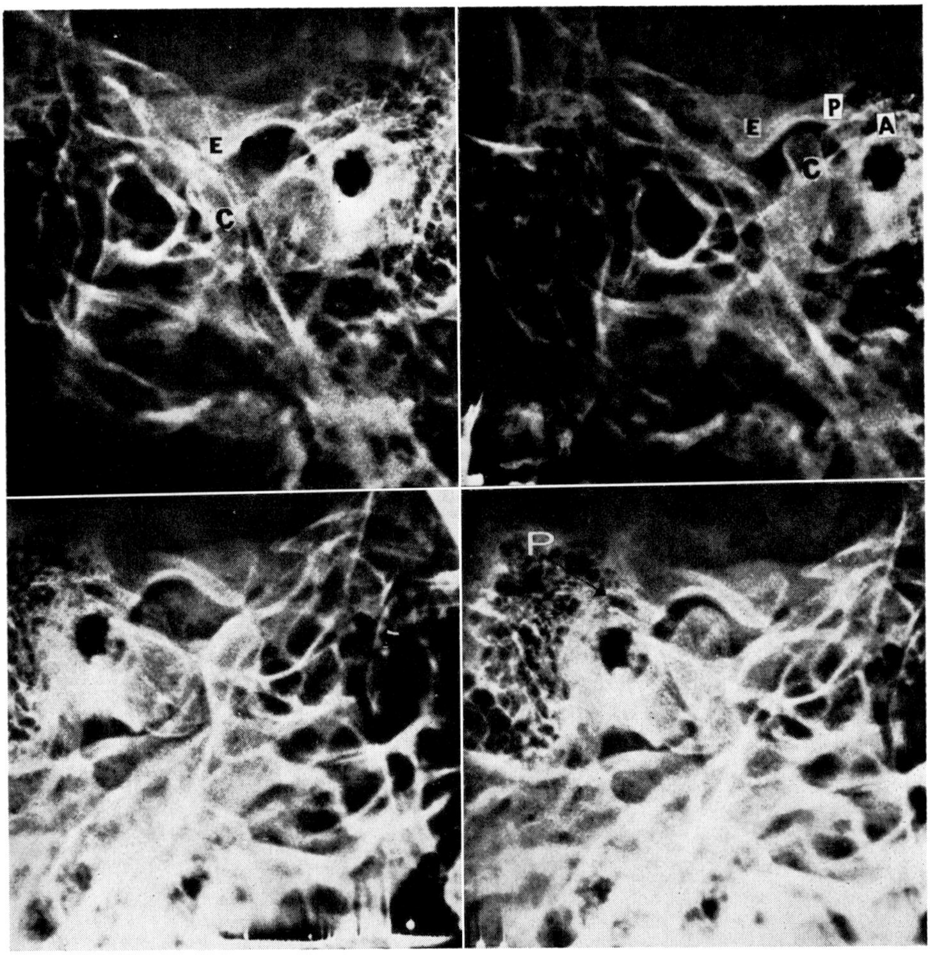

Fig. 10. Lateral Roentgenograms of normal occluded and opened temporomandibular joints of patient with normal dental occlusion. The occluded condyle (C) is in the center of the fossa about 5 mm. anterior to the periauricular bone and the petrotympanic fissure (P). The opened condyle is below the crest of the articular eminence (E).

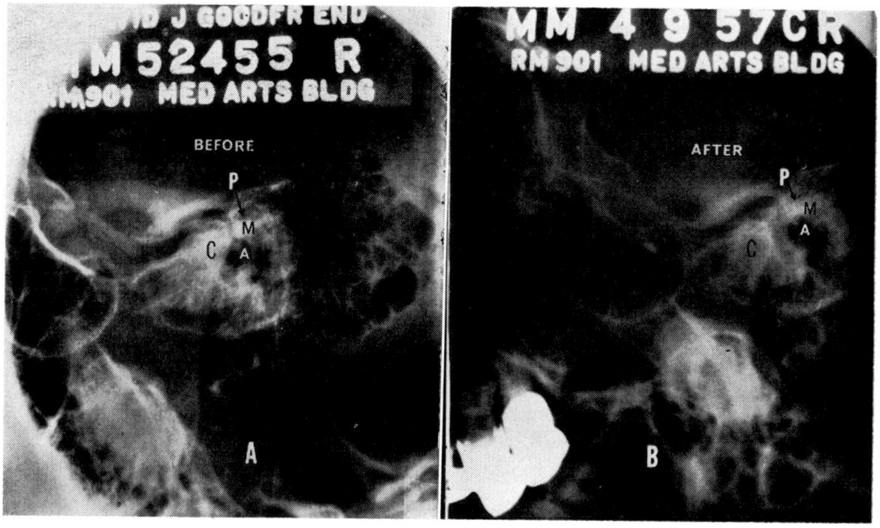

FIG. 11. *A:* Roentgenograms of the abnormal ear-joint region of a patient with abnormal dental occlusion and symptoms before dental corrective treatment. The condyle (C) is displaced superoposteriorly in contact with the petrotympanic fissure (P) and the auditory meatus (A) and malleus (M). *B:* Roentgenogram of same joint of same patient after dental treatment and relief of symptoms. The corrected condyle (C) is in the center of the fossa 5 mm. anterior to the periauricular bone, the petrotympanic fissure (P) and the malleus (M).

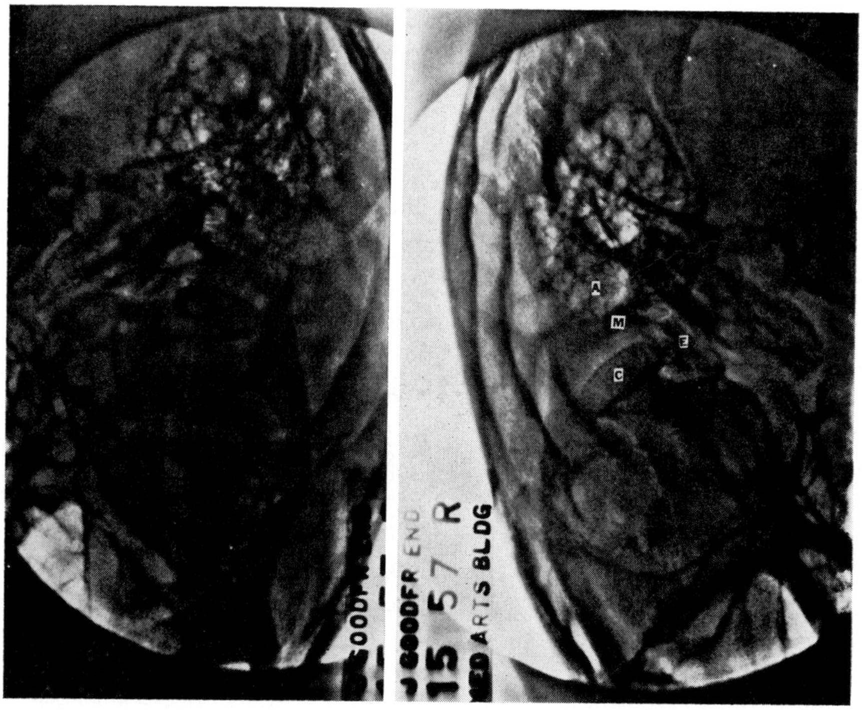

FIG. 12. Vertex roentgenograms of a patient with normal dental occlusion showing the olive-shaped condyle situated 5 mm. anterior and lateral to the meatus (A), malleus and middle ear (M), and the eustachian tube.

ders, hypertension, Meniere's disease, neurosis, and brain tumor on the basis of otologic, neurologic, internal medical and other work-up. These are shown by the following case reports:

CASE REPORTS

Case 1. A sheet metal worker, aged 49, had had progressive deafness for 6 years and tinnitus for 3 years. Paroxysmal attacks of dizziness, nausea, and vomiting started 2 years previously. The intensity of attacks increased until the night before admission to the University of Pennsylvania Hospital, when he had 3 severe attacks which finally resulted in loss of consciousness. Otoscopic findings were negative. Barany tests reported bilateral involvement, more marked on the left side. Neurologic diagnosis was Meniere's disease. Internal medical studies attributed the symptoms to focal infection.

Dental examination showed extreme attrition of teeth with many periapical infections and severe overclosure of occlusion, as shown by Figure 6A. Palpation and roentgenographs of the temporomandibular joints showed that the overclosed occlusion had displaced the condyles into pathogenic relations with the adjacent auditory structures and that this was worse on the left side. Infected teeth were removed and an autogenous vaccine made from the periapical granulomas. A full course of vaccine therapy did not relieve the symptoms. The occlusion was then corrected by overlays of the remaining posterior teeth to establish normal joint relations, as shown by Figure 6B. This relieved all symptoms within 2 weeks. The patient wore the overlays for 2 months, at which time they were replaced and duplicated by dentures. One year later, checkup indicated recurrence of slight dizziness. The occlusion was adjusted to equilibrate the mandible at the dental and temporomandibular articulations. This resulted in complete relief of all symptoms during a 2-year checkup period. Audiometric tests before and 2 years after dental treatment showed 8 per cent improvement of hearing in the right ear and 6 per cent improvement in the left ear. The tinnitus was improved to the point of being completely bearable and only recalled by questioning.

Case 2. A locomotive worker, 58 years of age, had a 5-year history of progressive deafness, more marked in the right ear. Nine months before being admitted to the University of Pennsylvania Hospital, he had a severe attack of dizziness, violent vomiting, and loss of consciousness. The attack was accompanied by severe pain in the upper right abdominal quadrant. He was taken to a hospital where his symptoms were attributed to calculous cholecystitis and where he was recommended for gallbladder surgery. The patient was well between attacks and rejected the recommendation. He

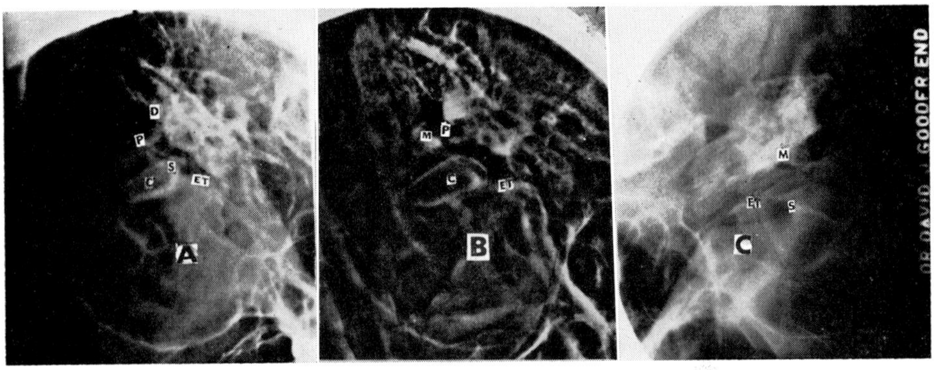

Fig. 13. Vertex roentgenograms of abnormal joint-ear regions of patients with abnormal dental occlusions and symptoms. *A* shows flattened displaced condyle (C) in contact with the petrotympanic fissure (P) with a spur (S) superimposed on the tympanic cavity and the eustachian tube (ET) *B* shows condyle (C) superimposed on the eustachian tube (ET). *C* shows a deformed condyle (C) with a spur (S) in traumatic contact with the meatus, middle ear and eustachian tube (ET).

had subsequent attacks without warning and was taken, unconscious, to the University of Pennsylvania Hospital, where the initial diagnosis was Meniere's disease and intestinal stasis. Otoneurologic studies indicated a vascular lesion or a tumor of the brainstem. This case was discussed in the medical seminar, where the choice of treatment was between intracranial surgery and a new set of dentures. His dentures, which had been made about the time he noticed deafness, were in traumatic occlusion and had overclosed his mandibular relationships by 12 mm. according to facial measurements. Palpation and roentgenographic studies of the temporomandibular joints showed displacement and traumatic movements of the condyles in pathogenic relationships with the adjacent auditory structures. New dentures were constructed that established harmonious dental occlusion and normal maxillomandibular and temporomandibular joint relationships. The patient had one severe attack of dizziness with the insertion of the new dentures and no recurrence of any of the symptoms during a 4-year period of postoperative observation. During this period he made an Atlantic Ocean crossing on a freighter without sea sickness or dizziness.

Case 3. A physician, aged 51 in 1953, had recurrent and severe paroxysmal attacks of dizziness, nausea, violent vomiting, loss of spinchter control, and loss of consciousness. Diagnostic studies by a team of specialists—including an otologist, neurologist, neurosurgeon, radiologist, internist, and gastroenterologist—concluded that the etiology was a left cerebellopontine angle tumor and recommended intracranial surgery. Dental examination showed extensive occlusal restorations. Palpation showed crepetic movements of the left temporomandibular joint and irregular movements of the mandible to the left side with opening of the jaw. He also had tinnitus, blocking, and deafness of the left ear. Temporomandibular roentgenographs and reproductions of his masticating system showed a traumatic dental occlusion and the left condyle in abnormal relation with the middle ear and eustachian tube. Treatment was confined to a two-stage dental correction of the occlusion and condyle malrelationships. The first stage of dental treatment consisted of cast metal overlays of the upper and lower, right and left bicuspid and molar teeth. These were constructed on the undisturbed underlying teeth with the understanding that if the overlays did not relieve the symptoms, they would be removed and the patient was to receive cranial surgery. The overlays restored equilibrium and there were no recurrences of symptoms by permanent tooth reconstructions which duplicated the occlusal relations of the overlays. The tinnitus gradually improved until complete elimination; the ear block was completely relieved and hearing improved. There have been no recurrences of symptoms during the past 12 years.

Case 4. In May 1954 a physics professor, aged 56, had an 18-month history of dizziness, pain, and pressure over the eyes; he had blurred vision that previous medical, otologic, and neurologic studies and treatment failed to relieve. Dental diagnosis showed a mutilated natural dentition with some missing teeth, some extruded and in cross-bite, and some depressed teeth. This obvious abnormal dental occlusion was associated with traumatic movements of the joint condyles, more marked on the left, and jerky jaw movements shifting to the left. The dental findings were rejected by the patient's family and medical and dental consultants, with the result that the patient was confined to a psychiatric institution for 1 year, during which he received 17 shock treatments without relief of his symptoms. In June 1955 the patient returned for dental correction of the overclosed dental occlusion. This treatment resulted in complete relief of all symptoms. There have been no recurrences since. The patient resumed his former teaching position.

Case 5. A single woman, aged 30, had six severe, yearly, paroxysmal attacks of dizziness, nausea, vomiting, and loss of consciousness since she was 11 years of age. The onset was related to orthodontia treatment which resulted in traumatic interlocking of her occlusion and was subsequently exacerbated by loss of the lower first molar tooth (Fig. 14A). She was unable to discern the source of sound and had constant left facial and ear pain. Her attacks usually occurred after eating, and she became completely dependent upon her mother's company, although she was employed as an art teacher. During this period she received extensive medical, psychiatric, and dental treatment. Despite the obvious malocclusion, the possibility of odontogenic etiology was not recognized by previous physicians and dentists.

Dental studies indicated that malocclusion and left joint trauma were the cause of symptoms. This was verified by temporomandibular joint roentgenograms, illustrated by Figure 15A, which showed that the left condyle was displaced and had a sharp spur on its medial surface. The abnormal occlusion was corrected by overlays of the posterior teeth, as shown by Figure 14B, that established normal relations of the condyle, as shown by Figure 15B. The initial phase of dental treatment completely relieved all symptoms and enabled the patient to discern the source of sound. The final phase of dental treatment is shown by Figures 14E and 14F. Roentgenograms, after this phase of treatment, showed that the corrected occlusion resulted in resorption of the spur and normal relations of the condyle, as illustrated by Figure 15C. There have been no recurrences of symptoms during an 8-year follow-up.

Case 6. A married woman, aged 62, had previously received two cranial operations at the Cleveland Clinic for suspected left and then right

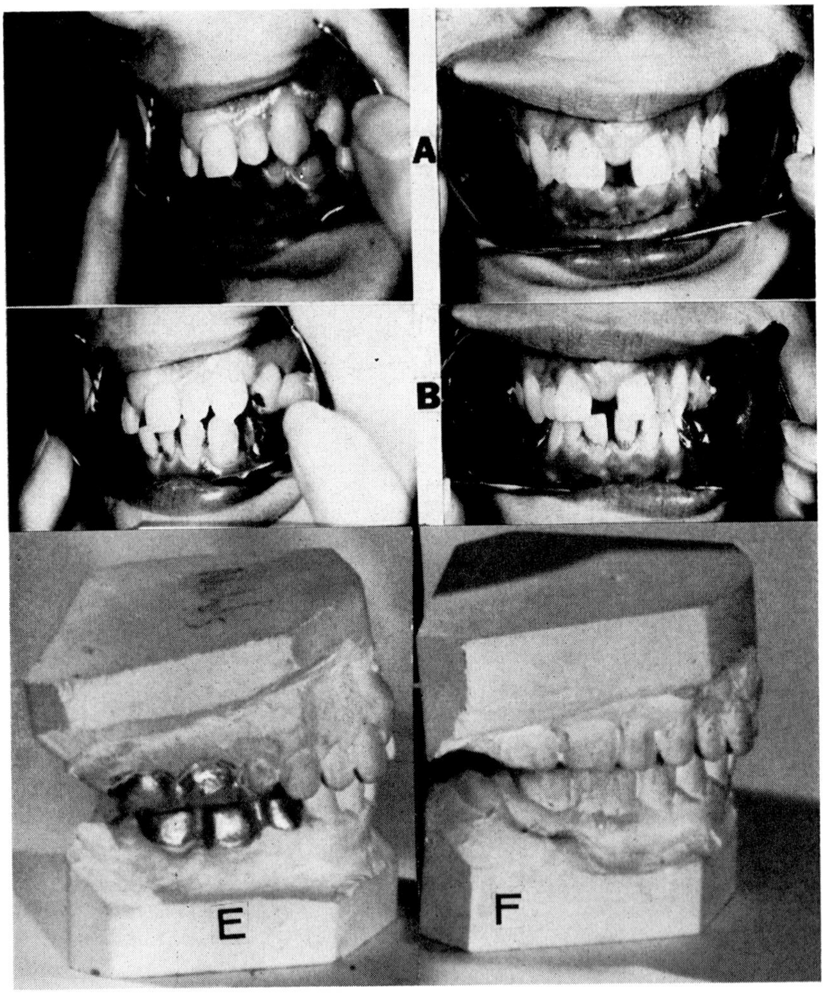

Fig. 14. *A:* Overclosed dental occlusion with posterior-superior displacement of mandible that was associated with symptoms of case 5. *B:* Corrected mandibular relations established by temporary overlays of upper and lower molar and dicuspid teeth, as shown by Figure E, that completely relieved all symptoms. *F:* shows permanent dental replacements which reproduced the relations of the overlays and prevented recurrence of symptoms.

cerebellopontine tumor as the cause of severe paroxysmal attacks of dizziness, nausea, vomiting, and loss of consciousness. These attacks had continued for 17 years, without recognition of possible dental occlusal etiology despite the obvious temporomandibular joint localization of symptoms. She had constant pain in the left side of her face and ear, and very limited movement of the mandible which shifted to the left. Although there was paresthesia of the left cheek, there was no evidence of paralysis. The cranial surgery did not relieve the dizziness and related symptoms which were subsequently attributed to cholecystitis and psychogenic etiology.

The dental occlusal abnormality was not obvious in this case. The patient had a complete natural detention with extensive gold inlay restorations, but the occlusion was interlocked by a deep overlap of the anterior teeth marked by a cupping out of the lingual surface of the uppers by the attrition of the lowers. This was most marked on the upper right canine tooth. Temporomandibular roentgenograms showed posterior-superior displacement of the occluded condyles which was worse in the left joint. The opened movement of the left condyle was severely limited. Diagnostic considerations of the occlusion and roentgenograms indicated odontogenic etiology of dizziness and related symptoms with the trigger zone localized to the left temporomandibular joint. This was attributable to reduced support of the left segment, and traumatic interlocking of the right and anterior segments of occlusion. The initial stage of dental treatment consisted of cast metal overlays of the bicuspid and molar teeth to establish normal maxillomandibular relations, harmony of lateral excursive occlusions, and normal relationships of the temporomandibular joints. The dental treatment completely relieved left facial and ear pain and gradually enabled the patient to open her jaw to normal extent. There were no recurrences of dizziness, nausea, vomiting, or loss of consciousness during the past 12 years of semiannual observations. During this period the patient has had an automobile accident, her husband died, and she has had bilateral mastectomy. Despite the severity of these psychological and physical traumas, there have been no recurrences of symptoms.

TREATMENT

Treatment of odontogenic dizziness and related symptoms requires cooperation of the physician and dentist. The patient suspects a grave etiology and does not readily accept

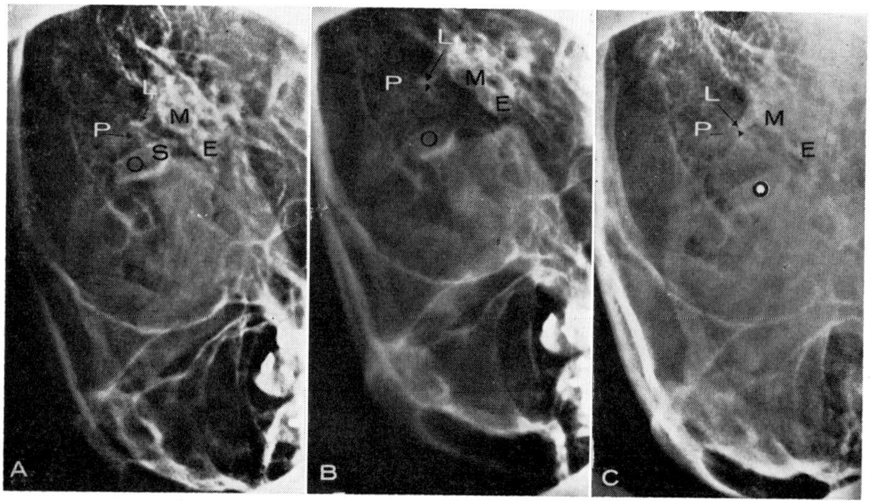

Fig. 15. *A:* Vertex roentgenogram of left joint-ear region of case 5 showing malformation and malrelations of condyle (O) and spur (S) with petrotympanic fissure (P), malleus (L), middle ear (M), and eustachian tube (E). *B:* Corrected relations of malformed condyle (O) by temporary overlays that relieved symptoms. *C:* Normal form and relations of condyle (O) with adjacent auditory and vestibular organs 1 year after dental treatment that prevented recurrence of symptoms.

the fact that his asymptomatic, abnormal dental occlusion may be a cause. It is important that the physician, dentist, and patient recognize that a previous abnormality may become a cause of the vestibular symptoms as the result of traumatic dentistry, reduction of occlusal support such as attrition and loss of teeth, bruxing and clenching habits, and traumatic dentistry. Also, the symptoms may be the result of increased vestibular sensitivity which may be due to psychological and somatic factors, including head injury, external traumas, traction, etc.

The dental treatment of these and other cases of odontogenic dizziness and related symptoms consists of reconstructing remaining teeth and replacing missing teeth to a harmonious occlusion that establishes nonpathogenic relationships of the temporomandibular joints in accord with the criteria of facial measurements, joint and muscle palpation, and temporomandibular roentgenography. The elimination of traumatic occlusion and repositioning of the joint condyles usually requires reconstruction of the occlusal surfaces of the upper and lower, right and left bicuspid and molar teeth to increase the intermaxillary space, at least sufficiently to allow clearance of lateral excursive movements of the teeth. Harmony of the reconstructed occlusal surfaces requires that they be smoothly regular on the same or an equivalent plane with the pathways of the temporomandibular joints, as shown by Figures 7 and 14. An important requirement of all dental treatment is that the initial stage be constructed on the undisturbed underlying teeth in order to provide for corrective adjustments and to permit the patient to resume his former occlusion in the event that the dental treatment does not relieve symptoms.

In cases with an adequate number of natural teeth, the treatment overlays are constructed of cast metal to plotted harmonious form and location, in harmony with the joint (Fig. 14E). These are cemented on the teeth and worn for at least 2 months to test their therapeutic effectiveness. As a rule, dizziness is relieved within a couple of weeks, but relief of tinnitus is gradual. Since there are natural remissions of paroxysmal attacks of dizziness, decision regarding the effectiveness of the overlay treatment should be delayed at least a few months.

When the overlays have relieved symptoms, they are replaced by permanent dental reconstructions that duplicate the height and occlusal relations of the overlays (Fig. 14F). If the overlays do not relieve symptoms, they may be adjusted or remade without disturbing underlying teeth. If they fail to relieve symptoms after adjustment, they are removed and the patient resumes his former occlusion or bite. The medical consultant may then assume that the dizziness is not attributable to odontogenic etiology.

Similar treatment procedures are followed in partial and complete edentulous cases, although the corrective indications are obviously the need for adequate dentures. This involves construction of partial dentures, as illustrated by Figure 7, and remaking old dentures, as illustrated by Figure 16.

RESULTS

The results of the documented treatment of the 105 patients in the Kelly-Goodfriend study show that dizziness was relieved by the dental correction of the temporomandibular malrelations and trauma, in cooperation with medical supportive therapy in 94 of 105 cases (89 per cent). Also, relief occurred in 83 per

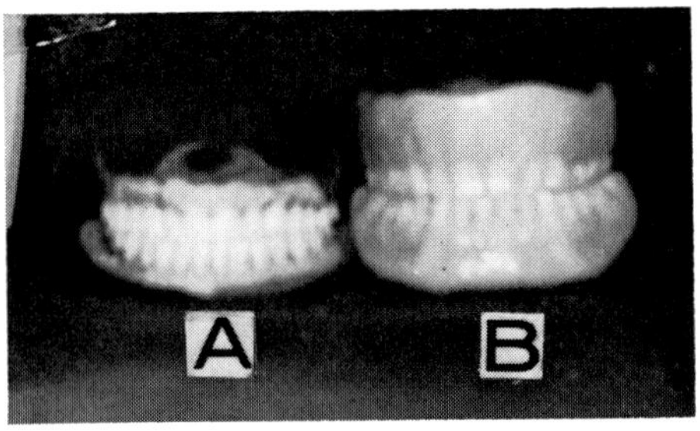

FIG. 16. *A:* Overclosed, traumatic dentures with hole in palate that were acceptable to patient after 47 years; patient had serious dizziness and related symptoms. *B:* Corrected dentures that increased dimension of maxillomandibular and temporomandibular relations and relieved symptoms.

cent of associated symptoms of light-headedness, blurring of vision, staggering gait, uncertainty of heights, nausea, vomiting, blackouts, and loss of consciousness. Eighty-three per cent of ear disorders were relieved or improved. All patients with temporomandibular joint dysfunction received relief. Sixty-four per cent of the patients having neuralgia were relieved by the dental-medical treatment.

Two years after the completion of this study, or 10 years after treating certain patients, questionnaires were sent to all patients. Forty-four patients responded to the questionnaire. These corroborated the favorable findings of the original protocols and showed that 83 per cent of the vertigo cases had no recurrence of dizziness and related symptoms. The therapeutic effectiveness of the corrective dental appliances was further tested by their removal in certain patients. Removal of the appliances returned the occlusions to their previous condition and usually resulted in recurrence of vertigo and other symptoms. These symptoms were relieved by replacing the appliances. This is illustrated by the experience of a woman 80 years of age who had symptoms of progressive deafness and tinnitus of 30 years duration. During the 2 years before the dental treatment she suffered from severe paroxysmal attacks of dizziness, nausea, vomiting, and blackouts. Her treatment consisted of maxillary and mandibular removable appliances. These relieved the vertigo and associated symptoms but failed to achieve patient acceptance. She returned the appliances and within 10 minutes had a severe attack of vertigo. The appliances were then reinserted and adjusted. This relieved the vertigo and the patient was able to go home unaided. She continued to wear the appliances without recurrence of the attacks of vertigo.

Most of the patients who rejected dental treatment continued to suffer from vertigo and associated symptoms. Some patients whose vertigo was relieved by dental-medical treatment, but whose habits of bruxing and clenching continued, subsequently complained of slight disorders of equilibrium and feared recurrence of vertigo. These were relieved by equilibrating adjustments of occlusion which usually required one short dental appointment.

The 105 cases treated in this study included two children with malocclusion of deciduous dentitions that were exacerbated by loss of teeth. One was considered a behavior problem because his attacks of vomiting followed the eating of tough foods. After thorough studies at a children's hospital the other was diagnosed as having abdominal epilepsy. Both were able to eat tough foods without attacks after dental overlays corrected the malrelationships of occlusion and the temporomandibular joints.

While many dental authorities consider that inadequate full dentures are not likely to be pathogenic to the temporomandibular joints, the findings of these studies show that they are likely to cause dizziness and related symptoms if the dentures overclose the mandibular relations and are in interlocking traumatic occlusion. Several elderly cases that were successfully treated in these studies had previously fallen during dizzy attacks; some had parkinsonian tremors, including the mandible, and one thought that he had paralysis of the legs after each meal. The response of these cases to dental treatment was as excellent as that of the younger patients, despite the extreme degree of correction that usually was needed with dentures worn for as long as 47 years, as illustrated by Figure 16.

Although there is a high percentage of frequency of dental occlusal causes of dizziness and related symptoms, there may be a high percentage of abnormal dental occlusions that do not cause these symptoms. This may involve host somatic and psychological susceptibility, as well as the physical factors that exacerbate preexisting pathogenic factors. Factors that exacerbate psychological susceptibility include persistence of symptoms despite extensive medical and dental diagnosis and treatment. Successfully treated cases include many who have had no psychiatric experience, while others were referred by psychiatrists or had had previous extensive psychiatric treatment. Relief of symptoms by dental treatment has aided patient response to future psychiatric therapy, and cooperative psychiatric therapy has contributed to the response of patients to dental treatment.

DISCUSSION AND CONCLUSION

It is important to consider the high percentage of relief of dizziness and related symptoms of the cases in the Kelly-Goodfriend study on the basis of their selection. These patients had no objective organic factors that indicated central nervous system etiology and all had dental occlusal abnormalities. All had diminished dimensions of the nose-to-chin segment of their faces and all had palpable crepitus of their temporomandibular joints. The surprising results indicate an early consideration of dental occlusal-temporomandibular joint cause in the diagnosis and treatment of dizziness and related vestibular, auditory, vagal, and ocular symptoms.

The percentage of dental malocclusions in the total population is extremely high. It increases with retrogressive deterioration of the dentition and with the age of patients. Studies of students of the Dental College of the University of Pennsylvania showed that 55 per cent had occlusal anomalies that could be associated with temporomandibular joint abnormalities. They had an average of 13 per cent greater hearing loss than those with normal dental occlusion. Studies of patients of the otology clinic of the Hospital of the University of Pennsylvania showed that 92 per cent had severe dental occlusal anomalies. These were shown by roentgenograms to have abnormal temporomandibular joint malrelationships.

The important factors of the early consideration and corrective treatment of dental occlusal and temporomandibular joint abnormalities of patients with dizziness and related symptoms are that the initial phase of dental treatment is diagnostic and reversible, that the dental treatment is completely harmless and without side effects, and that the least benefit that patients receive is improvement of their dentitions.

REFERENCES

1. Goodfriend, D. J.: Role of dental factors in cause and treatment of ear symptoms and diseases. J. Amer. Dent. Ass. 21: 204, 1934.
2a. Costen, J. B.: Neuralgias and ear symptoms associated with disturbed function of the temporomandibular joint. J.A.M.A. 107:252, 1936.
2b. Costen, L. B., Clair, M. H., and Bishop, G. H.: The transmission of impulses via the chorda tympani nerve. Ann. Otol. 60:591, 1951.
3. Cawthorne, T.: Modern Trends in Diseases of Ear, Nose and Throat. London, Butterworth & Co. Ltd., 1954.
4. Myrhaug, H.: Locale og perife symptomer ved kjevelleddsarthro, Finsk Tanal. Forhandl. 98, 1955.
5. Schwartz, L.: Disorders of the Temporomandibular Joint. Philadelphia, W. B. Saunders Co., 1959.
6. Perry, H. T.: Muscular changes with temporomandibular joint dysfunction. J. Amer. Dent. Ass. 54:644, 1957.
7. Goodfriend, D. J.: Deafness, tinnitus, vertigo and neuralgia. Arch. Otolaryng. 46:1, 1957.
8a. Kelly, H. T., and Goodfriend, D. J.: Vertigo attributable to Mandibular joint-bite abnormalities. J. Amer. Med. Coll. Dent. 24:182, 1927.
8b. Goodfriend, D. J., and Kelly, H. T.: Medical significance of equilibration of the masticating mechanism. J. Prosth. Dent. 10:197, 1960.
8c. Goodfriend, D. J., and Kelly, H. T., Temporomandibular joint criteria in dento-prosthetic rehabilitation. J. Amer. Dent. Ass. 60:7, 1960.
8d. Goodfriend, D. J., and Kelly, H. T.: A technic for balancing occlusion for the prevention and treatment of temporomandibular joint disorders. J. Prosth. Dent. 13:1130, 1963.
8e. Kelly, H. T., and Goodfriend, D. J.: Vertigo attributable to dental and temporomandibular joint disorders, J. Prosth. Dent. 14:159, 1964.
9a. Goodfriend, D. J.: Dysarthrosis and subarthrosis of the mandibular articulation. Dent. Cosmos 74:523, 1932.
9b. Goodfriend, D. J.: Symptomatology and treatment of abnormalities of the mandibular articulation. Dent. Cosmos 75:844, 947, 1106, 1933.
9c. Goodfriend, D. J.: Abnormalities of mandibular articulation. J. Amer. Dent. Ass. 21:204, 1934.

CHAPTER 16

Vascular Disturbances of the Peripheral Labyrinth

MARTIN SPECTOR

ANATOMY

Anson and Bast described the arterial supply as follows:

The internal auditory artery, a branch of the basilar artery, supplies the entire otic labyrinth. This artery passes through the internal auditory meatus and then divides into three branches. The first of these branches, the vestibular artery, supplies the vestibular nerve and parts of the saccule, utricle and semicircular ducts. The second branch, the vestibulocochlear artery, supplies the basal turn of the cochlea, the greater part of the saccule, the body of the utricle, the posterior semicircular duct, and parts of the lateral and superior semicircular ducts. The terminal, or the third branch, is the cochlear artery.

The venous drainage of the inner ear is primarily accomplished by two veins. These are the vein of the cochlear aqueduct and the vein of the vestibular aqueduct, following along the ductus endolymphaticus, according to Eggston and Wolff.

CLINICAL CONDITIONS

The pathologic and postmortem corroboration of many of the following syndromes is meager. It is presumed, by eminent authorities, that angiospasm and vascular occlusion may cause certain labyrinthine disturbances. The following syndromes and descriptions are gathered from the literature to illustrate the type of disturbance ascribed to occlusion of the vessels.

Occlusion of the Labyrinthine Division of the Vestibular Artery

Millikan et al. described this syndrome as follows:

These patients have an instantaneous onset of severe vertigo associated with nausea and vomiting without pain, tinnitus or hearing loss. The vertigo persists for many days to a week, totally incapacitating the patient. There is severe nystagmus on ocular rotation and during the weeks of gradual recovery, there is exacerbation of the nystagmus by lateral movement of the head. There are no symptoms or signs of any neurological dysfunction. When caloric studies are possible, such investigation reveals one dead labyrinth. This is a finding that appears to be permanent. Studies revealed that these patients did not develop signs of neurologic disease or recurrence of vertigo. It is postulated that a sudden occlusion of the labyrinthine division of the internal auditory artery is the only logical clinical explanation for the pathogenesis of the syndrome described.

Occlusion of the Vestibulocochlear Branch

Altman stated that the branch of the internal auditory artery most frequently occluded is the vestibular cochlear branch, which supplies the utricle and semicircular canals and also the basal cochlear turn causing a sudden drop in high tones. Shuster wrote: "The cochlear vestibular branch supplies the basal turn of the cochlea and the anterior vertical semicircular canal. When a patient, in the age of vascular thrombosis, develops sudden onset of vertigo, it may be due to involvement of the vestibular portion of this artery. Clinically, it may be noted that such a patient has a loss of the vestibular component from the vertical canals (to caloric) and at the same time, his hearing is markedly depressed in the high pitched sounds (basal turn of the cochlea)."

Vascular Interference

Kos described several syndromes which he ascribed to vascular interference. In one group, at ages 50 to 60, there was constant dizziness accentuated by movement. The patient felt worse in the morning and better by noon. Vestibular tests often showed hypoactivity. The hearing loss became progressively worse. There was a steamlike tinnitus. Kos described another type, occurring at 60 to 70 years of age, in which the patient developed an acute attack of severe vertigo and was completely incapacitated for 2 to 3 weeks. The hearing loss was complete if it was involved. There was numbness and tingling in the face. Nystagmus occurred to the opposite side. There sometimes was a pulling sensation to one side or a postural nystagmus.

Venous Obstruction

Perlman and Kimura studied the vestibular lesions produced by venous obstruction of the inferior cochlear vein in 38 guinea pigs. Rapid horizontal nystagmus to the unoperated side was evident, and the neck and trunk were twisted toward the operated side. By the third day, the nystagmus disappeared and circling movements had lessened. Histologic changes in the vestibular apparatus were less severe than those produced in the cochlea. The sensory cells of the vestibular end-organs were particularly affected, especially the saccule, and the utricle and cristae were less severely damaged. Marked perilymphatic hemorrhage followed by fibrosis and ossification was produced. New bone formation was most frequent in the canals. Even complete occlusion of the endolymphatic space in the superior canal was observed. Detachment and disintegration of the otolithic membrane were observed when there was extensive degeneration of the neural epithelium.

Free Blood in the Endolymph

Kelemen stated that free blood reaching the ampullar cupula—by injury, poisoning, or disease—acts in the manner of a specific poison against cupular tissue, whereas inflammatory secretion invading the endolymph can be resisted by the cupula for prolonged periods. Hemorrhage occurs with rare exceptions at the moment of trauma or during the prodroma of an infectious disease. Consequently, breakdown of the cupula is an initial phenomenon. Damage to the action of the respective crista is irreversible.

REFERENCES

1. Anson, B. J., and Bast, T. H.: *In:* Looseleaf Textbook, Otolaryng., Vol. I (Coates, Schenck and Miller, Eds.). Hagerstown, Md., W. F. Prior Co., 1960, p. 57.
2. Aubert, M.: Vertiges et Surdites D'Origine Vasculaire: Notes Anatomo-Cliniques et Therepeutiques. Paris, Masson and Cie, 1958.
3. Eggston, A., and Wolff, D.: Histopathology of the Ear, Nose and Throat. Baltimore, Williams & Wilkins Co., 1947, p. 193.
4. Hilger, J. A., and Goltz, N. F.: Some aspects of inner ear therapy. Laryngoscope 61:695-716, 1951.
5. Kelemen, G.: Hemorrhage: a specific poison to tissue of ampullar cupulae. Arch. Otolaryng. 77:365-374, 1963.
6. Kos, C.: Study Course at American Academy of Otolaryngology, 1959.
7. Matson, R. E., and Creston, J. E.: Vascular supply of the inner ear. Arch. Otolaryng. 78:62-68, 1963.
8. Millikan, C., Siekert, R. G., and Whisnant, J. P.: The syndrome of occlusion of the labyrinthine division of the internal auditory artery. Trans. Amer. Neurol. Ass. 84:11, 1959.
9. Perlman, H. B., and Kimura, R.: Experimental obstruction of venous drainage and arterial supply of inner ear. Ann. Otol. 66:537-546, 1957.
10. Shuster, B.: Circulatory causes of vertigo. Eye Ear Nose Throat Monthly 38:562, 1959.

CHAPTER 17

Lesions of the Neck and Vertigo

BERNARD SANDLER

The most common neck lesions from a clinical point of view are cervical spondylosis and cervical sprain (whiplash). The vertebral artery is often indirectly involved. There are other lesions which can involve the neck, but we are here concerned chiefly with those conditions which may be associated with vertigo. Neoplasms of the upper cord may produce vertigo, but they are clinically a rare event.

CERVICAL SPONDYLOSIS

Clinicians have known for many years that pain in the shoulder, arm, and hand may follow compression of spinal nerve roots by osteophytes. The process causing osteophytosis has been commonly called osteoarthritis, hypertrophic arthritis, or degenerative arthritis. In the last 15 years, it has become clear[1-9] that cervical osteoarthritis or, more precisely, cervical spondylosis[10,11] is associated with myelopathy as well as radiculopathy. Cervical spondylosis has also been implicated as a cause of vertigo.[12,13] However, in spite of a fairly large literature, recent texts do not mention this possible relationship.[14-16]

Etiology

The spondylotic process has been well described by Logue,[8] Wilkinson,[9] Hadley,[10] Payne and Spillane,[17] Payne,[18] and Horwitz.[19] The central feature appears to be a degeneration of the intervertebral disc. With aging, trauma, and perhaps the stress of daily neck movement, there is an interference with diffusion of nutrients from the marrow of the vertebrae to the intervertebral discs. Subsequently, there is fibrillary change, dehydration, and fissuring of the disc material. The cartilaginous plates become fragmented and there is invasion of the disc by blood vessels. The degeneration begins in the annulus and continues as a fibrous tissue replacement of the nucleus pulposus. As the disc space narrows, there is an approximation of the vertebral bodies. Mobility and bulging of the annulus increases. This causes increased traction on the periosteum to which the annulus is attached and stimulates proliferation of bone along the margins of the vertebral bodies to produce osteophytes. In time, the osteophytes bridge the disc from above and below to form transverse bars or ridges.[6] When the disc space is severely narrowed, then osteophytosis may be stimulated directly by friction between bony margins of adjacent vertebrae.[10,20]

Payne[18] points out that the first macroscopic change in the intervertebral disc is a vertical or a horizontal displacement of the nucleus pulposus. Disc narrowing appears to be due to this displacement. One result of the narrowing is osteophyte formation at the uncinate process, which has been thought to be the site of a synovial joint. This area has been called the lateral intervertebral joint, the joint of Luschka, the uncovertebral joint, the covertebral joint, the neurocentral joint, the lateral interbody joint, hemiarthrosis intervertebralis lateralis,[21] and synovial half-joint.[18] The notion that this is a true synovial joint has been laid to rest by several authors.[10,17,18,22] This is an important distinction, because the term "spondylosis" does not include changes in the synovial apophyseal joints—similar though they may be to changes initiated by disc degeneration.[17]

Confusion has been compounded by the fact that spondylosis has different meanings. Brain[11] distinguishes between a herniation of the nucleus pulposus and a protrusion of the annulus fibrosus. Both, in his opinion, can lead to spondylotic changes. O'Connell,[23] however, makes a distinction between escape of disc material (both nucleus pulposus and annulus fibrosus) into the spinal canal at one level only, and degenerative changes at many levels. Logue[8] avoids the diffculty by stating that the hard transverse ridge of fibrocartilage, bone, and fibrous tissue is the entity implied by spondylosis. It is not incompatible with this definition to note that sometimes nuclear material may herniate through a tear in the annulus and in time becomes a calcified part of the ridge or bar.[17] *Acute* herniations of the nucleus pulposus into the spinal canal are excluded from the definition.

Spondylotic changes are usually seen at several levels. Changes at a single level occur in 20 per cent.[9] Bradshaw[24] calls these single-level abnormalities *focal spondylosis* and believes that they are caused by traumatic nuclear herniation. O'Connell[25] calls this condition *secondary spondylosis.* He reserves the term *primary spondylosis* for those degenerative changes *not* characterized by protrusion of the annulus or herniation of the nucleus into the spinal canal. He qualifies this definition by admitting that on occasion disc protrusion may occur. Bradshaw[24] considers spondylosis as osteophytosis of the vertebral rims and uncovertebral area with or without subluxation, whether this is a sequel to nuclear herniation, or desiccation and degeneration of the disc produced by aging. If we agree that disc degeneration entails some bulging and protrusion of the annulus fibrosus,[9,26,27] then apparent discrepancies in definition are resolved.

The causes of the intervertebral disc disturbance are not clearly known. Implicated (in addition to aging and trauma) are "insidious wear and tear" and abnormal fluid absorption by the nucleus pulposus,[18] "a metabolic process,"[6] failure of diffusion of nutrients from the vertebral marrow to the disc,[17] congenital anomalies,[28] and occupational trauma.[20,26]

LESIONS INVOLVING TISSUES OF THE NECK

From a clinical point of view cervical spondylosis is by far the most important lesion of the neck. However, trauma to the vertebrae[29] (presumably *not* producing concussion), avulsed nerve roots,[30] trauma to the joints,[31] lesions of the neck muscles,[32-34] cervical adenopathy,[35] and involvement of the vertebral artery[36,37] have all been implicated as causes of vertigo.

Barré[38] believed that headache and other symptoms associated with cervical spondylosis arose because of irritation of the vertebral sympathetic plexus, which is in close proximity to the vertebral artery. Since 1926, when his paper was published, the number of European publications on this so-called posterior cervical sympathetic syndrome has been legion. Barré's pupil, Lieou,[39] mentioned a host of symptoms, including vertigo —in effect a good description of vertebral-basilar artery insufficiency. Laskiewicz[36] claims that spondylosis irritates the periarterial neural plexus in the wall of the vertebral and basilar arteries. This eventually, he believes, leads to spastic contraction of the vessels, thickening of the intima, and narrowing of the lumen. This in turn leads to edematous conditions in the inner ear. Again the emphasis is on sympathetic irritation rather than arterial compression. Sandström[37] considers the cervical syndrome to be the result of a mild, intermittent cerebral ischemia in the territory of the vertebral artery. Spondylosis (or osteochondrosis, as he calls it) causes compression of the vertebral artery on head rotation but also possibly causes sympathetically provoked contraction. He states that poor collateral circulation through the circle of Willis is probably the chief cause of the syndrome. It is significant that he admits that nystagmus provoked by rotation of the head may be due to neck reflexes rather than involvement of the vertebral artery.

Maran[40] discusses the case of a 48-year-old man who straightened up suddenly and became dizzy after bending over to lock his car. An orthopedic collar gave dramatic relief. X-rays revealed osteoarthritis of the cervical spine and presumably there was no evidence of vertebral-basilar artery insufficiency. In a special test of atlanto-occipital motion, the patient was unable to recognize less than $6\frac{1}{2}°$ of neck turning. Normals recognized $\frac{1}{4}°$ of turning. The author interprets this as a loss of proprioception but cannot relate this to the osteoarthritis. Here we find an implication that there is a cause of vertigo other than arterial compression or sympathetic irritation.

Stoddard[31] writes that in most cases of vertigo which he had seen there was evidence of joint fixation and subluxation. He is certain that manipulation relieves vertigo in many cases of neck injury involving cervical joints. However, tinnitus cannot be explained on the basis of a neck lesion exclusive of involvement of the vertebral artery.

Rebattu and Lesne[29] report the case of a 31-year-old woman who developed vertigo on a sudden movement of the head. She also complained of tinnitus in the right ear, blurring in the right eye, and stiffness of the neck. Radiographic examination revealed a subluxation of the fourth cervical vertebra on the fifth and cervical kyphosis. Traction and a Minerva plaster jacket removed all symptoms except for mild visual trouble for which no opthalmologic reason could be found. The authors do not explain the etiology, but it appears to be a rather good history for vertebral artery encroachment as a result of the subluxation.

Decher et al.[30] describe cases of avulsed cervical nerve roots (C_4-T_1) resulting from motorcycle and other accidents. Eight of ten cases suffered vestibular damage which the authors attribute to sympathetic nervous system involvement. However, they were careful to raise the question of damage as a result of concussion, neck reflex changes, and injuries to cervical muscles.

The paper of Ryan and Cope[44] brings a glimmering of light to the problem. They present cases of cervical spondylosis, trauma to the head and neck, and cases treated by cervical traction. The cases receiving traction had cervical spondylosis, but the cases of trauma did not. In these three groups, vertigo was elicited by bending the neck, not merely positioning the head in space. If the traction was sudden, vertigo was elicited. Gentle traction did not produce vertigo. In addition, when the head and neck were immobilized, bending maneuvers did not elicit vertigo. Vertebral artery involvement was ruled out on the basis that these cases did not have widespread involvement of the central nervous system, but only vertigo and nystagmus. Involvement of the cervical sympathetic plexus was also ruled out. The authors contend that stimulation of this system would certainly produce more widespread disturbances than vertigo alone.

Indeed, because of the host of symptoms described in the Barré-Lieou syndrome, it seems likely that several etiologically distinct conditions may have been improperly considered to be the result of sympathetic irritation. These conditions may range from Meniere's disease on the one hand to neurasthenia on the other.[13] Although it is possible that sympathetically provoked vascular contractions in the vertebral artery may play a role, there is no experimental proof. Spasm in vertebral angiography is known to occur; however, Ryan and Cope[44] conclude that derangement of the tonic neck reflexes is the cause of this type of vertigo. Any condition such as osteoarthritis, neck traction, injection of fluid into neck structures, and trauma causes damage to cervical muscles and ligaments and so alters the tonic neck reflexes. They emphasize that the neck reflex center is high in the cord (C_1-C_3). Consequently, the majority of cases of spondylosis (which involves chiefly the lower cervical roots) do not present with vertigo. Damage to muscles and ligaments alter proprioceptive impulses. Pain and edema temporarily cause splinting of the neck. When healing begins and stretching of neck structures take place, false information is transmitted to the cerebellum and vestibular nuclei. As healing continues, more stretching is needed to produce vertigo, until finally no amount of stretching produces it.

Stretch injury of the second cervical nerve root and the great occipital nerve is said by Seletz[45] to give rise to severe headache and retro-orbital pain. It is of interest that vertigo is not mentioned as a symptom.

Braaf and Rosner[46] studied over 1000 cases of whiplash injury. They explain the vasomotor and sensory changes they observed as a consequence of nerve root irritation and reflex involvement of the sympathetic nervous system. How this would relate to vertigo is certainly vague.

In the four cases of cervical adenopathy described by Mayoux,[35] there were both infectious and carcinomatous lesions. It was postulated that the vertigo produced came about from pericarotid sympathetic plexus irritation or pressure on the carotid bulb. The mechanism is not explained.

Travell[33] has made much of myofascial trigger areas—areas of tenderness in muscles which produce pain referred to areas some distance away from the trigger zone. Thirty-two cases are described in whom attacks of loss of balance and dizziness were treated successfully by ethyl chloride spraying and procaine infiltration of trigger areas in the sternocleidomastoid muscle. Once again, a proprioceptive disturbance is postulated, arising this time from abnormal impulses in this muscle. Painful motion of the neck is said to be caused by other trigger areas in the trapezius and levator scapulae muscles. Although we believe Travell deserves credit for her work on referred pain and the myofascial syndrome, one must treat with caution statements that there was a *low* incidence of osteoarthritis of the cervical spine or that abnormal neurologic signs were absent *as a rule*. In addition, we are told that five patients complained of intermittent tinnitus. There is a nagging doubt here that the vertigo may have had other causes.

1. Abnormal discharges from proprioceptive receptors in the sternocleidomastoid, the chief balancing muscle of the head, misinform the brain as to the position of the head during changes in posture. Presumably, tonic neck reflexes which help maintain equilibrium are altered.
2. The barrage of impulses which reaches the central nervous system produces reflex vasospasm in areas of the vestibular apparatus, brainstem, and cerebellum. Vasospasm may involve the end artery supplying the crista of the horizontal semicircular canal.

Gray[32] also believes that localized lesions of cervical muscles may cause vertigo. Radiographic examination was not routinely done in his cases. However, two of them did have spondylitis (spondylosis). He claims that galvanic stimulation over the lesions in the cervical muscles with 2-3 milliamperes of current produced symptoms because of the action of the afferent impulses on a hyperexcitable posture reflex center. The hyperexcitability is thought to be a result of stress or possibly autonomic disturbance. The neck lesion will cause vertigo only when it involves afferent nerve fibers in the upper three cervical segments.

THE VERTEBRAL ARTERY

It is apparent from the discussion so far that involvement of the vertebral artery is frequently the cause of vertigo. The ways in which lesions or attitudes of the neck affect this artery has not always been clear. (Powers' work[47] is discussed in Chapter 13, "Neurosurgical Aspects of Vertigo," of this book.

The effect of the head position on flow through the vertebral and carotid arteries has been studied in various ways. Toole and Tucker[48] examined changes in flow of water from a reservoir through the arteries of cadavers. Rotation, lateral flexion, and flexion-extension of the neck all caused marked change in flow. The authors postulated that the degree of head turning required to impair vertebral circulation may be small if, in addition to arteriosclerotic plaques and loss of vascular elasticity, there is also cervical osteoarthritis. Tissington-Tatlow and Bammer[49] described three patients with symptoms of vertebral artery insufficiency aggravated by head turning. The possible exacerbation of symptoms by osteophytic compression was mentioned. The intimate relationship between cervical spondylosis and vertebral artery insufficiency was very clearly defined by Sheehan et al.[50] in a study of 26 cases by angiography. The authors also raise the question (previously discussed by Hutchinson and Yates[51]) whether spondylotic compression may predispose to the development of arteriosclerotic plaques in the artery just beneath the site of compression. These latter authors have demonstrated clearly the pathology which may develop because of involvement of the cervical portion of the vertebral artery. Meyer et al.[52] point out that the cervical portion of the vertebral artery is a common site both of atherosclerotic change and compression by spondylotic exostoses. In short, two factors are operating in concert to the detriment of the patient. Bauer et al.,[53] in another arteriographic study, noted tortuosity and kinking of at least one major blood vessel (particularly during rotation of the head) in approximately one-quarter of a series of 75 cases. They demonstrated that rotation of the head caused stenosis of a vessel by (1) compression of the vertebral artery against the lateral masses of the atlas, (2) kinking of the first portion of the artery, and (3) compression by spondylotic spurs. Maslowski[54] emphasized the importance of head position as a factor causing stenosis of the artery. Hardin and his colleagues[21] demonstrated that spondylotic compression of one vertebral artery may be particularly dangerous in the face of congenital absence of the other. Ford's case[55] shows the vulnerability of the vertebral artery as a result of a defect in the odontoid process and excessive mobility of the second cervical vertebra. Compression of the vertebral artery at the C_1 intervertebral foramen and at the occipital condyle is cited by Schneider and Crosby[56] when dislocation of the atlas occurs. Hadley[10] presents histologic proof of the actual compression of the vertebral artery by the spondylotic process.

We have presented ways in which certain neck lesions involve the vertebral artery. Wilkinson[9] suggests that since the vertebral arteries themselves supply the vertebrae and joint capsules, any interference with blood supply through them may hasten cervical spondylosis. This brings the problem full circle: cervical spondylosis → compression of the vertebral artery → ischemia to the vertebrae and joints → acceleration of spondylosis.

CERVICAL SPRAIN ("WHIPLASH" INJURY)

This is so common an occurrence as to merit special attention. It is an extension-flexion injury of the cervical spine which ranges in severity from mild soft tissue damage to decapitation. Symptoms are a result of root, disc, vertebra, or cord damage as well as involvement of the vertebral artery.[72] Soft tissue injury is the most frequent result. Neurotic complaints, especially where litigation is involved, are very common. Vertigo may be due to concussion, involvement of the vertebral artery, or to changes in the attitude of the head and neck brought about by soft tissue injury. There may be hemorrhage, edema, scar formation, and loss of elasticity in the soft tissues. The chief findings are tenderness and spasm of cervical musculature, limitation of motion of the cervical spine, and loss of cervical lordosis.[73] Early treatment consists ideally of rest, horizontal traction, analgesics, and muscle relaxants. One should stress the tremendous range of involvement—from very mild to very severe.

For mild cases, very little or nothing in the way of treatment may be required. All patients who complain after a reasonable treatment period are not neurotic. Indeed they may have real cause for complaint, such as ruptured interspinous ligaments and scar formation. Settlement of litigation does not relieve the pain in these cases and cervical fusion may be of great benefit.[74]

Application of heat in the immediate post-traumatic period may add to the edema and discomfort if hemorrhage has taken place. Ice packs for 24 to 48 hours may prove very helpful. Local procaine infiltration may also give marked relief.

THE NECK, PROPRIOCEPTION, AND CERVICAL NERVES

That vertigo is one of the symptoms resulting from vertebral artery involvement is plain from the preceding discussion. The mechanism by which vertigo is produced in affections of tissues of the neck is not so clear-cut. Spector[57] and Peele[58] note that proprioceptive impulses are important in maintenance of normal orientation in space or equilibrium. The impulses coming from the neck are especially significant, since it is information obtained through the position of the head and eyes which the patient interprets.

"Clinicians have known for a long time that certain types of upper cervical (especially C_3) cord lesions (for example syringomyelia or irritation of the ventral funiculi of the spinal cord by pressure) may produce, along with other defects, a nystagmus."[61] It seems likely that when nystagmus is present, vertigo is not far behind.

McCouch et al.[62] found that tonic neck reflexes in labyrinthectomized, decerebrate cats were abolished only when cervical nerve roots C_1-C_3 were sectioned at their exit from the ligaments, even though muscular and cutaneous branches were left intact. They reasoned that the upper cervical joints were the site of receptors necessary for retention of tonic neck reflexes. They further reasoned that proprioceptors in muscle were not important since section of muscle and muscle nerves did not produce a diminution of the reflex.

Philipszoon and Bos[63] found that they had to cut the spinal cord of rabbits below the occipital foramen before nystagmus produced by neck torsion could be abolished. A rotatory nystagmus could still be produced after cord section by stimulation of the semicircular canals. Here, a clear distinction is noted between the nystagmus produced by change in neck position and that produced by change in the labyrinth. The work seemed to support the possibility that vertigo and nystagmus could be elicited in patients with cervical disorders and normal labyrinths.

Bos[64] contends that irritation of posterior nerve roots C_1-C_4 is sufficient explanation of complaints of vertigo in cervical arthrosis. The relationship between the cervical nerves and the vestibular system has been demonstrated, but it is difficult to come to conclusions about humans on the basis of rabbit experiments. As evidence of the relationship between cervical arthrosis and vertigo, the author presents the cases of three young judo experts with vertigo, positional nystagmus and arthrosis, and normal labyrinths. However, cases are described without arthrosis or vertigo but with cervical nerve irritation. Certainly the problem of concussion, as well as arthrosis, should be evaluated as a possible cause of the vertigo. What is not always clear either is the level of arthrosis. If we accept the theory of irritation of C_1-C_3 or C_4, then the arthrosis must be at a high enough level to affect these nerves. It should be remembered that spondylosis (arthrosis) involves chiefly the lower cervical segments.

Cohen,[65,66] working with monkeys and baboons, found that section of dorsal roots C_1-C_3 produced widespread deficit in balance and orientation very similar to the deficit in bilaterally labyrinthectomized animals. He concluded that loss of proprioception from the neck might be a cause of vertigo and disorientation. Again we must infer that vertigo develops. (We cannot prove it since it is entirely subjective. That is, the patient must tell us he is suffering from it; we cannot see it.) Certainly vertigo is not an invariable concomitant of ataxia or nystagmus.

Davis[13] did not see nystagmus in his cases. He claims that upper cervical root compression due to osteoarthritis (spondylosis) and postural strain causes vertigo of a mild transient type and a severe form with unsteadiness of gait. He also states that vertigo may follow minor trauma to the neck and shoulder girdle. He cites the following as evidence for a cervical etiology: (1) striking response to cervical traction and exercises as shown by the immediate effect on the attack and the prevention of recurrences; (2) close relation between attacks and abnormally held attitudes of the cervical spine; (3) high incidence of other motor and sensory manifestations of cervicodorsal radiculitis; (4) absence of clinical manifestations of intracranial disease, cerebral arteriosclerosis, and disturbances of the labyrinth.

Psychologists have perhaps unwittingly thrown some light on the problem. Wapner et al.,[67] in a study of visual perception of verticality, found that electrical stimulation of the right or left sternomastoid muscle caused a shift in verticality to the side opposite the stimulation. The same authors[68] found that when the body was tilted 15 degrees or more from the vertical, apparent verticality of objects was shifted to the opposite side. The inference is clear that changes in neck and body position (whatever the cause) are related to one's sense of orientation.

In cases of post-traumatic headache, Wolff[75] was able to induce vertigo by lifting the head from the prone position or pressing upon tender tissues near the base of the skull. Procaine injection into these areas made reproduction of vertigo impossible. Campbell and Parsons[76] produced listing and giddiness by injection of hypertonic saline solution into the neck. They thought these were caused by spread of excitation among cranial nerve nuclei and tracts of the upper cervical cord and brainstem. They believed also that stimuli arising in periosteum, ligaments, muscles, blood vessels, and connective tissue could cause sustained muscular contraction which would aggravate the original pain of the post-traumatic headache. Procaine infiltration removed the pain, both local and referred, to the head.

One cannot escape the observation that head and neck pain and vertigo occur concomitantly. A patient may awaken with a headache because of an unnatural position of the head on the pillows. This may be accompanied by vertigo which is aggravated by stooping.[77] A medical student who keeps his neck in an unchanged position for many hours while studying may be aware of headache and vertigo simultaneously. Massage and active motion usually cause improvement. Traction is of help here because it really brings tissues of the neck back into a normal alignment.[78] Again we must assume on the basis of evidence cited that prolonged abnormal attitudes give rise to noxious stimuli.

TREATMENT

Although the literature is replete with information on the treatment of cervical spondylosis and other neck lesions, the treatment of vertigo presumably produced by these lesions is scant indeed. Davis[12,13] recommended posture and neck exercise and cervical traction, although he could not explain why these were effective.

If we begin with the premise that abnormal attitudes of the neck (and subsequently vertigo) may be produced by lesions of cervical structures such as muscles, vertebrae, ligaments, soft tissues and nerves, then any therapy directed toward the correction of these abnormal attitudes should be helpful. Postural exercise and traction have been successful in reducing symptoms related to cervical spondylosis. In this regard it is interesting to recall Ryan and Cope's cases,[44] in whom vertigo was triggered by traction. They remark, however, that slow, nonjerky traction did not produce symptoms.

Jackson[71] has outlined very concisely the chief modes of treatment for what she calls the cervical syndrome. They comprise heat, massage, traction, anesthetic infiltration, correction of posture, immobilization of the neck, a cervical contour pillow, drugs, and psychotherapy. Since we must treat the cause rather than the symptoms, all the methods of treatment have a place. However, from a practical point of view, traction, procaine infiltration into tender or painful areas, and immobilization are the most important.

It is difficult to explain how immobilization of the neck and traction are both beneficial in vertigo. In an acute episode, perhaps immobilization and drugs used for motion sickness may be the logical treatment. As the disturbance becomes less severe, traction and exercise to maintain normal attitudes of the neck seem indicated. As pointed out by Ryan and Cope[44] and Davis,[13] traction may aggravate symptoms. It should be carried out slowly without jerking. Both continuous and intermittent traction have been used.[69,70] Intermittent treatment is better tolerated by the patient.

The mode of traction is controversial. Some physicians believe that a few pounds applied horizontally for several hours at a time is the answer. This may be logical for an acute injury in which immobilization is indicated. In cervical spondylosis without acute root symptoms, heavy traction (even up to 100 pounds) for 1 or 2 minutes continually or 5 to 10 minutes intermittently is more effective. This may be carried out in the vertical position and does not require hospitalization. The use of a collar should be considered with caution. The purpose is to immobilize because of a relatively acute injury. Once the lesion begins to heal, the patient should be weaned from his collar in spite of short periods of discomfort. Exercises consisting of flexion, extension, lateral flexion and rotation are indicated to keep the neck supple and to prevent postural changes brought about by injury and scar. Movement of the shoulders in all planes is also of benefit in order to prevent loss of range in the shoulder girdle, which often complicates neck lesions.

CONCLUSION

Before one states categorically that vertigo may be produced by lesions of the neck, the question of vascular or labyrinthine disease must be ruled out. The evidence presented does support the contention that vertigo may arise from neck structures by way of afferent nerve irritation. Caution about etiology must be maintained until more work is done on the problem.

REFERENCES

1. Brain, W. R., Northfield, D., and Wilkinson, M.: Neurological manifestations of cervical spondylosis. Brain 75:187, 1952.
2. Allen, K. L.: Neuropathies caused by bony spurs in the cervical spine with special reference to surgical treatment. J. Neurol. Neurosurg. Psychiat. 15:20, 1952.
3. Yuhl, E. T., Hanna, D., Rasmussen, T., and Richter, R. B.: Diagnosis and surgical therapy of chronic midline cervical disk protrusions. Neurology 5:494, 1955.
4. Clarke, E., and Robinson, P. K.: Cervical myelopathy; a complication of cervical spondylosis. Brain 79:483, 1956.
5. Braham, J., and Hertzberger, E. E.: Cervical spondylosis and compression of the spinal cord. J.A.M.A. 16:1560, 1956.
6. Odom, G. L., Finney, W., and Woodhall, B.: Cervical disc lesions. J.A.M.A. 166:23, 1958.
7. Nugent, G. R.: Clinicopathologic correlations in cervical spondylosis. Neurology 9:273, 1959.
8. Logue, V.: Cervical spondylosis. *In:* Modern Trends in Diseases of the Vertebral Column (R. Nassim and H. J. Burrows, Eds.). London, Butterworth & Co., Ltd., 1959, p. 174.
9. Wilkinson, M.: The morbid anatomy of cervical spondylosis and myelopathy. Brain 83:589, 1960.
10. Hadley, L. A.: The Spine. Anatomico-Radiographic Studies. Development and the Cervical Region. Springfield, Ill., Charles C Thomas, Publisher, 1956., p. 125.
11. Brain, R.: Spondylosis. The known and the unknown. Lancet 1:687, 1954.
12. Davis, D.: A common type of vertigo relieved by

traction of the cervical spine. Ann. Intern. Med. 38:778, 1953.
13. Davis, D.: Radicular Syndromes with Emphasis on Chest Pain Simulating Coronary Disease. Chicago, The Year Book Publishers, Inc., 1957, pp. 183-200.
14. DeWeese, D. D.: Dizziness. An Evaluation and Classification. Springfield, Ill., Charles C Thomas, Publisher, 1954.
15. Alpers, B. J.: Vertigo and Dizziness. New York, Grune & Stratton, 1958.
16. Grinker, R. R., Bucy, P. C., and Sahs, A. L.: Neurology. Springfield, Ill., Charles C Thomas, Publisher, 1960.
17. Payne, E. E., and Spillane, J. D.: The cervical spine. An anatomicopathological study of 70 specimens (using a special technique) with particular reference to the problem of cervical spondylosis. Brain 80:571, 1957.
18. Payne, E. E.: The cervical spine and spondylosis. Neurochirurgie 1:178, 1959.
19. Horwitz, T.: Degenerative lesions in the cervical portion of the spine. Arch. Intern. Med. 65: 1178, 1940.
20. Schmorl, G., and Junghanns, H.: The Human Spine in Health and Disease, American Edition 1 (translated and edited by S. P. Wills and L. S. Gain). New York, Grune & Stratton, 1959, pp. 186-197.
21. Hardin, C. A., Williamson, W. D., and Steegmann, T. A.: Vertebral artery insufficiency produced by cervical osteoarthritis spurs. Neurology 10:855, 1960.
22. Orofino, C., Sherman, M. S., and Schechter, D.: Luschka's joint. A degenerative phenomenon. J. Bone Joint Surg. 42-A:853, 1960.
23. O'Connell, J. E. A.: Involvement of spinal cord by intervertebral disk protrusions. Brit. J. Surg. 43:225, 1955.
24. Bradshaw, P.: Some aspects of cervical spondylosis. Quart. J. Med. 26:177, 1957.
25. O'Connell, J. E. A.: Discussion on cervical spondylosis. Proc. Roy. Soc. Med. 49:202, 1956.
26. Brain, R.: Discussion on cervical spondylosis. Proc. Roy. Soc. Med. 49:197, 1956.
27. McRae, D. L.: Asymptomatic intervertebral disc protrusion. Acta Radiol. 46:9, 1956.
28. Clarke, E., and Little, J. H.: Cervical myelopathy. A contribution to its pathogenesis. Neurology 5:861, 1955.
29. Rebattu, J-P., and Lesne, G.: Syndrome cochleovestibulaire en rapport avec une subluxation cervicale par mise en traction. J. Franc. Otorhinolaryng. 11:1091, 1962.
30. Decher, H., Rohr, H., and Unterharnscheidt, F.: Der Einflus von traumatische cervicalen Wurzebausrissen auf den Hör und Gleichgewichtsapparat. HNO 7:365, 1958-1959.
31. Stoddard, A.: Letter to editor regarding vertigo. Brit. Med. J. 2:1043, 1952.
32. Gray, L. B.: Extra labyrinthine vertigo due to cervical muscle lesions. J. Laryng. 70:352, 1956.
33. Travell, J.: Referred pain from skeletal muscle. The pectoralis major syndrome of breast pain and soreness and sternomastoid syndrome of headache and dizziness. New York J. Med. 55:331, 1955.
34. Weeks, V. D., and Travell, J.: Postural vertigo due to trigger areas in the sternocleidomastoid muscle. J. Pediat. 47:315, 1955.
35. Mayoux, R.: Quelques Notions Nouvelles sur le Vertige. Méthodes d'Exploration de l'Appareil Vestibulaire. Paris, Masson et Cie, 1953.
36. Laskiewicz, A.: Cervical spondylosis and the ear. Acta Otolaryng. 51:403, 1960.
37. Sandström, J.: Cervical syndrome with vestibular symptoms. Acta Otolaryng. 54:209, 1962.
38. Barré, J. A.: Sur un syndrome sympathique cervical postérieure et sa cause frequente. L'arthrite cervicale. Rev. Neurol. 45:1246, 1926.
39. Lieou, Y. C.: Syndrome Sympathique Cervical Postérieur et Arthrite, Chronique de la Colonne Vertébrale Cervicale: Etude Clinique et Radiologique. Strasbourg, Schuler & Mink, 1928.
40. Maran, A. G. D.: Cervical vertigo—report of a case. J. Laryng. 77:1032, 1963.
41. Rebattu, J. P., and Bonnefoy, J.: Le vertige et le nystagmus de position dans les arthroses cervicales. Rev. Otoneuroophtal. 35:129, 1963.
42. Omitted in proof.
43. Omitted in proof.
44. Ryan, G. M. S., and Cope, S.: Cervical vertigo. Lancet 2:1355, 1955.
45. Seletz, E.: Trauma and the cervical portion of the spine. J. Int. Coll. Surg. 40:47, 1963.
46. Braaf, M. M., and Rosner, S.: Whiplash injury of the neck: symptoms, diagnosis, treatment and prognosis. New York J. Med. 58: 1501, 1958.
47. Powers, S. R., Jr., Drislane, T. M., and Nevins, S.: Intermittent vertebral artery compression: a new syndrome. Surgery 49:257, 1961.
48. Toole, J., and Tucker, S.: Influence of head position on cerebral circulation. Studies on blood flow in cadavers. Arch Neurol. 2:616, 1960.

49. Tissington-Tatlow, W. F. T., and Bammer, H. G.: Syndrome of vertebral artery compression. Neurology 7:331, 1957.
50. Sheehan, S., Bauer, R. B., and Meyer, J. S.: Vertebral artery compression in cervical spondylosis. Arteriographic demonstration during life of vertebral artery insufficiency due to rotation and extension of the neck. Neurology 10:968, 1960.
51. Hutchinson, E. C., and Yates, P. O.: Cervical portion of the vertebral artery. A clinicopathological study. Brain 79:319, 1956.
52. Myer, J. S., Sheehan, S., and Bauer, R.: An arteriographic study of cerebrovascular disease in man. I. Stenosis and occlusion of the vertebral-basilar arterial system. Arch. Neurol. 2:27, 1960.
53. Bauer, R., Sheehan, S., and Meyer, J. S.: Arteriographic study of cerebrovascular disease. II. Cerebral symptoms due to kinking, tortuosity and compression of carotid and vertebral arteries in the neck. Arch. Neurol. 4:119, 1961.
54. Maslowski, H. A.: Symposium on myelopathy in cervical spondylosis. The role of the vertebral artery. J. Neurol. Neurosurg. Psychiat. 23:355, 1960.
55. Ford, F. R.: Syncope, vertigo, and disturbances of vision resulting from intermittent obstruction of the vertebral arteries due to defect in the odontoid process and excessive mobility of the second cervical vertebra. Bull. Hopkins Hosp. 91:168, 1952.
56. Schneider, R. C., and Crosby, E. C.: Vascular insufficiency of brain stem and spinal cord in spinal trauma. Neurology 9:643, 1959.
57. Spector, B.: Neuroanatomic mechanisms underlying vertigo and nausea. Bull. New Eng. Med. Center 10:145, 1948.
58. Peele, T. L.: The Neuroanatomic Basis of Clinical Neurology, 2nd ed. New York, McGraw-Hill Book Co., Inc., 1961, p. 245.
59. Omitted in proof.
60. Omitted in proof.
61. Crosby, E. C., Humphrey, T., and Lauer, E. W.: Correlative Neuroanatomy of the Nervous System. New York, The Macmillan Company, 1962, pp. 157-158.
62. McCouch, G. P., Deering, I. D., and Ling, T. H.: Location of receptors for tonic neck reflexes. J. Neurophysiol. 14:191, 1951.
63. Philipzoon, A. J., and Bos, J. H.: Neck torsion nystagmus. Pract. Otorhinolaryng. 25:339, 1963.
64. Bos, J. H.: On Vestibular Nystagmus without Causative Endolymph Displacement. Amsterdam, Drukkerij Cloeck En Moedigh N. V., 1962, pp. 41-55.
65. Cohen, L. A.: Mechanisms in body balance and orientation. Conn. Med. 24:500, 1960.
66. Cohen, L. A.: Role of eye and neck proprioceptive mechanism in body orientation and motor coordination. J. Neurophysiol. 24:1, 1961.
67. Wapner, S., Werner, H., and Chandler, K. A.: Experiments on sensory tonic field theory of perception: I. Effect of extraneous stimulation on the visual perception of verticality. J. Exp. Psychol. 42:341, 1951.
68. Werner, H., Wapner, S., and Chandler, K. A.: Experiments on sensory-tonic field theory of perception. II. Effect of supported and unsupported tilt of the body in the visual perception of verticality. J. Exp. Psychol. 42: 1951.
69. Harris, R.: Traction. *In:* Massage, Manipulation and Traction (Sidney Licht, Ed. New Haven, Conn., Elizabeth Licht, Publisher, 1960, Chap. 12.
70. Rogoff, J. B.: Intermittent traction. *In:* Massage, Manipulation, and Traction (Sidney Licht, Ed.). New Haven, Conn., Elizabeth Licht, Publisher. 1960, Chap. 13.
71. Jackson, R.: The Cervical Syndrome, 2nd ed. Springfield, Ill., Charles C Thomas, Publisher, 1958, pp. 135-174.
72. Stuck, R. M.: Whiplash injuries. S. Dakota J. Med. 14:385-390, 1961.
73. Eck, D. B.: Flexion-extension injury of the cervical spine. J. Med. Soc. New Jersey 57: 300-306, 1960.
74. Janes, J. M., and Hooshmand, H.: Severe extension flexion injuries of the cervical spine. Proc. Mayo Clin. 40:353-369, 1965.
75. Wolff, H. G.: Headache and Other Head Pain, 2nd ed. New York, Oxford University Press, 1963, p. 631.
76. Campbell, D. G., and Parsons, C. M.: Referred head pain and its concomitants. Report of preliminary experimental investigation with implications for the post-traumatic "head'" syndrome. J. Nerv. Ment. Dis. 99:544, 1944.
77. Seydell, E. M.: Indurative or myalgic headache. Arch. Otolaryng. 32:860, 1940.
78. Neuwirth, E.: Headache and facial pains in cervical discopathy. Ann. Intern. Med. 37: 75, 1952.

CHAPTER 18

Systemic Medical Causes of Dizziness

ALBERT J. FINESTONE

A vast number of clinical abnormalities can result in vertigo. In an effort to simplify the medical consideration of this and to do more than just compile a list of diseases, the various causes will be grouped into pathophysiologic entities.

VASCULAR FACTORS

Vessel Wall

Any pathologic state of the vessel wall, vessel tone, or vessel contents which interferes with the circulation to areas responsible may result in the symptoms of vertigo.

Arteriosclerosis

Arteriosclerosis is certainly among the most important causes to be considered. The specific cerebral vascular syndromes are considered elsewhere. The vertigo in cerebral arteriosclerosis is not usually paroxysmal, but is frequently positional, related to standing or bending. Even though the arteriosclerosis is frequently disseminated, the clinical discovery of this may be difficult, as patients may have vertigo due to cerebral vascular arteriosclerosis without obvious evidence of arteriosclerotic disease elsewhere. However, the clinician should guard against labeling the vertigo in an older person as being due to arteriosclerosis; he should first make a careful clinical evaluation and consider all the other possible causes. This is of utmost importance since the diagnosis of vertigo due to cerebral arteriosclerosis is a diagnosis of exclusion without arteriography.

Hypertension

Vertigo may also occur in hypertension, but its exact mechanism is obscure. There are many patients with a significant degree of hypertension without symptoms, particularly those referable to the central nervous system. It has been observed that many of these patients, when informed of their blood pressure elevation, then developed headaches, "dizziness," light-headed episodes, and a "heavy head." This sequence has suggested to some observers that these symptoms with hypertension are functional. However, there are a group of hypertensive patients who have "light-headed episodes" probably on an organic basis; the exact mechanism is obscure. Of course, specific vascular lesions secondary to the hypertension can produce vertigo if the vessels in the proper anatomic area are involved.

In Bechgaard's (1946) series of 1038 outpatients[7] who at first examination had a blood pressure of 160/100 or a systolic of 180 mm. or above, 65 per cent complained of no symptoms referable to the central nervous system; 18 per cent complained of dizziness, 15 per cent of headaches, and 25 per cent of sequelae of cerebral vascular lesion.

The exact mechanism of vertigo in hypertension is unclear, but it is not an uncommon symptom in patients with hypertension, particularly elderly patients in the benign phase. It is probably due to organic vascular lesions in the labyrinth or its nerve connections. It is important to emphasize that severe hypertension may be unassociated with symptoms and that many of the symptoms with hypertension, particularly of a mild degree, may be psychoneurotic in origin.

Vessel Contents

Red Blood Cells

Polycythemia Rubra Vera. An increase in blood viscosity and decreased blood flow can certainly result in vertigo and dizziness. These symptoms are not uncommon in this condition. Secondary polycythemia may also result in these symptoms, again by the same mechanism. Here the added factor of decreased oxygenation may be a factor.

The Anemias. Regardless of etiology, anemia may result in vertigo and dizziness. A detailed discussion of all the anemias is not in the sphere of this presentation.

Platelets

In essential thrombocytosis there is a marked increase in platelets which predisposes to small thrombosis, and if the proper anatomic site is involved, dizziness may result.

Protein Abnormalities

Protein abnormalities can produce dizziness. These symptoms have been reported in Waldenstrom's macroglobulinemia. In this syndrome, hyperglobulinemia and associated macroglobulinemia is a characteristic finding. This is a chronic debilitating illness, primarily affecting males in the older age group. Weakness, weight loss, and a bleeding tendency are usually present. Lymphadenopathy and hepatosplenomegaly are frequently noted. (The Sia water test, which consists of the formation of a white flocculus, following addition of a drop of the patient's serum to a test tube filled with distilled water, is a useful screening test.)

Neurologic signs have been found in about 25 per cent of the reported cases. Among the neurologic syndromes noted were encephalopathy, peripheral neuropathy, strokes, and subarachnoid hemorrhage. Vestibular dysfunction as a neurologic complication was generally noted with the encephalopathic type.

Blood Volume Disturbances

In these clinical situations, the vertigo problem may be overshadowed by the primary condition producing the blood volume abnormality. However, for purposes of simplification they may be considered under the following general headings. In these situations, there may be excessive output of fluid and electrolytes.

Profuse Sweating. For any reason, profuse sweating may lead to dehydration and produce disturbances of balance. Heat exhaustion can be considered in this category, but this is certainly not the entire physiologic explanation of this syndrome. With exposure to high temperatures, there is a dilation of the peripheral vessels which greatly increases the vascular space. If physical work is also performed, the cardiac output may be inadequate to meet the needs of increased muscular, skin, and cerebral circulation, and symptoms result. Salt depletion and dehydration predisposes to to this syndrome. In this situation the patient is sweating profusely and the prognosis is satisfactory as compared to the grave prognosis in heat stroke, in which there is a breakdown in heat elimination.

Burns. In extensive burns of the skin there may be great losses of extracellular fluid.

Gastrointestinal Tract Losses. Vomiting and diarrhea from any etiology may cause fluid and electrolyte losses. Also, fistulous tracts from the gastrointestinal tract to the exterior may be responsible for large losses. Examples would be bile fistulas, pancreatic fistulas, and ileostomy. The dumping syndrome results from rapid gastric emptying, particularly after partial gastrectomy, but also after vagotomy and gastroenterostomy or pyloroplasty. Food, which is hypertonic, enters the small intestine rapidly to produce a movement of extracellular fluid from plasma to achieve isotonicity and therefore decreases effective circulating blood volume. This in turn may cause dizziness.

Renal Abnormalities. Renal abnormalities of many different etiologies may result in dehydration. In chronic renal disease, in which there is an inability to form a concentrated urine, dehydration may occur if an adequate intake of fluid cannot be maintained.

Endocrine Abnormalities. Here the prime example would be uncontrolled diabetes mellitus, in which there are large losses of fluid and electrolytes. In diabetes insipidus, there is a deficiency of antidiuretic hormone, which results in excretion of large volumes of dilute urine. Dehydration will occur only if intake of water is impaired.

Neurologic Abnormalities. In this category, orthostatic hypotension is the clinical syndrome where, on standing, there is a profound fall of systolic blood pressure. Normally, there is little or no difference in pressures in these positions. If the fall is a significant amount, dizziness or syncope may result. At times, this syndrome may be idiopathic with no evident cause. It may also follow prolonged illness or confinement to bed for a considerable period of time. It has also been reported to be one of the complications of space travel and prolonged weightlessness. It may also occur with diabetes mellitus, apparently secondary to a neuropathy of the autonomic nervous system. Other neurologic abnormalities, such as tabes dorsalis and syringomyelia, may produce this syndrome. Surgical sympathectomy and treatment with ganglionic blocking agents may be complicated by orthostatic hypotension.

Metabolic Abnormalities. Under this heading, it would be convenient to consider the hyperventilation syndrome. On standing, forced ventilation may cause a fall in arterial blood pressure. This may be sufficient to cause dizziness or even fainting, since cerebral blood flow is decreased. Also, the hypocapnea produced by hyperventilation causes a reduction in the cerebral blood flow. This syndrome is a very common cause of dizziness and light-headedness. It is almost always secondary to emotional problems. In addition to dizziness, chest tightness and tingling in the hands frequently occurs. The patients may not be aware of hyperventilation, but may only state that they cannot "get a deep breath." Superficially, chest distress and "shortness of breath" might resemble cardiac problems, but a careful history will distinguish the two. Detailed questioning will reveal the "shortness of breath" to be sighing respirations. It is quite helpful to reproduce the symptoms in the patient by hyperventilation. Further, the relief of the symptoms by rebreathing into a paper bag to avoid the losses of carbon dioxide may be helpful in treatment. A variety of the hyperventilation syndrome may be considered under the clinical picture of neurocirculatory asthenia, where, in addition, there is a considerable degree of heart consciousness.

CARDIAC FACTORS

Any pathologic state interfering with cardiac output and therefore causing impairment in cerebral blood flow must be considered a cause of vertigo. Usually, the central nervous system symptom, however, is not the major presenting symptom, but the clinician must be aware that vertigo or light-headedness may herald a primary cardiac problem. A convenient method to consider these various cardiac causes follows.

Mechanical Obstruction

Aortic Stenosis. In this clinical situation, a characteristic murmur will be heard. Also, the relationship of onset of symptoms to sudden position changes is helpful. However, elderly patients often have an aortic systolic murmur and only a vague relationship of symptoms to position, and it may therefore become increasingly difficult for the aortic vascular lesion to be labeled as the cause of vertigo or light-headedness. Also, it must be remembered that the classic criteria of aortic stenosis—such as dyspnea, syncope, angina, pulse pressure narrowing and easily recognizable left ventricular hypertrophy on x-ray and ECG—occurred with regularity only in the most severe cases.

Primary Myxoma. Primary myxoma of the left antrum should be suspected in any patient with "mitral stenosis" who presents unusual features such as positional attack of syncope or cyanosis.

Idiopathic Hypertrophic Subaortic Stenosis. This may produce dizziness by the same mechanism of aortic stenosis.

Pulmonary Infarction. It is rare for central nervous system symptoms to prevail as the major symptoms of pulmonary infarction, but it can occur, given the proper clinical situation. For example, in a postoperative elderly patient, dizziness and apprehension can be the alarm to herald a pulmonary infarction.

Muscle Factors

Any pathologic entity that interferes with pumping action of the heart may result in the symptom of vertigo or dizziness, since cerebral blood flow is compromised.

Myocardial Infarction. Dizziness may be a symptom of myocardial infarction, but it is not a common one. Usually, other associated clinical features are present, such as chest pain, sweating, apprehension, etc. However, it would be worthwhile for the clinician, seeing a middle-aged man who has vertigo or dizziness and who is sweating with some apprehension, to consider myocardial infarction as well as Meniere's syndrome in the differential diagnosis. Thus, it appears that the symptoms of vertigo and dizziness might be called "the great imitator," as syphilis and tuberculosis were called in past years.

Myocarditis. Myocarditis of any variety may also cause central nervous system symptoms (for the same reasons as myocardial infarction) and should also be considered in the different diagnosis.

Pericardial effusion. If large enough, pericardial effusion can also interfere with cardiac output and might be considered in this same category.

Rhythm Disturbances

Any arrythmia may produce vertigo and dizziness. Any significant alteration in rate or rhythm which impairs cerebral blood flow will produce dizziness or vertigo. A detailed description of all disorders of this type will not be considered here. When a physician is confronted with a patient who has dizzy episodes, the diagnosis of an arrythmia may be most difficult, since at the time of examination regular rhythm may be present. However, the patient may state that the dizzy episode is associated with detectable changes in cardiac rhythm. Some of the arrythmias may be unassociated with cardiac disease and may be due to such causes as tobacco, coffee, or emotional disturbances.

A complete classification of arrythmia is obviously beyond the scope of this presentation. However, certain aspects of this problem deserve emphasis. From the practical standpoint in considering if an arrythmia is responsible for a problem in vertigo, it is worthwhile to think in terms of 2 factors: Is the rhythm regular or irregular? Is it unusually rapid or unusually slow?

Tachycardias which are regular include (1) sinus tachycardia, (2) paraxysmal atrial tachycardia, (3) ventricular tachycardia, and (4) atrial flutter with 1:1 response. Irregular tachycardias include (1) atrial fibrillation, (2) atrial flutter with varying block, and (3) sinus tachycardia with numerous premature beats.

Bradycardias with regular rhythm include (1) sinus bradycardia, (2) nodal rhythm, (3) severe partial heart block with constant degree of block, and (4) complete heart block. Irregular bradycardias include (1) sinus bradycardia with marked sinus arrythmia or frequent premature beats, and (2) partial heart block with frequent dropped beats or changing degree of block.

Irregular rhythms with normal heart rate include frequent premature beats, atrial fibrillation with ventricular rate slowed by digitalis, sinus arrythmia, and partial heart block with dropped beats.

Sinus tachycardia, in which the rate does not go over 100/min., is usually not associated with dizziness. Sinus bradycardia, on the other hand, may definitely be associated with dizziness or faintness. Sinus arrythmia associated with marked bradycardia may be associated with dizziness, but sinus arrythmia alone is not associated with symptoms. Sinus arrest denotes a pause in cardiac rhythm due to a transient failure of the sinus node to initiate an impulse, and it may be associated with dizziness if the pause is sufficiently long.

Premature beats are very common and many persons with them are unaware of their presence. When the symptoms are present, they are frequently related to the compensatory pause and may be associated with dizziness. The paroxysmal tachycardias—such as paroxysmal atrial tachycardia, atrial flutter, and atrial fibrillation—are also frequently associated with dizziness.

Disturbances in conduction may be associated with dizziness. Sinoatrial block is a disturbance in the transmission of impulse from the sinoatrial node to the atria. This disturbance may be secondary to digitalis intoxication or vagal stimulation, due to a sensitive carotid sinus. Usually, no associated symptoms are present, but if the pause in the heart beat is prolonged, dizziness may occur.

Atrioventricular block is due to impairment in conduction from atria to ventricle. This is not an uncommon disorder of heart beat. In complete heart block with a slow ventricular rate, dizziness is not an uncommon symptom. This is more frequently present if a degree of cerebral arteriosclerosis is present. Also, in complete heart block the symptoms may be worse with exercise, since the ventricular rate does not increase with exercise.

With regard to the carotid sinus syndrome, syncope is usually the resultant clinical situation. These attacks are reproduced by pressure over the carotid sinus. In normal persons, only a slight reduction in pulse rate and blood pressure occurs. However, in certain people, usually those past middle age and especially those with hypertension or arteriosclerosis, the carotid sinus becomes hypersensitive. In these subjects, the slightest pressure may induce dizziness or syncope. Carotid sinus hypersensitivity may result in (1) drop in blood pressure, (2) cardiac slowing, cardiac standstill, or heart block with or without ventricular standstill, or (3) reflex cerebral ischemia. Each of these reaction types can cause syncope. It is worthwhile to note that in a study from the Cleveland Clinic[10] of 510 patients with syncope, only 15 had a hypersensitive carotid sinus. These figures indicate that this is not a very common consideration in a patient with syncope or dizziness. Finally, the test for carotid sinus hypersensitivity should be performed with caution in patients with vascular disease, since "strokes" may result.

METABOLIC FACTORS

Any etiologic factor causing hypoglycemia may produce dizziness or vertigo among its symptoms. Since many factors may cause a depression of blood glucose, it is well to remember that hypoglycemia is a symptom, not a disease. In hypoglycemia, 2 groups of symptoms may occur and the dizziness or vertigo may be related to both. Symptoms may result from hypoglycemia and also from an increase in epinephrine. Also, increase in secretion of epinephrine results in tachycardia, anxiety, sweating, pallor, and rise in blood pressure. Dizziness may again be associated on this basis. It is important to recognize the relationship of the symptoms to hunger and its possible improvement with food.

The signs of hypoglycemia are partly due to the central effects of the low blood glucose and partly to an increased secretion of epinephrine. A convenient classification of hypoglycemia follows.

Etiology of Hypoglycemia (Partially adapted from Williams[12])

1. Deficient food supply
   a. Starvation
   b. Excessive elimination
      (1). Diarrhea or malabsorption
      (2). Lactation
      (3). Losses in urine-proteinuria, glycosuria

c. Hyperutilization—severe exercise, fever, thyrotoxicosis
d. Abnormal metabolism — certain derangements of metabolism (for example, leucine-induced hypoglycemia)

2. Hepatogenic disorders
   a. Primary hepatogenic disorders
      (1). General hypofunction. In this situation, the basic problem is a decreased ability of the liver to form glucose. Examples are cirrhosis and hepatitis.
      (2). Glycogen storage disease. In this group of diseases, there is an excessive accumulation of glycogen in this tissues, due to a deficiency of certain enzymes involved in glycogenolysis. Von Gierke's disease is an example.
   b. Secondary hepatogenic disorders. In this group, hypoglycemia results from decreased hepatic glucogenesis.
3. Hypersecretion of insulin
   a. Neoplasm of beta cells. These cells may either be benign or malignant. Lightheadedness was found in 30 per cent of a group of 193 patients with insulinomas.[3] The intravenous tolbutamide tolerance test has been an important addition to the available procedures in establishing this diagnosis.
   b. Functional hypoglycemia. These patients frequently are tense and have associated emotional problems. In this situation, hypoglycemia does not occur with fasting. Symptoms frequently occur several hours after eating, particularly high carbohydrate feedings. Loss of consciousness does not usually occur. Some patients who have had a gastric resection or gastroenterostomy may experience hypoglycemic attacks. It is believed that the gastric surgery allows rapid passage of glucose into the small intestine with rapid glucose absorption; this, in turn, stimulates increased insulin secretion and results in hypoglycemia.
4. Drugs
   a. Excess insulin. This is probably the most common cause of hypoglycemia.
   b. Other agents
      (1). Sulfonylureas. Apparently the chief action of these drugs is to stimulate increased production of insulin. Hypoglycemia can occur with any of these drugs, but it is more common with chorpropamide (Diabinese), apparently due to its longer half-life.
      (2). Biguanides (DBI)
      (3). Other drugs—antergan, neoantergan, pyribenzamine, salicylates, etc.
5. Early diabetes mellitus. Seltzer and his co-workers[9] reported that mild untreated diabetes mellitus is frequently associated with periodic, symptomatic, spontaneous hypoglycemia and that symptoms of hypoglycemia occurring 3 to five hours after meals may represent the earliest clinical manifestation of diabetes in many cases.

No medical consideration of dizziness would be complete without a brief word about the psychiatric aspects of this problem. This subject of course will be covered in more detail in Chapter 23, "Psychiatric Aspects of Vertigo." Fleming[4] found that true vertigo may be emotional. Weiss and English[11] noted that even in the majority of organic cases, emotional factors were important. Therefore, these factors indicate that evaluation of the dizzy patient requires a careful consideration of both the organic and emotional factors.

REFERENCES

1. Best, C. H., and Taylor, M. B.: The Physiological Basis of Medical Practice. Baltimore, The Williams & Wilkins Co., 1961.
2. Conn, J. W.: Aldosteronism in man. J.A.M.A. 183:775-781, 871-878, 1963.
3. Crain, E. L., Jr., and Thorn, G. W.: Functioning pancreatic islet cell adenomas. Medicine 28:427, 441, 1949.
4. Fleming, B.: The Psychiatric Aspects of Dizziness & Vertigo. Thesis, Temple Medical School, Philadelphia, 1960.

5. Friedberg, C. K.: Diseases of the Heart, 2nd ed. Philadelphia, W. B. Saunders, 1956.
6. Logothetis, J., Silverstein, P., and Coe, J.: Neurologic aspects of Waldenstroms macroglobulinemia. Arch. Neurol. 3: 564-573, 1960.
7. Pickering, G. W.: High Blood Pressure. New York, Grune & Stratton, 1955.
8. Pyke, D. A.: Disorders of CHO Metabolism. Philadelphia, J. B. Lippincott, 1962.
9. Seltzer, H. S., Fajans, S. S., and Conn, J. W.: Spontaneous hypoglycemia as an early manifestation of diabetes mellitus. Diabetes 5: 437, 1956.
10. Wayne, H. H.: Syncope. Amer. J. Med. 30:418-438, 1961.
11. Weiss, E., and English, O. S.: Psychosomatic Medicine, 3rd ed. Philadelphia, W. B. Saunders, 1957.
12. Williams, R. H.: Diabetes. New York, Paul B. Hoeber Inc., 1960.
13. Zatuchni, J., Shenkin, H., and Fisher, H.: Arteriography in so-called cerebral embolism. Amer. J. Med. Sci. 24:468-473, 1961.

CHAPTER 19

Infections Outside the Labyrinth Causing Dizziness

Viral and Focal Infections, Herpes Zoster, and Syphilis

Martin Spector

VIRAL INFECTIONS

Acute systemic infections may precipitate or be accompanied by vertiginous episodes. The traditional name for such an episode has been acute toxic labyrinthitis. The modality assumed for this has been a subclinical labyrinthitis or localized neuritis of the vestibular nerve; however, the modality may well be an encephalitis. Pantazopoulos and Constantinides reported cases of vertigo which they ascribed to brainstem infection. These cases were accompanied by symptoms or signs denoting brainstem involvement as well as an infectious process. Their course was benign. Such entities are covered more completely under toxic labyrinthitis and the neurologic section.

Vestibular Paralysis

Hart reported cases of vestibular paralysis secondary to viral infection. In several of his cases, influenza was confirmed. He wrote:

> The typical history of the group is as follows: sudden onset of vertigo, nausea, and vomiting, usually on awakening, occurring from one to three weeks after the onset of a viral infection, most commonly of the upper respiratory type. The vertigo is aggravated by sudden movements, and on attempting to walk there is marked disequilibrium, with a tendency to fall to the affected side. Occasionally hearing is affected on the same side, as revealed by tinnitus and some degree of sensorineural loss. . . . Examination at this time usually reveals a spontaneous nystagmus toward the normal ear, and on positional testing there may be seen an increase in its intensity in certain positions, with a proportional increase in the vertigo. This is quite marked in the supine position, and in the lateral positions the nystagmus and vertigo are usually more marked with the affected ear undermost. . . . Some days later, sudden movements will still produce vertigo, and the postural element often persists for some weeks, with or without positional nystagmus. . . . After the disappearance of the spontaneous nystagmus, it may still be possible to evoke a type II (direction fixed) positional nystagmus in the same direction and in the positions which previously caused an increase in the intensity. . . . The caloric tests reveal a hypoexcitability of the affected side. . . . There is but a single episode of severe vertigo and the vestibular signs are unilateral distinguishing this from vestibular neuronitis.

Mumps, Measles, Typhus, etc.

A single attack of vertigo (often associated with deafness) has been reported from mumps, measles, or typhus, in addition to the respiratory infections. Bilateral loss of vestibular function may result from typhus or encephalitis. A hearing loss is associated in most cases.

Rinaldi reported the case of a 42-year-old woman who suffered a vestibular crisis on the right side, and 20 days later she developed mumps. The cochlear function was not affected. Positional vertigo was present, and there were no signs of intracranial involvement.

FOCAL INFECTION

The role of focal infection has not been looked upon with as much favor in recent years as formerly. It is most difficult to judge whether a focal infection is merely coincidental; even the fact that vertigo clears after treatment of the infection is not conclusive. The course of Meniere's disease, in particular, is so erratic that the abeyance of the vertigo is not absolute proof that treatment of a focal infection produced the cure. To illustrate this difficulty in judgment, a case of endolymphatic hydrops is presented which fulfilled all the diagnostic criteria. Episodes of vertigo on different occasions seemed related to bouts of suppurative maxillary sinusitis on the same side as the affected ear. However, episodes of vertigo occurred in the absence of sinusitis. Furthermore, alleviation of the sinusitis did not prevent further vertiginous attacks in this case. Wilson stated that he has never been certain in his own mind that a focus of infection caused vertigo. "Could it not actually be a stress reaction to the infection?" In the literature the most commonly blamed foci have been tonsillitis, sinusitis or periapical tooth abscesses.

The role of bacterial toxin in the origin of Meniere's disease, even without acute or chronic reactions, has been emphasized by Godlowski. He urged a careful study of all potential sources of infection—such as the throat, nasal and paranasal cavities, mouth, prostate, vagina, cervix, and adnexae — as primary sources of the factors which cause osmotic disequilibrium in the organism in terms of inactivation of hyaluronidase.

Lenke reported a 62-year-old man who had a marked inner ear deafness, first in one ear and then in the other, accompanied by vertigo at the beginning. He was found to have a cyst in one antrum, and after removal of the cyst there was a return of hearing and improvement of vertigo. Vertigo is certainly not a usual accompaniment of the ordinary attack of sinusitis.

Goodyear reported several cases of dizziness with sphenoid infection in which the sensation was a movement from side to side or the feeling that the sidewalk was coming up. Williams reported that Thornwaldt abscess in the nasopharynx caused recurring vertigo with inner ear deafness which was cleared by surgery of the Thornwaldt abscess. He reported two cases. The examiner should not confuse the sensation of stuffed nose and clouded head (which is the usual complaint with sinusitis) with dizziness. On several occasions, the author has noted a persistent imbalance which was readily cleared by antral wash.

Northington, in Fowler's textbook, described in one case a unilateral vestibular disorder associated with a suppurative maxillary sinusitis. He ascribed another case to chronic prostatitis. A third case was an acute vestibular disturbance without any cochlear symptoms, cleared by irrigations of a suppurative right sphenoid sinus. Northington added, "Infections of the sphenoid sinuses are associated more frequently with vestibular disorder than that of any other of the nasal accessory sinuses."

Role of Infections in Vestibular Neuronitis

Dix and Hallpike reported that vestibular neuronitis is usually preceded by infection, frequently of the nose or pharynx. They thoroughly examined 50 of 100 patients in their series for symptoms of infection and established manifest sinusitis or tonsillitis in 12 patients and a very probable infection in 23 cases; only in 15 cases was there nothing indicative of infection. The other 50 cases were examined less thoroughly for infection, but they found at least 8 cases of sinusitis and 14 with a history of manifest infection immediately before the onset of vertigo. The occurrence of infection immediately before the onset of vertigo was considered an essential feature in vestibular neuronitis.

Pfaltz reported that among 25 cases of vestibular neuronitis vertigo began with infection, and after the infection had been cured, the subjective condition improved in 17 patients. Sinusitis was established in 13 cases and this was the most common infection; tonsillitis or urinary tract infection was found in others. Aschan and Stahle reported 10 cases. Three of the patients had acute respiratory infection at the initial phase of the disease; one had enteritis. No infection was detected in 4 patients. The authors believed that no direct bacterial or viral component was involved but that a toxic or allergic process played a part.

Lumio and Haho tried to elucidate the role of infection in the etiology of vestibular neuronitis in 40 patients. Both the patient's own report of an infection and the examination were taken into consideration. Ten patients reported that vertigo had begun without preceding infection, and the others reported that infection had preceded vertigo. By the time a patient sought treatment for vertigo, the infection had been alleviated in 16 cases, but examination revealed objective signs of infection in 14 cases. The time lapse from infection to onset of vertigo was 2 to 10 days with a mean of 5 days. Twenty cases of vertigo began while the infection was still active. In 10 cases, there was a healthy period of several days between the infection and vertigo. Lumbar puncture was negative in 12 patients in whom it was performed. They found a common cold in 14, tonsillitis in 6, sinusitis in 5, urinary tract infection in 2, enteritis in one, infectious mononucleosis in 1, and suppurating wound of the hand in 1. The diagnosis of sinusitis was confirmed by roentgenography. The most important part of therapy was considered to be treatment of the infectious focus with antibiotics and topical measures. The onset of vertigo was preceded by an infection in exactly three-fourths of the patients. It was localized in the upper respiratory tract in 26 out of 30 cases.

HERPES ZOSTER

The geniculate form of herpes zoster oticus has been subdivided from the least extensive type: (1) herpes oticus alone, (2) with facial palsy, (3) facial palsy and auditory symptoms, and (4) the most severe type with facial palsy and auditory and labyrinthine symptoms. The zoster zone was described by Hunt to be afflicted with the vesicular lesion of herpes, and this included the tympanic membrane, external auditory canal, and lateral surface of the auricle.

Welsh and Welsh presented the case of a 74-year-old man with pain in the right ear, sudden deafness, vertigo, and severe instability on walking. He also developed a facial palsy, pain in the throat, hoarseness, and dysphagia. He had a vesicular lesion over the top of the head and right side of the pharynx. There was severe perceptive deafness in the right ear. One month after the attack had abated, an ice water caloric test demonstrated no activity in the right ear.

Pampus reported that in the acute stage, in addition to the herpetic vesicles in nearly all cases, paralysis of the facial nerve is seen. The cochlear and vestibular nerves were affected in about fifty per cent of his patients. Occasionally, involvement of other cranial nerves such as the abducens and hypoglossus was noted, but these cleared completely. Lesions of the facial, cochlear, and vestibular nerves presented only a partial tendency to improve, depending upon the degree of severity. Sequelae persisted in at least half of the patients, disturbance of the vestibular nerve being especially intense.

Sarcoidosis

Jepson reported sarcoidosis which simulated neurinoma of the acoustic nerve. All four of his patients had perceptive hearing loss and dizziness. The complaints varied in severity from time to time.

SYPHILIS

Syphilis may cause vertigo, often with deafness. In congenital syphilis the fistula symptom is common, due to erosion of the bony wall. Eggston and Wolff wrote:

> The most commonly observed pathological

change in the temporal bone in cases of chronic syphilis is the more or less complete obliteration of the lumen of the semicircular system with bone. This type of pathological alteration has not been observed in the cochlea by the authors. All stages of the disease are to be found in the vestibular labyrinth, from an early proliferative periostitis (endostitis) through fibrosis of the perilymphatic tissue to deposition of dense bone within the canals. Earlier stages of the disease cause the contour of the canal lumen to be irregular and motheaten in appearance. These vestibular changes apparently progress so slowly that the individual compensates for them and is not aware of the lesion.

As to the clinical course, Christie wrote:

When a young adult complains of a profound degree of deafness, with or without giddiness at first, the probable cause is syphilis, especially if the onset has been sudden and the progress rapid. In the acquired form, the ear may be involved early, even before the primary chancre has disappeared, but as a rule the time of onset is toward the end of the secondary stage. One or both ears may be affected and the disease is rapidly progressive. The deafness and tinnitus may be accompanied by giddiness, nausea and nystagmus or deafness may be the only sign. In the inherited form, both ears are affected and the deafness appears suddenly sometimes along with severe vertigo. The time of its appearance like that of interstitial keratitis is between 7 and 16 years of age.

"In tabes and general paresis, Krassnig usually failed to detect anomalies of the labyrinth, while Eagleton observed in tabetics an early reduction of the vestibular reaction to turning," wrote Spiegel.

REFERENCES

1. Aschan, G., and Stahle, J.: Vestibular neuritis. J. Laryng. 70:497, 1956.
2. Christie, J. F.: Syphilitic infections of the ear. M. Press. & Circ. 147:362, 1938.
3. Dix, M. R., and Hallpike, C. S.: The pathology, symptomatology and diagnosis of certain common disorders of the vestibular system. Proc. Roy. Soc. Med. 45:341, 1952.
4. Eggston, A. A., and Wolff, D.: Histopathology of the Ear, Nose and Throat. Baltimore, Williams and Wilkins Co., 1947, p. 436.
5. Godlowski, H.: Meniere's disease. Eye Ear Nose Throat Digest, July 1965, p. 63.
6. Hart, C.: Vestibular paralysis of sudden onset, from probably viral etiology. Ann. Otol. 74: 33-44, 1965.
7. Jepson, B.: Neurootological symptoms in sarcoidosis. Pract. Otorhinolaryn. 24:361-371, 1962.
8. Lumio, J., and Haho, J.: Vestibular neuronitis. Ann. Otol. 74:264-270, 1965.
9. Northington, P.: Extraneous infections. *In:* Medicine of the Ear (E. P. Fowler, Jr., Ed.). New York, T. Nelson and Sons, 1948, pp. 532-536.
10. Pampus, H., et al.: Herpes zoster oticus, clinical aspects and prognosis. Fortschr. Neurol. Psychiat. 30:506-524, 1963.
11. Pantazopoulos, P. E., and Constantinides, A. S.: Infectious conditions of the brain stem masquerading as a labyrinth syndrome. Ann. Otol. 74:194-202, 1965.
12. Pfaltz, C.: Diagnosis and therapy of vestibular neuronitis. Pract. Otorhinolaryng. 5-6:454, 1955.
13. Rinaldi, L.: Boll. Mal. Orecch. 76:388-396, 1958.
14. Stahle, J., and Terens, S.: Paroxysmal positional nystagmus. Ann. Otol. 74:69-82, 1965.
15. Welsh, L. W., and Welsh, J.: Herpes zoster involving the head and neck. Laryngoscope 72:653-662, 1962.

Cogan's Syndrome

Henry L. Williams

Cogan's syndrome may be rightfully included among the episodic vertigos. In the typical case the onset may be signaled by complaints referred to either the ears or the eyes. There are, however, atypical examples of the condition in which disorders of hearing predominate sometimes almost to the exclusion of eye symptoms. In some instances, which still seem classifiable as atypical examples of Cogan's syndrome, the disorder approaches the clinical picture of the condition described by Sheehy under the classification of "rapidly advancing hearing loss of the younger age group" and is now termed "Sheehy's syndrome." It is interesting to note that the first case reported in the literature of a syndrome consisting of nonsyphilitic interstitial keratitis associated with vestibuloauditory symptoms was reported as "Meniere's disease complicated by recurrent interstitial keratitis."

In 1945 Cogan reported 4 cases with typical nonsyphilitic interstitial keratitis associated with vestibuloauditory symptoms and identified the case of Mogen and Baumgartner (mentioned above) as the same condition.

In 1960 Cody and Williams reviewed the literature of Cogan's syndrome and added 4 typical cases and 2 atypical examples of this disease entity. They found it evident that the vestibuloauditory symptoms occurred with greater regularity than did the interstitial keratitis. It seems probable that had the symptom complex not been identified by an ophthalmologist, the term "episodic vertigo with audiovestibular deterioration and associated with various ophthalmologic disorders" might have been adopted. This would have been more descriptive of the clinical pattern usually revealed than the term suggested by Cogan.

Cogan's syndrome may herald its onset by either an attack of severe rotatory vertigo with rapidly deteriorating hearing or complaints referred to the eyes, although the first type of onset is the more common. The vertigo usually terminates in a few hours, but the hearing loss tends to persist for an extended period and is usually bilateral. A sudden remission may then occur in the hearing loss and it may suddenly return to a nearly normal level. The patient may have forgotten that he or she ever had a hearing loss when, with another episode of vertigo, a severe hearing loss accompanied by a persistent tinnitus may recur. In spite of the remissions, the general tendency is for the hearing to progress steadily downward until both auditory and vestibular function is completely lost. When present, the interstitial keratitis is usually bilateral and is also characterized by rapid remissions and exacerbations and may or may not lead eventually to diminution of visual acuity.

Cody and Williams concluded from an analysis of their own cases and those reported in the literature that Cogan's syndrome was not a nosologic entity but was merely one manifestation of a systemic disease. They felt, from the available evidence, that this systemic disease is panarteritis nodosa, one of the "collagen" or autoimmune disorders. It is thus related to many syndromes once considered separate entities, such as idiopathic midline granuloma (Wegener's granulomatosis), Libman-Sacks' syndrome, temporal arteritis, dermatomyositis, Loeffler's syndrome, and thrombotic thrombocytopenic purpura. As the volume of literature on the respective autoimmune diseases grows, it is increasingly evident that we are not finding a clearer differentiation between one and the other, but that we are discovering more and more overlapping on the histologic, clinical, and experimental levels.

The relatively good prognosis and the frequent failure of muscle biopsy to yield a diagnosis are shown by these authors not to be serious objections to the hypothesis that Cogan's syndrome is nothing more than a localized manifestation of panarteritis nodosa.

Williams was the first to suggest that adrenal cortical steroids might be effective in relieving the symptoms of collagen (autoimmune) disease on the basis that it seemed to be a type of allergic disorder. The glucocorticoids still seem to be the only medication that offers any chance of amelioration in these disorders, although the response is limited and unpredictable. However, Burnet has recently stated that the glucocorticoids are a logical medication in one of these conditions.

To secure the best results, the glucocorticoid preparations should be started early, given in full dosage until a full remission of symptoms has been obtained, then gradually decreased to a maintenance dose which must be estimated by the response of the patient, and continued for 2 or 3 months. The medication should be gradually terminated and the attending physician must be prepared to resume therapy at the first indication of a return of symptoms.

REFERENCES

1. Cogan, D. G.: Syndrome of nonsyphilitic interstitial keratitis and vestibuloauditory symptoms. Arch. Ophthal. 33:144, 1945.
2. Mogan, R. F., and Baumgartner, C. J.: Meniere's disease complicated by recurring interstitial keratitis. West. J. Surg. 42:628, 1934.
3. Cody, D. T. R., and Williams, H. L.: Cogan's syndrome. Laryngoscope 70:447, 1960.
4. Williams, H. L.: Lethal granulomatous ulceration involving the midline facial tissues. Ann. Otol. 58:1013, 1949.

CHAPTER 20

Drugs and Toxins Causing Vertigo

MARTIN SPECTOR AND
HAROLD WILF

MECHANISMS OF ACTION

It has been postulated that medications or toxins which alter the blood flow to the head, either by altering the cardiac output or the autonomic control of the small vessels supplying the vestibule, may produce effects on vestibular function. Toxic agents which result in anemia or hypoxia may cause vertiginous symptoms. Circulating agents interfering with the enzyme metabolism of nerve endings or electrolytes of the body fluids may influence the function and physical integrity of the statokinetic system. It is interesting to note that the salicylates, quinine, and streptomycin drugs are all products of plant metabolism. It has been suggested that they interfere with the enzyme system of the sensory elements. Measurable effects directly on the central vestibular connections by sedatives, tranquilizers or antimotion sickness drugs have been reported. Some drugs primarily show toxicity on either the cochlear or vestibular system, but many affect both systems. The cochlea seems to be initially and predominantly more involved than the vestibular apparatus in general. This is ascribed to the more recent phylogenetic development of the cochlea. The route of action of the drugs seems to be by way of the cerebrospinal fluid to the perilymph or by way of the vascular system to the stria vascularis and then to the endolymph. Some toxic drug effects are also known to be transmitted to the fetus in utero, resulting in vestibular abnormalities. Also, toxicity has been demonstrated by osmosis or absorption through the oval or round window for drugs locally administered into the middle ear.

The cristae of the semicircular canals seem less resistant than the maculae of the utricle and the saccule. The external hair cells are more sensitive than the internal hair cells of the organ of Corti, according to animal experiments.

MEDICATIONS

Streptomycin

Incidence

Northington observed 56 patients with bilateral vestibular paralysis from streptomycin who had received a daily dose of 2.5 to 3.2 Gm. streptomycin. Toxic effects usually occurred during the second week of administration. Only one had impairment of hearing. Among 50 patients who received a daily dose of 1 Gm. streptomycin for 75 consecutive days, only one experienced neurotoxic effects. Thomas reported that patients receiving 2 Gm. streptomycin daily were four times as likely to become dizzy as those receiving 1 Gm. per day. The effects were much more severe in those over 45 years of age. In the mild cases, the dizziness cleared after 4 weeks. The mean date of onset of dizziness with 2 Gm. daily was the 22nd day, but the mean date of onset with 1 Gm. daily was the 45th day. Linden Wallner studied patients who had received 2 Gm. streptomycin per day, and 79 per cent of these developed subjective complaints. In a group who had received 1 Gm. per day, 45 per cent had symptoms. None of the patients had any hearing loss. No case, with complete loss of function by caloric test, was found to improve. Of the 53 patients receiving 2 Gm. per day, 21 developed absence of caloric responses. This group received streptomycin for 4 months. Of the 40 patients receiving 1 Gm. per day for 4 months, 6 developed absent caloric responses. All the patients with depressed or absent caloric responses had complained of symptoms during treatment.

Pathology

Ruedi found that (1) the cristae and maculae displayed a distinct reduction of sensory epithelium, and that (2) the degeneration of sensory cells was accompanied by a loss of sensory hairs beginning with a loss of single hairs. Berg administered exceedingly large doses of streptomycin to cats in order to find the site of the lesion responsible for the vestibular dysfunction. In all the animals, postrotatory nystagmus finally became extinct. The time required for this varied according to the total amount of streptomycin administered. Berg found marked degenerative changes in the sensory epithelium of the crista ampullaris, macula utriculi, and macula sacculi in his animal studies. The brain and vestibular nuclei showed no definite pathologic changes. Berg concluded that the primary effect was on the sensory epithelium of the labyrinth with slight, presumably secondary, changes of the vestibular ganglion. Degeneration in the organ of Corti was only found in one animal which had received tremendous doses.

Symptoms and Signs

Northington reported the symptoms after streptomycin. A few hours after the appearance of the initial complaints (mainly dizziness on movement in bed, sensation of fullness in the head, noises in the ears, headache, nausea, and vomiting), patients experienced inability to maintain customary posture and gait, along with jumbling of distant visual objects. All complaints increased in severity, but usually for only a few days. In the acute stage, the patients with the greatest disability were unable to stand and walk unsupported; in patients less severely affected, ability to maintain a standing position was faulty, especially when the body was tilted in any direction. Regression from this peak occurred even when streptomycin therapy was continued. Some amelioration of intensity of symptoms took place over a few days and was usually followed by several months of slow and gradual improvement in posture, gait, vision, and diminution of dizziness. The headache was diffuse and not localized and usually subsided before the end of the acute stage, but in some cases it lasted several months, occurring in periodic attacks. Tinnitus was a very common symptom; the tinnitus was intermittent and subsided soon in most of the patients who did not acquire any impairment of hearing. In some patients, the tinnitus was very annoying. Although neither nausea nor vomiting was common, even in the acute stages, in occasional patients this was so distressing as to be the reason for discontinuing streptomycin therapy soon after it was begun. Spontaneous nystagmus was not seen with the eyes in the primary position, and when seen on rare occasions it was on lateral fixation. The Romberg test revealed only slight swaying in no specific direction.

The usual course in which the initial symptoms of headache, aural noises, and vomiting subsided soon after the onset was in contrast to that of slow regression of the symptoms of dizziness, disturbance of gait and posture, and jumbling of visual objects. The dizziness was a sense of false motion, a feeling of being compelled to continue movement of the body in the direction in which the head was tilted, chiefly to the face-up or face-down positions, as well as the sensation of continuing on the course in which the subject was walking after turning the head in a different direction. As soon as the patient stopped walking, the dizziness disappeared. In the chronic stage, when improvement in gait was considerable, the patient was likely to bump into a nearby object in passing, having the sensation of being drawn to it. After the patient was able to walk straight with good ability, if he turned his head to change his course, he could not execute the maneuver with precision. The disability was comparable to that of excessive use of alcoholic beverages. The gait was characteristic, with feet wide apart. When blindfolded, the patient had great difficulty walking on irregular surfaces; the steps were broad and hesitant.

Books could be read with ease, but objects appeared to run together and lose detail on movement of the head, especially when walking or riding in an automobile. In order to see clearly, the patient had to stand still. This was observed equally well with monocular as with binocular vision. These disorders were regularly accompanied by a bilateral loss of vestibular reaction to both rotatory and caloric tests; the loss was total in some patients and the degree of response was usually proportional to that of the clinical disability. Another finding reported by Northington was that after rotation there was no response, when the responses after caloric tests were still good; that is, a rotatory test usually detected changes before the caloric test. Optokinetic tests were normal. After 4 years, patients who had minimal symptoms attained complete recovery. A few patients with complete bilateral vestibular paralysis recovered to the degree found on bilateral ablation of vestibular receptors; there was a lasting disturbance for precision in locomotion in the dark, especially if the patient attempted to swim or dive without the aid of vision. None of Northington's patients exhibited symptoms which would indicate impairment of function of neurologic elements other than that of the eighth cranial nerve.

Other Antibiotics

Dihydrostreptomycin, kanamycin, and neomycin have their primary and predominant effect on the cochlear apparatus and a lesser and later effect on the vestibular system. The effects of these drugs are increased by poor renal function, which increases the body retention of the drugs in regard to dosage.

Harbert wrote: "Neomycin injected intramuscularly has been reported to cause deafness in patients with renal disease in as short a time as one to two weeks on as low as one gram daily. In individuals with good kidney function, neomycin may be tolerated as long as three to six weeks without evidence of deafness." In two cases studied histologically by Lindsay in 1960, after neomycin there were no changes in the vestibular apparatus. Fields, in a review of neomycin ototoxicity, remarked: "Vertigo is not a common symptom of early neomycin toxicity, and in many cases, does not appear at all." He reported a case resulting from colonic irrigation with neomycin; the patient developed severe deafness but never had vertigo. Caloric testing with ice water revealed bilateral labyrinthine function with a decreased response on the right.

Harbert reported that isoniazid can produce tinnitus, vertigo, and ataxia, but not in the doses usually administered. Hawkins wrote that kanamycin, so far as the vestibular system is concerned, shows itself less ototoxic than streptomycin. He studied toxicity in cats. Polymyxin B has been demonstrated to have a very marked toxic effect on the vestibules of guinea pigs.

Aspirin and Quinine

Aspirin and quinine appear somewhat similar in their toxic effects and are therefore discussed together in the literature. The literature indicates that quinine and salicylates rarely cause dizziness. However, quinine is said to aggravate dizziness already present.

Symptoms may be precipitated by either an overdosage or idiosyncrasy to the drugs. Shea felt that toxicity was less likely from small amounts of quinine ingested over a long period of time than from excessively large amounts ingested over a short period. On the other hand, Kapur emphasized that otoxicity from salicylates was often due to an idiocrasy. In an idiosyncrasy, the time intering between the administration of acetylicylic acid and the onset of symptoms usu- is short, the minimal recorded time being minutes and the longest being 2 hours. th symptoms from excessive dosage of icylates, the symptoms usually fade when salicylates are discontinued. Tinnitus, ring loss, and dizziness may be manifested ether from toxicity or they may be maniited separately.

Waltner reported a woman who ingested) five-grain tablets of acetylsalicylic acid l developed hearing loss, tinnitus, and rerent sensations of unsteadiness. The unadiness and hearing loss were temporary. loric tests performed by the Hallpike meth- showed no vestibular disturbance. Kapur orted the case of a 13-year-old boy who veloped hearing loss plus dizziness after 3 lets of aspirin. The dizziness lasted 3 days. e Hallpike caloric test showed hypofuncn of both labyrinths.

Shea reported that a very consistent feae of quinine toxicity "is a bizarre and disbing tinnitus characterized by a variety of unds, especially the sound made by electric res arcing and other such bizarre sounds." Although excessive aspirin or quinine dur- pregnancy has been reported to cause ngenital deafness, there is a dearth of rerts of congenital vestibular disturbance due quinine or salicylates.

Barbiturates

Aschan reported that barbiturates produce sitional nystagmus. This was not as easily produced as the nystagmus occurring after ohol. Patients who demonstrate a spontanes positional nystagmus on electronystaggraphy are often found to have taken barturates during the previous evening. Any tient who demonstrates a spontaneous posinal nystagmus and has no other abnormalis of labyrinthine function should be suscted of having taken barbiturates recently. a series in Sweden, 68 per cent of patients in this category had a positive blood barbiturate level. To illustrate, Aschan et al. found positional nystagmus Type II in a patient who had ingested a very large dose of barbiturates 10 days previously. They reported weak positional nystagmus. After exclusion of all medication, positional nystagmus could not be confirmed at reexamination a few days later.

Opiates

The nystagmus from opium is a vertical nystagmus downwards. Morphine has been reported to produce a significant decrease in vestibular response but there was an increase in nausea. Demerol also produces a vertical nystagmus.

Other Drugs

Dilantin, Tridione, antitoxins, mercury, gold, sulfonamides, and mephenesin are among the drugs also reported to affect the labyrinth. Most drugs affect the auditory apparatus before they affect the vestibular endorgan, so tinnitus is usually the first symptom. The toxic effect may persist. Indocin occasionally causes prolonged dizziness; a side-to-side sensation or propulsion has also been reported with indocin.

Many medications may cause temporary dizziness and the effects wear off shortly after the medication is withdrawn. This includes many sedatives, tranquilizers, hypnotics, strong analgesics, and antihistamines. With these effects, the patient must be particularly warned against driving an automobile. Although not a medication, excessive salt intake has been reported to precipitate attacks of endolymphatic hydrops.

TOXINS

Alcohol

Alcohol intoxication results in positional alcoholic nystagmus which follows a specific pattern related to the concentration of the blood alcohol. This subject has been extensively studied by Aschan, Bergstedt, and

Stahle. The following discussion has been culled from their work.

Alcoholic nystagmus is a typical positional nystagmus Type I in which, after administration of alcohol in a single dose, two distinct phases can be distinguished. A maximum blood alcohol concentration of no more than .02 per cent in their experiments was enough to release both phases of positional alcoholic nystagmus. Aschan, Bergstedt, and Stahle recorded by electronystagmography after subjects consumed 100 cc. of Swedish schnapps.

The first phase of the gaze nystagmus is at the peak of the alcoholic concentration. The primary nystagmus always jerks in the direction of the gaze (to the right in gazing or head turning to the right; to the left in gazing or head turning to the left). This positional alcoholic nystagmus (PAN), phase I, beats to the right in the right lateral position and to the left in the left lateral position. It appears in an average of 31 minutes and disappears about 207 minutes after consumption of alcohol. This gradually diminishes after the peak of the alcohol concentration is past but may be reinstituted quantitatively by the ingestion of additional alcohol.

Phase I is followed by an intermediate period lasting 102 minutes (average), during which no nystagmus can be recorded. Then the secondary phase occurs in which the direction of the nystagmus is just opposite to that of the primary phase. In phase II (PAN II), the nystagmus is to the left in the right lateral position and to the right in the left lateral position. This second phase begins about 5 hours and 45 minutes after drinking, and the nystagmus changes so that in the right lateral position there is a nystagmus to the left, and in the left lateral position it beats to the right. It is of importance that PAN II may not occur until after all alcohol has disappeared from the blood. PAN II always persists for several hours after all alcohol has disappeared from the blood. PAN II, therefore, constitutes a sign of the state commonly known as a "hangover." This nystagmus is greatest when the hangover symptoms are greatest. The intensity of the nystagmus during PAN I, PAN II and the duration of PAN II were significantly correlated to the quantity of alcohol consumed.

Alcoholic intoxication with blood alcohol concentration above 40 mg. per cent changes a spontaneous nystagmus to a positional nystagmus. If there is ingestion of more alcohol during the secondary stage, there is a 15 to 20 minute latency period and then the primary curve is superimposed on the secondary curve. If both labyrinths are destroyed, no positional alcoholic nystagmus can be induced, even though all other signs of intoxication hangover do occur. Even if only one labyrinth is working, both phases of alcoholic nystagmus in both directions are obtained. It is interesting to note that phase II of the alcohol-induced nystagmus only occurs in man; it has not been seen in either rabbits or monkeys.

Carbon Monoxide

Aschan, Stahle, and Terens reported vertigo and nystagmus in cases of carbon monoxide poisoning. In one case, with a long history of exposure to carbon monoxide, the patient developed rapidly increasing vertigo, obviously dependent upon the position of the head. Nystagmography revealed transitory direction changing positional nystagmus of type III. These curves showed marked similarity to benign paroxysmal positional nystagmus. Schullenberg reported that vestibular symptoms varied greatly with carbon monoxide intoxication and that real vertigo was rare but nystagmus was frequent. Hearing impairment was more common in his experience than vestibular disturbances.

Miscellaneous Toxins

Diamant studied arsenical compounds (such as sodium arsanilate), thiurams, sulfides (such as antabuse), and nitrogen mustards. He administered intracarotid injections into guinea pigs. He reported that the nitrogen mustards, sodium arsanilate, and the arsenicals had an appreciable destructive effect; sodium arsanilate probably had a large peripheral effect, while nitrogen mustard, in addition, caused a destruction of the vestibular nuclei.

Diamant also used the nerve gases, tabun and sarn (which are cholinesterase inhibitors), to produce vestibular syndromes of central origin. The nerve gases act strongly upon the cholinesterases but cause no histologically verifiable lesions. He stated that Miehlke found that ammonia induced a vestibular disturbance in one case, and in an experimental investigation observed that the primary lesion was probably localized to the vestibular nuclei of the brain stem.

Phosphoric esters are largely used by fruit growers in disinfestation of plants. Vigi reported the history of 5 patients with labyrinthine symptoms of vertigo and nystagmus and signs of peripheral labyrinthine hyporeflectivity. The recovery of the patients occurred within a few days. Ferreri and Zina treated rabbits daily with aniline for 90 days and found some lesions of the vestibular apparatus. They concluded that aniline is toxic to the labyrinth.

Tobacco, formaldehyde, and insecticides are reported to cause dizziness. Nicotine causes nystagmus which is spontaneous and vertical in direction. Carbon disulfide, the aniline dyes, lead, phosphorous, etc., can cause tinnitus, deafness and vertigo. Another reported incitant is air embolism in caisson disease. Roentgen ray therapy has been reported to cause hyperexcitability of the labyrinth. Wodak reported several cases of vertigo due to heat from the hot air used in permanent waves or in very hot occupations. He claimed the heat affected the central vestibular checking mechanisms. Other toxins which have been reported as instigators of dizziness include methyl (wood) alcohol, oil of chenopodium, chloroform, and the heavy metals.

REFERENCES

1. Aschan, G., Bergstedt, M. and Stahle, J.: Nystagmography. Acta Otolaryng. Suppl. 129:54, 1956.
2. Aschan, G., et al.: Positional alcohol nystagmus changes after labyrinth destruction. Confin. Neurol. (Basel) 24:80-102, 1964.
3. Berg, C.: Toxic effect of streptomycin on the eighth cranial nerve. Ann. Otol. 58:448, 1949.
4. Diamant, H.: Toxic action of some compounds on the inner ear and vestibular connections. Arch. Otolaryng. 67:546-552, 1958.
5. Falbe-Hansen, J.: Clinical and experimental histological studies or effects of salicylates and quinine on the ear. Acta Otolaryng. Suppl. 44, 1941.
6. Fields, R. L.: Neomycin ototoxicity. Arch. Otolaryng. 79:67-70, 1964.
7. Harbert, F.: Collected Letters of Otolaryngology, Series X:118, 1965.
8. Hawkins, J.: The ototoxicity of kanamycin. Ann. Otol. 68:698-718, 1959.
9. Kapur, Y. P.: Ototoxicity of acetylsalicylic acid. Arch. Otolaryng. 81:134-138, 1965.
10. Northington, P.: Vestibular paralysis by streptomycin. Arch. Otolaryng. 52:381-396, 1950.
11. Ruedi, L.: Streptomycin in otology. Laryngoscope 61:623-630, 1951.
12. Shea, J., Jr.: Collected Letters of Otolaryngology, Series X:56, 1965.
13. Stahle, J., and Terens, S.: Paroxysmal positional nystagmus. Ann. Otol. 74:69-82, 1965.
14. Thomas, J. A. B.: The toxic effect of streptomycin on the eighth cranial nerve. J. Laryng. 65:472, 1951.
15. Wallner, J.: Otologic effects of streptomycin therapy. Ann. Otol. 58:111-116, 1949.
16. Waltner, J. G.: Effect of salicylates on the inner ear. Ann Otol. 64:617-622, 1955.

CHAPTER 21

Etiologic Classification of Vertigo in Children

HENRY W. BAIRD, III

True vertigo is a rare presenting symptom in the pediatric age group. Occasionally, a child will describe a sense of rotation or movement, but often he or his parents have difficulty in distinguishing dizziness from a transient loss of consciousness. The table on page 249 lists the etiologic classifications of vertigo in children.

REFERENCES

1. Alpers, B. J., and Yaskin, H. E.: The Bruns' syndrome. J. Nerv. Ment. Dis. 100:115, 1944.
2. Alpers, B. J.: Vertiginous epilepsy. Laryngoscope 70:631, 1960.
3. Basser, L. S.: Benign paroxysmal vertigo of childhood (a variety of vestibular neuronitis), Brain 87:141, 1964.
4. Behrman, S.: Vestibular epilepsy. Brain 78:471, 1951.
5. Behrman, S., and Wyke, B. D.: Vestibulogenic seizures. Brain 81:529, 1958.
6. Craig, W. McK., Dodge, H. W., and Ross, P. J.: Acoustic neurinomas in children: report of two cases. J. Neurosurg. 11:505, 1954.
7. Cramer, F., and Kimsey, W.: The cerebellar hemangioblastomas. Arch. Neurol. Psychiat. 67:237, 1962.
8. Crowe, S. J.: Meniere's disease. Medicine 17:1, 1938.
9. Dix, M. R., and Hallpike, C. S.: The pathology, symptomatology and diagnosis of certain common disorders of the vestibular system. Proc. Roy. Soc. Med. 45:341, 1952.
10. Everberg, G.: Paroxysmal vertigo with nystagmus and parotid swelling. Arch. Otolarng. 72:610, 1960.
11. Ford, F. R.: Diseases of the Nervous System in Infancy, Childhood and Adolescence. Springfield, Ill., Charles C Thomas, 1959.
12. Greer, M., and Schotland, D.: Abnormal hemoglobin as a cause of neurological disease. Neurology 12:114, 1962.
13. Harrison, M. S.: Vertigo in childhood. J. Lary 76:601, 1962.
14. Harrison, M. S.: Epidemic vertigo—vestibu neuronitis. Brain 85:613, 1962.
15. Henningen, E. J.: Epidemic vertigo. Uges Laeg. 1935, p. 1285.
16. Holt, G. W.: Epidemic neuromyasthenia: sporadic form. Amer. J. Med. Sci. 249: 1965.
17. Margolis, M. P.: Sickle cell anemia. Medic 30:357, 1951.
18. Miller, R., anod Raven, M.: Epidemic nau and vomiting. Brit. Med. J. 1:1242, 1936
19. Ombredanne, I. M., and Aubrey, M.: Menier disease. Bull. Soc. Pediat. 38:193, 1941.
20. Pederson, E.: Epidemic vertigo. Brain 82:5 1959.
21. Penfield, W., and Erickson, T. C.: Epilepsy a the Cerebral Circulation. Springfield, Charles C Thomas, 1941.
22. Revilla, A. G.: Neurinomas of the cerebel pontine angle. Bull. Hopkins Hosp. 20: 2 1947.
23. Ruchel, A.: Epidemic Vertigo. Ugeskr. La 1936, p. 45.
24. Russell, J. R., and Bucy, P. C.: Meningiomas the posterior fossa. Surg. Gynec. Obst. 9 183, 1953.
25. Serrins, A. J., Hanson, R., and Chandler, J. Cogan's syndrome. Arch. Otolaryng. 785, 1963.
26. Snyder, C. H.: Epileptic equivalents in childr Pediatrics 21:308, 1952.
27. Stevens, T.: Cogan's syndrome. A.M.A. Ar Neurol. Psychiat. 71:337, 1954.
28. Sorensen, H.: Meniere's disease in a seven ye old girl. J. Laryng. 73:346, 1956.
29. Tinney, W. S., Hall, B. E., and Griffen, H. Central nervous system manifestations polycythemia vera. Ann. Intern. Med. 1360, 1940.
30. Wilson, T. G.: Diseases of the Ear, Nose a Throat in Children. New York, Grune Stratton, 1962.

	Age of Onset	Associated Signs or Symptoms
1. Infection		
Serous labyrinthitis "Active suppuration" inner ear Viral illness (following measles, chickenpox, etc.)	Variable	Evidence of disease elsewhere.
2. Presumed infection or "toxin"		
Vestibular neuritis	Variable	May be associated with blackout episodes. No cochlear disease evident. One attack may be followed by unsteadiness up to 5½ months.
Epidemic vertigo	Variable	Associated with evidence of encephalitis. Caloric responses normal; hearing normal.
Toxin (Drugs—streptomycin, Dilantin, aspirin, quinine, etc.)		Usually follow prolonged use.
3. Meniere's Disease	?	May be a defect in a portion of the carotid blood supply rather than a true degenerative disease. If it occurs in children, then in 2nd decade.
4. Tumor	Variable	Brainstem lesions or posterior fossa tumor. May be paroxysmal; other evidence of cranial nerve defect usually present. Sarcoma at base of skull has been reported.
5. Convulsive disorder	Variable	EEG may be helpful. Psychomotor seizures in young adolescents (temporal lobe syndrome) most difficult to distinguish.
6. Migraine	Variable after age 2	Family history.
7. Functional	Over 4 years	Other evidence of phobic reaction on psychometric studies. Examination not remarkable otherwise.
8. Benign paroxysmal	Less than 4 years usual	Episodes of dizziness rarely more than 2 minutes. No loss of consciousness. EEG normal. Nystagmus may be present. Severe canal paresis.
9. Other conditions in which vertigo has been described:		
Foreign body against tympanic membrane		
Sickle cell disease "S.S." disease = hemoglobin S and hemoglobin C		
Head trauma		
Cholesteatoma		
Syringobulbia		

CHAPTER 22

Allergic Aspects of Vertigo

WILLIAM H. WILSON

The clinical manifestations of an abnormal vascular reaction to allergic stress may be catastrophic if they evolve from a congenitally predisposed labyrinth which is responding as a shock organ. Instrumental in the severity of the symptomatic response is the end arterial type of vascularization of the vestibular apparatus and cochlea, plus the very nature of the responding sensory organ. The resulting symptoms depend upon the labyrinthine components involved in the ischemic process.

Embarrassment of the circulation of the stria vascularis may be responsible for purely cochlear manifestations in the form of an early pitch dysacusis which may later develop into a sensorineural hearing loss. If the resulting endolymphatic biochemical and/or physical changes extend to the maculae and cristae, vertigo ensues. A symptom complex of dysacusis, sensorineural hearing loss, and vertigo stemming from a disorder of the capillary bed of the stria vascularis may deserve classification as Meniere's disease.

We may also postulate the possibility of arteriolar dysfunction of the vestibular branches of the internal auditory artery when we observe a patient experiencing episodic vertigo of end-organ origin without cochlear symptoms. Arteriolar-induced ischemia might involve one or more of the maculae and cristae.

Vasospasm involving penetrating branches of the basilar artery which supply the vestibular nuclei may also be responsible for episodes of vertigo. The possibility of vertigo from involvement of the equilibrial cortex has also been suggested.

The clinical manifestations of vascular labyrinthine dysfunction may thus be classified into three groups: (1) cochlear, (2) cochlear and vestibular, and (3) vestibular. A fourth group of central vascular dysfunction must also be considered.

The fact that abnormal vascular responses to stress are a local manifestation of systemic disease is well documented elsewhere in this volume. Food-induced migrainous episodes were referred to by Vaughan[1] as being due to a localized sensitization of the temporal artery which acted as a shock organ. Mention was made of a local predisposition so to react. A high percentage of patients experiencing episodic vertigo of end-organ origin give a personal or family history of migraine or one of the other vasomotor neuroses. When an aberrant labyrinthine vascular response takes place in these individuals, it may be assumed there has been a change in the capacity to react of the predisposed shock tissue.

The capability of arteriolar and metarteriolar spasm to persist following an initial stimulus is explainable by Lorente de No's[2] description of the summating effect of the internuncial neurone reflex arc. Williams[3] theorized that an antigen circulating in the blood stream could also act as a continuing stimulus to the initial abnormal vascular response to stress. Such an antigen could also have a summating effect in raising a synaptic subthreshold stimulus to a responsive level.

The consideration of episodic vertigo as an allergic reaction of the labyrinthine system has appeared in the literature at intervals since Duke[4] in 1923 reported two cases of Meniere's disease in which relief could be obtained by the avoidance of foods to which the patient gave a positive intracutaneous test. In each case he was able to reproduce an attack of vertigo during a period of remission by injecting an extract of the offending food intracutaneously. Symptoms were also reproduced by eating of the offending foods. Vogel,[5] Proetz,[6] Dohlman,[7] Criep,[8] Dean,[9] Derlacki,[10] and Shambaugh[11] have, among others, documented the role of foods in selected cases of episodic vertigo.

Vertiginous patients whose symptoms are precipitated by the ingestion of food are not prone to develop hay fever or perennial nasal allergy, in my experience. An attempt to classify a vertiginous patient as allergic by searching for a history of nasal allergy will only result in the repeatedly established opinion that allergy seldom plays a role in labyrinthine dysfunction.

I have found flatulent abdominal distention or bloating the most frequent symptoms and signs in episodic vertigo aside from those actually labyrinthine in origin. Any known food intolerance should be considered significant in classifying patients if the vertigo is due to an abnormal vascular response to stress, episodic or postural in character, and of end-organ origin.

The failure to associate labyrinthine symptoms with food intolerances is due largely to the failure on the part of the physician to realize that digestive disorders and vertiginious attacks may have a common etiological denominator. The generally unfortunate experience of the medical profession in attempting to determine specific food hypersensitivities by reliance on skin whealing response has also been a factor in this disassociation.

A searching history must be taken on all patients, with particular attention being paid to potential exogenous stress factors. Inquiry must also be made as to possible endocrine disorders, attention being directed toward the possibility of adrenal insufficiency, hypothyroidism, euthyroid hypometabolism, functional hypoglycemia, and ovarian dysfunction.

A family as well as personal history of allergy is of importance, but frequently unobtainable. Patients rarely associate their vertigo or gastrointestinal distress with a given food. This is due to the masking effect so well described by Rinkel.[12] Many individuals suffering from intermittent episodes of flatulent abdominal distention may deny its existence until questioned extensively.

A history of excessive fatigue, even after a light meal, must be considered of particular significance in selecting patients with possible food hypersensitivities. An account of episodes of nuchal pain and rigidity of undetermined origin must be regarded as highly suggestive of food intolerances. The more readily recognized cough or headache, particularly when nocturnal, should also be respected as a salient symptom in patient classification.

When the history leads to the suspicion of an allergy to food, further interrogation may aid materially in narrowing a suspected reflex excitant to two or three possibilities. Alcoholic beverages which, taken in moderation, cause headache or bloating should direct the search toward cereal grains or yeast. An intolerance for beer is of particular significance. Drowsiness following the drinking of one glass of beer is highly suggestive of a hypersensitivity. A known penicillin allergy should also lead to the suspicion of an allergy to yeast and other ferments.

A history of a diathesis toward gastroduodenal ulcer should lead to questioning regarding a Sippy regime at some previous time. The repetitious use of any one food is known to produce an intolerance to it in certain individuals. In this congenitally predisposed group, the frequent use of cow's milk in years past may be responsible for a persisting hypersensitivity to its protein. Many patients intolerant of milk will be aware of gastric distress only after eating ice cream. This is considered to be due to a concomitant cold-food response.

Frequent use of, and particularly a craving for, a specific food should lead to suspicion of its possible role in vertigo. For example, the use of coffee 3 or more times per day should enroll it for investigation. A history of frequent ingestion in past years also should not be overlooked.

When ingestants are suspected as excitants, but a specific offender is not suggested by the history, certain common foods should be considered first. The following foods are known to be common allergens: wheat, corn, milk, egg, yeast, coffee, chocolate, beef, potato, tomato, and pork. To this list should be added any frequently used ingestant.

Through the intelligent observation of Rinkel,[13] in recent years we have acquired two highly reliable methods of determining food intolerances: the deliberate provocative feeding test, also known as the challenge test, and the still more recent intracutaneous provocative food test.

In testing by the provocative feeding technique, the food is eliminated in its entirety for 4 days. The morning of the fifth day note is made of all signs and symptoms present before testing. Three to 4 hours after breakfast a generous amount of the food to be tested is ingested in its pure form. The patient is observed closely for 1 hour for any change in signs and symptoms. If no reaction develops, he is then fed a further quarter portion of the test food. Close observation should continue for another 30 minutes. The test food is also included in the evening meal if the midday feeding proves negative. Symptoms that occur during the night and upon arising are also to be taken into consideration.

As an adjunct to the observed symptomatic response to the deliberate provocative feeding test, Rinkel employed serial total leukocyte blood counts. This particular technique was developed by Vaughan.[14] Counts were made just prior to the ingestion of the test food and 20, 40, and 60 minutes postprandial. A relative leucopenia of 10 per cent or more for any one count was considered as indicative of a positive test. The far greater importance of the observed symptomatic responses must be kept in mind in evaluation of such testing.

Rinkel et al.[15] recently described the provocative intracutaneous food test. Testing is initiated by placing 0.10 cc. of a 1:5 dilution* of the food extract concentrate into two separate sites on the lateral side of the arm. The patient is observed for 10 minutes for any change in symptom pattern. If no change is observed, 0.02 cc. of a 1:125 dilution of the same food extract concentrate is then injected. Observations are continued for an additional 10 minutes. Further details and the technique of administering neutralizing doses are outlined in the original paper.

Positive reactions to provocative intracutaneous testing generally occur within 10 to 15 minutes after the injection of the antigen. In some instances there may be a delayed reaction occurring as late as 2 to 3 hours after the injection.

Employment of either method, if accurately executed, will disclose major food excitants in certain selected cases of episodic vertigo. Although there is no technique for the determination of food hypersensitivity that is completely reliable, there is a high degree of accuracy in diagnosis when using these techniques. Questionably positive reactions obtained by one method can be substantiated or disproved by use of the other.

In testing patients with episodic vertigo and dysacusis when it is suspected they are precipitated by foods, a positive test frequently produces an ear response. This is true of both the feeding and the intracutaneous injection techniques. The patient may experience an increase in, or return of, a sensation of fullness in the ear, tinnitus, diplacusis, and hearing loss. A mild vertiginous episode may also be precipitated. A Romberg test should be done before and after all provocative testing.

In many instances, however, the reaction to the provocative test may appear in areas other than the inner ear. Systemic signs and

*Diluent = 0.4 per cent phenol in normal saline.

symptoms may occur independent of, or in association with, a labyrinthine response. The immediate state of readiness of the predisposed labyrinth to respond to an excitant is felt to be a major determining factor in the production of a labyrinthine response.

In patients with episodic vertigo, the chest and nasal symptoms, so frequently provoked in the individual with respiratory allergy, rarely occur. The most common extralabyrinthine response is that of extreme lassitude or allergic fatigue. Gastrointestinal distress in the form of burning, bloating, or cramping is not uncommon. Nuchal aching and stiffness may occur and some patients may complain of numbness of a hand or arm. Occasionally there is muscle cramping in one or more of the extremities. Itching, general chilling, and facial flushing may sometimes be seen.

Foods proved to be offenders should be completely eliminated from the diet, including all of their products. If the patient does not show signs of definite improvement within a 10-day period, other ingestants should be suspected. Persisting systemic food symptoms such as described above are of particular importance in formulating a continuing approach to the problem. The possibility of concomitant endocrine dysfunction must always be considered.

After a complete elimination of a proved food excitant for 9 months, the food may be reintroduced into the diet on a rotation basis. The food is generally allowed at one meal every third day. If symptoms do not recur after several months, the program may be liberalized to one meal every second day. Consideration of the introduction of a second eliminated food should also be entertained at this time. Some individuals can eventually tolerate former offenders once a day.

When the possibility of an antigenic summation effect is suspected, the investigation of possible food excitants should not be embarked upon lightly. The patient must be fully informed as to what the complete elimination of a major food entails. Only then is he capable of deciding if his complaint warrants the dietary deprivations inherent in the final culmination of such a program.

Decision is not difficult for the vertiginous patient. Only in the case of dysacusis without vestibular involvement need the physician point out the possibility of the complete triad of Meniere's developing if the pathological labyrinthine response is not reversed. Alfaro[16] has stressed the recognition of these early cases of endolymphatic hydrops.

Considerable guidance is essential in the selection of permissible foods. Less imaginative patients require a maximum of instruction and encouragement. The help of a well-versed dietician is invaluable.

The patient should be instructed to follow the "diversified rotary" diet developed by Rinkel, since the possibility always exists that new sensitivities will develop from too frequent use of any one food. This is particularly true with the group of cereal grains when wheat is eliminated from the diet. If good clinical results are obtained, the patient may be more easily persuaded to adhere to the program. The loss of concomitant symptoms further enhances patient cooperation. Realization by the patient that he may return to a more normal dietary regime at some future time is of additional help in gaining cooperation.

CASE REPORTS

To illustrate two types of labyrinthine stress reactions precipitated by foods, three exemplary cases are presented. The first two cases suggest ischemia of a portion of the vestibular apparatus without cochlear involvement; the third dysfunction of the capillary bed of the stria vascularis with dysacusis and extension of the biochemical endolymph changes to involve the maculae and cristae.

Case 1: A 33-year-old woman was first seen in March 1964 with a complaint of intermittent episodes of severe vertigo with accompanying vomiting. There had been an interval of 1 year between her first and second attacks, but during the past 4 years the episodes had occurred every

4 to 8 weeks. Severe attacks lasted about 12 hours, but she described her balance as very poor for several additional days. The past year she felt she had never been completely free of giddiness.

A fullness and tinnitus in both ears preceded attacks of vertigo. The patient had been unaware of a hearing impairment, hyperacusis, or diplacusis. She had noted that her hands and feet would frequently swell 1 or two days prior to the onset of vertigo. Accompanying this was an occipital soreness for which she had seen a chiropractor on numerous occasions. Excessive fatigue had been an additional problem for over a year. This was much worse for several days following a period of vertigo.

The patient's mother had experienced sensations of vertigo on several occasions in the past. A maternal uncle and his daughter gave a similar history to that of the mother's. The patient gave a history of migraine headaches, but had been free of them for over 5 years. A history of a diathesis toward ulcer was unobtainable.

Ice cream was known to cause abdominal bloating if eaten in excess. Too much coffee had upset her stomach on occasions. She drank coffee on an average of 3 times a day. The patient volunteered that she was certain that the excessive use of either grapefruit or orange had produced several attacks of vertigo. Chocolate was known to produce headache. The patient was not known to be allergic to penicillin.

The otolaryngological examination was essentially negative. Pure tone and speech audiometry were normal. Bithermal caloric testing gave responses within normal limits. An intradermal provocative test for cow's milk was made because of the history of occasional gastric distress from ice cream. Ten minutes after injecting a 1:5 dilution of milk concentrate the patient experienced definite gastric distress. This was followed shortly by fullness in the ears, stiffness of the neck, and true vertigo. Extreme lassitude soon became an additional complaint. A 1:15,625 dilution of cow's milk concentrate was then injected intracutaneously in an attempt to neutralize the provocative response. In 20 minutes the patient was much more comfortable. In 30 minutes she was free of complaints, due either to the neutralizing effect of the last injection or to a normal rapid fading of the response to the provocative test.

Further testing was undertaken the same day because the patient traveled a great distance for office visits. A provocative intradermal test was made for beef because of the occasional cross sensitivity with cow's milk. The test was negative. Wheat and egg also proved negative. An intradermal provocative test with coffee produced fullness in the ears, vertigo, gastric distress, stiffness of the neck, and excessive fatigue.

The patient was sent home on a diet which completely eliminated all cow's milk, citrus fruits, coffee, and chocolate. She returned in October 1964 and reported that she had been free of symptoms for 5 months. One month prior to her return visit she had again noted fullness in the ears and stiffness of the neck. Two weeks later she experienced an attack of vertigo. Close questioning revealed an actual craving for chocolate for several months. She admitted eating it at frequent intervals. She had been completely faithful to her diet otherwise. The return of chocolate to her diet was felt to be the cause of this remission.

A letter in late April 1965 reported that her exacerbation in the fall of 1964 subsided as soon as she stopped eating chocolate. On Christmas she had eaten a salad containing Mandarin oranges and had become vertiginous shortly after. She remained uncomfortable for the remainder of the day. Otherwise, she had been completely free of vertigo, neck stiffness, and allergic fatigue.

At a later date the trial return of one food at a time on a planned rotation is contemplated. It is not deemed advisable at this time.

Case 2. A 39-year-old woman was seen in November 1963 because of a complaint of postural vertigo and an intermittent feeling of fullness in her left ear of 6 months duration. She had been awakened in the night on two occassions with spontaneous vertigo accompanied by severe nausea. Looking up produced a definite sense of vertigo, while looking down would cause distress on occasions. She had been unaware of a hearing impairment or dysacusis. Abdominal bloating had been a problem for several years, particularly before menstrual periods. She had noted that drinking cow's milk would cause bloating at intervals. Extreme fatigue was frequently experienced following her noon meal.

The otolaryngological examination was essentially negative. A modified Kobrak caloric test gave a normal response. An Aschan type III positional nystagmus was demonstrable with the patient supine and the head turned to the left while hyperextended. The nystagmus was directed to the left. Pure tone and speech audiometry were normal.

An intradermal provocative test for cow's milk produced gastric distress, excessive salivation, and coryza within 15 minutes. Testing was discontinued and the patient instructed in the complete elimination of cow's milk and all milk products from her diet.

Two weeks later she reported that her postural vertigo was much improved but that the feeling of fullness in her left ear had been worse since her husband undertook painting the interior of the house.

When she returned to the office 1 month after her initial visit she was free of fullness in the ear. She no longer was aware of postural vertigo and had not experienced abdominal bloating before or during her last menstrual period. Postprandial fatigue had ceased.

The patient was not seen again until May 1964. She had been completely free of vertigo, bloating, and fullness in the ear. It was suggested that in another 3 months she attempt the ingestion of milk one time every fifth day.

In November 1964 she reported that during the summer she had inadvertently ingested milk in foods on two occasions. The first time she experienced a frontal headache and the second time moderate bloating accompanied by a sense of giddiness. She had not reintroduced milk into her diet for this reason. Except for these two episodes she had been completely free of symptoms.

On her next office visit in May 1965, the patient reported an excellent 6 months. Minimal bloating had been experienced premenstrually on two occasions, but she had been completely free of postprandial fatigue, fullness in the ear, and vertigo. Positional nystagmus and postural vertigo were not demonstrable. The reintroduction of cow's milk in her diet once every fifth day was again suggested.

The patient was contacted 2 months later and was able to relate an apparent tolerance for cow's milk. She was advised to increase the frequency of its use to one time every third day.

Case 3. A 53-year-old woman was first seen in June 1963 because of a complaint of staggering

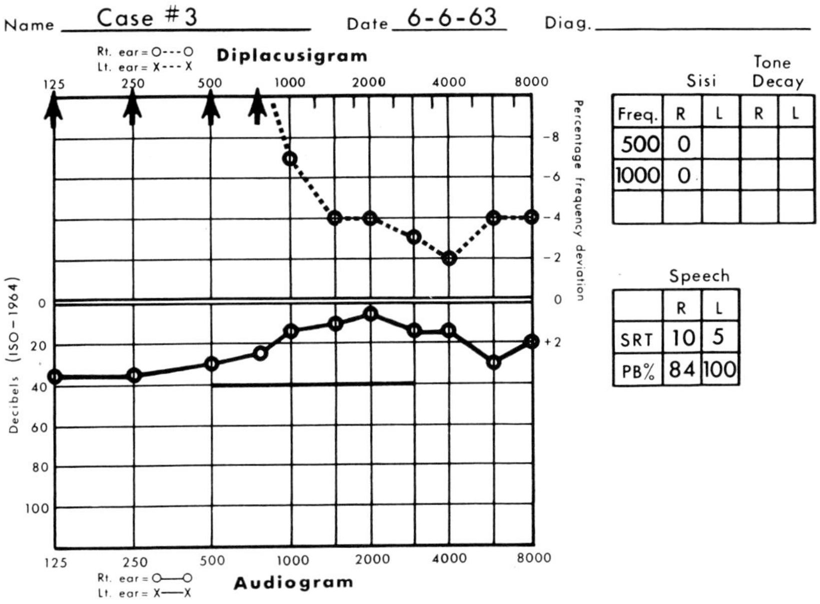

FIG. 1. *Case 3.* Diplacusigram and audiogram. The diplacusigram is recorded above and the audiogram below the common zero reference line. Diplacusimetry accomplishes binaural frequency balance in diplacusis, measuring the percentage of deviation detectable in the abnormal ear at given frequencies. The normal or better ear is used as a reference.

on walking for 18 months. She dated her complaint from an episode of vertigo associated with nausea, right ear pressure, and a roaring tinnitus. Her nausea had returned the past month, as had an intermittent fullness and tinnitus in her right ear. There was a tendency to weave toward the right on walking. Loud sounds were very irritating to her right ear.

A gallbladder x-ray series had been done the previous winter because of the patient's tendency to bloat to the point of increasing her girth several inches. These studies were negative. She also gave a history of fluid retention necessitating diuretics at times.

A hysterectomy had been performed at 27 years of age. She had been on oral estrogens at intervals since that time. One grain of thyroid extract per day had also been taken for several years.

The patient volunteered that onions and cabbage distressed her. Beer caused complete "head blockage." She was also aware that blended whiskeys and wine caused gastric and nasal symptoms.

The otolaryngological examination, including vestibular testing, was essentially negative. Pure tone audiometry showed a 25 to 35 decibel rise in threshold in the bass frequencies in the right ear. The discrimination score was 84 per cent on the right and 100 per cent on the left. A diplacusigram, executed according to the technique developed by Albers,[17] showed a 10 to 14 per cent frequency deviation through 750 cycles per second in the right ear. At 1000 cycles the deviation was 7 per cent. At 1500 cycles and higher the deviation ranged between 2 and 4 per cent.

An intradermal provocative test for yeast was made during her first visit because of her history of distress from brewer's yeast. Fifteen minutes after 0.10 cc. of a 1:5 dilution of yeast concentrate was injected, she became very sleepy. She reported later that she had a severe episode of vertigo the night of the yeast test and was more vertiginous for several days. Yeast and all products of fermentation were eliminated from her diet. Cabbage and onion were also eliminated because of the history that both caused gastric distress at intervals.

The patient was still vertiginous when she returned 11 days later, although she had been very faithful to the diet. Frequently used foods were then considered as offenders. Provocative intradermal testing was done with wheat and milk extracts. Both were negative. Egg gave a questionably positive reaction. The patient was asked to recheck egg at home by the deliberate provocative feeding technique. With this test

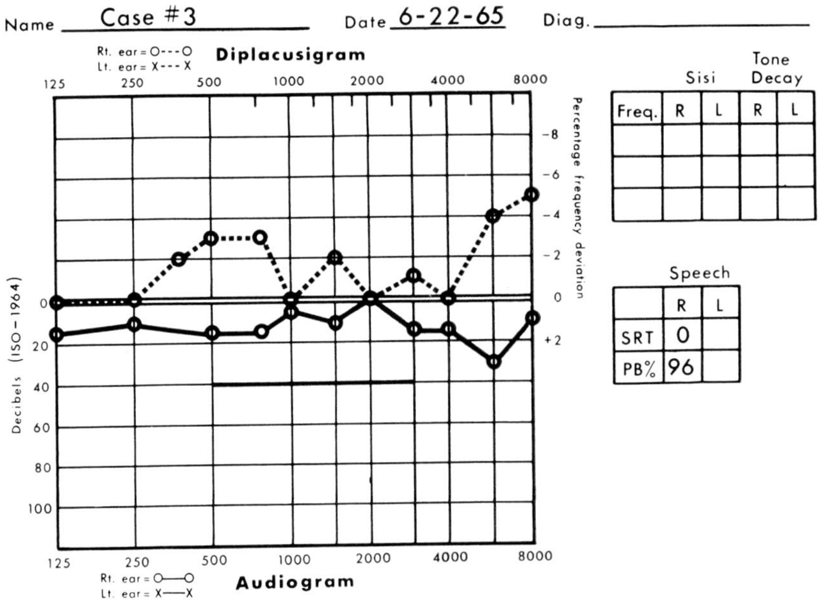

FIG. 2. *Case 3.* Diplacusigram and audiogram.

she developed right upper quadrant pain and bloating.

With the additional elimination of egg she was appreciably improved upon her return 10 days later. Some persisting positional vertigo led to the testing of beef and tomato by the provocative intradermal technique. The beef test was negative but marked gastric distress followed the tomato injection. Tomato was added to her list of foods to be eliminated.

Two months after her initial visit she was completely free of bloating and experienced positional vertigo only when under considerable stress. Her pure tone audiometric curve had returned to normal and there was marked improvement in her diplacusigram.

In May 1964, 11 months after her first visit, she reported that she was symptom free except for a recent moment of unsteadiness when getting out of an automobile. Egg was returned to her diet at one meal every third day.

In February 1965 she reported that she was completely free of symptoms. She had not felt the need for diuretics for almost a year. Tomato was returned to her diet once every third day.

In June 1965 the patient was still free of vertigo and bloating. She was tolerating both egg and tomato on an every third day rotation. It was not felt advisable to add yeast to her diet at this time.

SUMMARY

Two concepts have been reviewed: (1) An abnormal labyrinthine vascular response to stress may cause episodic vertigo. (2) Antigens circulating in the blood stream may act as excitation factors in labyrinthine vascular dysfunction.

The recognition of extralabyrinthine signs and symptoms has been stressed as being essential in the classification of patients experiencing episodes of vertigo precipitated by allergic excitants.

Means of detecting specific food hypersensitivities by history and provocative food testing have been outlined.

Three case histories have been presented, exemplifying labyrinthine reactions to stress precipitated by foods.

REFERENCES

1. Vaughan, W. T.: A theory concerning the mechanism and the significance of the allergic response. *In:* Medical Papers Dedicated to Henry Asbury Christian (R. T. Montoe, Ed.). Baltimore, Waverly Press, 1936, pp. 711-737.
2. Lorente de No, R.: Analysis of the activity of the chains of internuncial neurons. J. Neurophysiol. 1:207-244, 1938.
3. Williams, H. L.: Meniere's Disease. Springfield, Ill., Charles C Thomas, 1952, p. 224.
4. Duke, W. W.: Meniere's syndrome caused by allergy. J.A.M.A. 81:2179-2181, 1923.
5. Vogel: Die Beziehungen des Menierеschen Krankheit zur allergishen Disposition und zu anderen Reizzustanden des vegetativen Nervensystems. Z. Hals-Nasen Ohrenheilkunde 29:175-177, 1931.
6. Proetz, A. W.: Allergy of the middle and internal ears. Ann. Otol. 40:67-76, 1931.
7. Dohlman, G.: Menieresche Krankheit auf allergisher Basis. Acta Otolaryng. 27:245-248, 1939.
8. Criep, H. L.: Allergic vertigo. Penn. Med. J. 43: 258-262, 1939.
9. Dean, L. W., Jr.: Meniere's syndrome and allergy. Int. Clin. 3:231-234, 1941.
10. Derlacki, E. L.: Non-surgical management of Meniere's disease. Laryngoscope 64:271-284, 1954.
11. Shambaugh, G. E., Jr.: Meniere's disease, Diagnosis and management. Texas J. Med. 58: 70-74, 1962.
12. Rinkel, H. J.: Food Allergy, Springfield, Ill., Charles C Thomas, 1951, pp. 10-11.
13. Rinkel, H. J.: Food Allergy, Springfield, Ill., Charles C Thomas, 1951, pp. 124-142.
14. Vaughan, W. T.: Food allergens. III. The leukopenic index, preliminary report. J. Allergy 5:601, 1934.
15. Rinkel, H. J., Lee, C. H., Brown, D. W., Jr., Willoughby, J. W., and Williams, J. M.: The diagnosis of food allergy. Arch. Otolaryng. 79:71-79, 1964.
16. Alfaro, V. R.: Discussion of Williams, H. L., and Corbin, K. B.: The differential diagnosis of vertigo. Tr. Amer. Otol. Soc. 46: 297, 1958.
17. Albers, G. D.: Diplacusis. To be published in Proceedings VIII International Congress of Oto-rhino-laryngology, 1965.

CHAPTER 23

Psychiatric Aspects of Vertigo

PAUL SLOANE

Vertigo is a common symptom in all forms of neurosis, particularly in those states which are characterized by emotional tension. Actually, the incidence of vertigo as a functional disorder is far greater than its occurrence as a result of organic states. Psychogenic vertigo is very often transient and as such has little clinical significance, but in many instances may be evidence of a deep-seated emotional conflict that warrants further study.

At one time objective vertigo (the sensation of movement of objects rather than of the patient himself) was considered to be typical of organic disease. It has been observed, however, that such sensations may also occur in emotionally disturbed states and therefore do not constitute the basis for a clear distinction between organic and psychogenic disorders. In addition, the objective manifestations of both types of conditions may be similar, although they are quantitatively more severe in organic cases.

When vertigo occurs in neurosis, it is frequently accompanied by anxiety, either as a primary or secondary symptom. Anxiety as a form of severe tension, for instance, may give rise to vertigo by disturbing the patient's psychic balance. Vertigo, on the other hand, produces loss of the normal feeling of control and stability with a resulting sense of emotional insecurity and anxiety.

NATURE OF PSYCHOLOGICAL SYMPTOMS

The ego, functioning as the executive of the personality, helps to mediate between the needs of the individual and his relationships to society, the outside world, and his conscience. It thus coordinates and organizes the various perceptions that enter the mind both from within and without. If it functions properly, the end result of its activity is to establish order and stability in the mind.

Neurotic symptoms arise as the result of unconscious emotional conflicts—i.e., those of whose existence the patient is not aware. Such conflicts take place between two warring parts of the personality: the instinctual (sexual and aggressive) drives which are seeking expression, and the forces of the conscience working through the ego. The instincts in question are those which are socially unacceptable because of moral, ethical, or esthetic reasons, and on that account are pushed back into the unconscious mind. Under normal circumstances the ego succeeds in keeping these impulses under repression. They may, however, increase in strength as the result of overstimulation, severe frustration, or physiological accession of energy, as in puberty or menopause. They then threaten to break through into consciousness by overpowering the defenses of the ego. This threatened breakthrough creates a state of alarm or anxiety, since any reaction to the impulse on the part of the individual would jeopardize his relationships with other people. Anxiety is thus a signal of danger and calls forth further psychological defense mechanisms. If the forces of the forbidden wishes and the forces of conscience are equally matched, neither can win and a compromise is reached between them. The compromise, which solves the conflict and relieves the anxiety, constitutes the neurotic symptom. In the symptom the patient's need to obtain gratification is pacified by a limited fulfillment of the unconscious desire, but this is accompanied by punishment in the form of neurotic suffering.

Vertigo may be a symbolic representation of a mental idea in the form of a physical feeling in the hysterical conversion symptom. In these instances, it is a sign of emotional insecurity and dependency on others, and expresses the desire to cling or lean on someone for support. The physical support that the patient seeks is an outward expression of his psychological need. In this sense, the concept of vertigo becomes a language which is expressed, not by words, but by means of a body symptom. Properly translated the symptom would therefore mean "I want to lean on you," or "I need your protection." This is also the idea behind the symptom when it occurs in association with various phobias, in which case the patient behaves like a helpless child in the face of unconscious sexual or aggressive wishes.

Vertigo may frequently also result from emotional tension. Any emotional conflict which produces psychic disequilibrium is likely to be expressed in terms of physical disequilibrium. This is related to the fact that the vestibular apparatus, by acting as the unifying center for centripetal impulses from a number of sources, and exerting direct influence on postural tonus, contributes to the psychological image of one's own body. As a result of the reciprocal relationship which exists between this psychic image and the vestibular apparatus, changes in the psychic sphere produce equilibratory disturbances, while alterations in vestibular function produce similar disturbances in the psyche. The existence of vertigo thus indicates some change in the integrating or organizing function of either the vestibular apparatus or the ego.

Psychogenic vertigo may be caused by the ego's inability to coordinate conflicting motor and sensory impulses—for instance, when some traumatic event or sudden change in the general life situation upsets a previous good state of emotional adjustment. This may occur as a result of a highly charged emotional situation, either sexual or aggressive, which threatens to upset the patient's relationship to those people who are important to him.

Since vertigo is a very distressing and threatening symptom, it may have the effect of paralyzing all physical and psychological activity. From this point of view it is well calculated to lead to a withdrawal from intolerable anxiety or conflict. This becomes particularly evident when the vertigo is followed by loss of consciousness. Both vertigo and loss of consciousness may therefore be the ego's way of abdicating when the warning signal of anxiety fails to induce an adequate mobilization of the psychological defenses against the instinctual drives. This was well illustrated in the case of a young woman who suffered from a fear of fainting in crowds. When confronted by a sexually stimulating thought or impulse, she would complain of a knot in the back of the neck as if a hand were gripping her. This was followed by tenseness of the entire body, dizziness, and lightness of the head. The patient then started to move her hands and legs in order to break up the tension, but if this failed and the tension increased, she would lose consciousness. Awaking from the syncopal attack, the patient complained of feeling tired but she was relaxed. She stated that this resembled the state of relaxation which she experienced following coitus with orgasm, and, indeed, following a fainting attack she was aware of the presence of increased vaginal secretion. The fainting was therefore not only an expression of withdrawal, but also a hysterical symptom which had the significance of a coitus equivalent.

CLINICAL OCCURRENCE OF VERTIGO

Vertigo may occur in a wide variety of psychological conditions and is not specific for any one. Where it does not occur as a symbolic hysterical conversion symptom, it is the result of dammed-up tension which may be caused by a diversity of factors. Since not everyone reacts to strain with vertigo, we must postulate a distinct character type to account for its appearance under these conditions, provided a constitutional factor, such as abnormal sensitivity of the vestibular apparatus, can be ruled out. The character type is represented by the individual who must lean on others for maintenance of his self-esteem, the so-called passive-dependent individual. These people are characterized by feelings of inferiority, unworthiness, and guilt. They depend for their self-confidence on the affection, encouragement, or approval of others. They have particular difficulty in manifesting anger or engaging in aggressive acts, primarily because such reactions might alienate people and cause them to withdraw their support.

A woman who was an obsessional neurotic and who had been brought up in a rigid home felt that she had to marry a man to whom she had permitted sexual liberties, even though no intercourse had occurred. She considered herself to be superior to her husband and felt that she might have married a man of higher caliber if she had not been intimidated by her dependency on her mother and fear of the latter's disapproval. She managed to displace her resentment from her mother to her husband. After her husband had a coronary attack, she developed fantasies of his death and her subsequent marriage to someone else. At such times she would develop intense anxiety associated with vertigo. Her fantasies about his death were unconscious and were brought out only during the course of psychotherapy. All that appeared on the surface were expressions of chronic dissatisfaction and resentment against him. The death wishes had to be repressed because of their violent nature, but the violence was expressed by the anxiety and vertigo which represented a fear of her own dissolution.

Another patient, a young girl, began to suffer from agoraphobia after she had read a newspaper account of a man who had broken into a house and raped a girl. Her fear of going out alone was associated with the unconscious fear of being exposed to temptation. Later the anxiety began to occur when she was alone at home. When she was in the presence of a sexually attractive man, even though she was not aware of having any sexual interest in him, she would develop anxiety accompanied by vertigo. Interestingly enough, when she became conscious of her sexual feelings during the course of her psychotherapy, the vertigo disappeared. This indicates that only unconscious ideas can produce symptoms; once they become conscious they lose their power to do so. The explanation for this lies in the fact that ideas which are unconscious have no way of being discharged by thinking, feeling, or action; therefore, inner tension is built up. Once they become conscious they are in a position to find discharge, if in no other way but verbal expression.

Attacks of vertigo have also been described as occurring under the following situations of tension: Resentment associated with unsatisfactory sexual relations with one's mate; hostility against an exacting employer; damming up of sexual urges after cessation of masturbation; anger against a parent who did not permit a grown child to become independent; sexual rejection by a husband while at the same time the patient's desire was being fired by contact with a friend who regaled her with stories of her extramarital affairs; financial success in a man in whom success gave rise to guilt-feelings and fear of some imminent danger; following a serious operation on the patient's wife; feelings of anxiety and despair following financial or other failure; in the case of a masculine woman, when her domination of the family was threatened; hearing over the phone of the death of a friend on whom the patient was dependent for business; in a woman who was disturbed by the divorces of her two children when she herself was feeling guilty about having had an extramarital affair; when a man was to take over for his superior who had been taken ill; a man who returned home from work one day and found his father dead on the couch in the living room.

Attacks of vertigo which have all the characteristics of Meniere's disease (paroxysmal attacks of vertigo, impairment of hearing, and tinnitus) can be connected with unbearable conflicts. In such cases the vertigo tends to occur during episodes of strain and pent-up tension which may or may not be associated with some discharge in explosive outbursts.

DIAGNOSIS

Cases of vertigo are very common in psychiatric practice in association with anxiety tension states. In these instances, however, vertigo is merely one symptom among many, although it may be the main complaint. Other common symptoms are palpitation, shortness of breath, fatigue, gastric distress, insomnia, profuse perspiration, and tremulousness. Emotional outbreaks are frequently observed in cases of vertigo, but these may be secondary and are related to fear of deafness or recurrence of attacks and to the annoying tinnitus.

The greatest difficulties in diagnosis arise in those patients who are referred initially to the otologist because of the suspicion of organic disease. Since the otologist is attuned to thinking in terms of organicity, it may not, as a matter of course, occur to him to think of psychogenic factors. The question, however, may be suggested by any of the following features: if thorough clinical investigation fails to reveal any evidence of organic disease; if the patient is vague in his description of symptoms or presents a multiplicity of complaints with shifting of emphasis from one symptom to another; if a severe attack of vertigo is preceded by an acute situation of emotional stress; or if anxiety-producing situations are followed by exacerbations of vertigo.

Vertigo in these instances is connected with distressing conflicts. It tends to occur during periods of strain where there is a release of pent-up feelings, particularly anger. It should be remembered that the type of vertigo, whether subjective or objective, is not conclusive, since either type may occur in both organic and psychogenic cases. Psychogenic vertigo may also be related to position and be accompanied by loss of equilibrium. The objective manifestations differ only in that they are quantitatively more frequent and intense in organic cases. There may be a close relationship to the clinical picture of migraine, since in both migraine and vertigo the same vascular changes may occur. Cases of Meniere's disease of a psychogenic nature have been described.

After the patient has had a chance to describe his symptoms and tell his story in his own way, one may start to ask relevant questions. Of particular significance are the circumstances of the initial attack or special features which are recurrent. Is the attack likely to occur in relation to certain people, in a particular place, or under particular circumstances? One patient, for instance, would get an attack whenever he was aggravated by his employer and was afraid he would explode in anger. In the case of a woman, the vertigo occurred whenever her husband, who suffered from premature ejaculation, would disappoint her in the sexual act, leaving her full of resentment against him.

Particular attention should be paid to the patient's personality, his manner of responding to typical stressful situations, his adjustment to his family, marital situation, and occupation, as well as anything unusual in his past adjustment which might be reflected in his current relationships. The fact that a patient may vehemently deny that he has emotional problems, or feel offended that it should be suggested, does not necessarily mean that such problems do not exist. On the contrary, the very vehemence of his denial may be taken as an indication that psychological problems are present.

THERAPEUTIC ASPECTS

What approach can the otologist or general practitioner use in dealing with patients in whom psychological factors are operative? One cannot expect to uncover all the complicated findings in such cases. It would furthermore not be wise for anyone but an experienced psychiatrist to become too involved in dealing with emotional problems. On the other hand, a psychiatrist may not always be available and the referring physician himself may have to manage the problem.

It is a good general rule for the physician to be a sympathetic and attentive listener. After convincing himself that no organic disease exists, he should be frank with the patient and convey this information to him. In an unhurried, conversational way he may then ask him whether he had been under any emotional strain at the time of onset of his symptoms. If patients are encouraged to talk, they may reveal material which will yield considerable understanding of their problems. The physician's understanding and friendly attitude may in itself have a therapeutic effect, particularly if it enables the patient to express himself freely, thus providing an outlet for pent-up emotions. The physician should be content to deal only with problems which the patient presents voluntarily. He should not attempt to probe too deeply or offer psychological interpretations. A good rule in psychiatry is that when in doubt, do nothing. If an obvious emotional problem exists, the physician may try to guide the patient in a friendly, reassuring manner by pointing out common sense ways of avoiding situations that give rise to tension and of seeking more healthy outlets for his energies. In any case, the patient can be reassured by being told that he has no serious underlying disease and by emphasizing the possibility of recovery if the causes of his emotional tension are dealt with.

Part IV. Treatment

CHAPTER 24
Medical Treatment

The Episodic Vertigos

Henry L. Williams

When a patient presents himself to a physician with dizziness or vertigo as a chief or major complaint, the physician should remind himself that this sensation is a symptom rather than a disease. It seems probable that failure of the physician to try to make certain what type of sensation the patient is experiencing accounts for some of the dissatisfaction as to the results obtained by medical treatment.

Therapeutic nihilists deny that there is an effective treatment for any type of dizziness, disequilibrium, or vertigo. They ascribe apparent good results from treatment to placebo effect. It has lately become medically fashionable to decry and disparage the placebo effect. This, at times, seems to have reached a point at which there is some evidence that the wish to appear scientifically oriented in medicine has introduced a bias in the reporting of therapeutic results which may even have penetrated studies conducted by the double-blind technic. There is, after all, nothing criminal in achieving results through the medium of the placebo effect. Patients consult the physician for relief of symptoms. They are usually not interested in a controversy as to why the symptomatic relief occurred.

In the episodic vertigos medical treatment is directed toward relief of symptoms. All that should be reasonably expected of medical treatment of any variety of episodic vertigo is either that it should produce a remission of symptoms for a certain period or that it will control the symptoms and signs as long as it is continued. I know of no one who pretends that a medicament or other form of medical therapy is available which will abolish the underlying physiopathologic defect. Therefore, in treating a patient with episodic vertigo, attempts at improving the general health of the patient should not be neglected, whether this includes correction of physical habits, nutritional faults, or endocrine dysfunctions. Relatively simple disorders may cause dizziness or vertigo. This is usually the case when dizziness is an incidental complaint, but more rarely if dizziness is the principal reason the patient consults the physician.

Dizziness and vertigo may be defined as unreal sensations of movement or hallucinations of movement, or sometimes mere impressions of dysequilibrium. Although a severe rotatory vertigo usually indicates involvement of the labyrinth, such vertigo may also be seen with lesions of the brainstem, especially in instances of sudden vascular disturbance to the vestibular nuclei and their tracts and, in rare instances, in central vertigo. Labyrinthine irritation, however, may cause other hallucinatory sensations of movement. Although sensations of dysequilibrium may be caused by aberrations of the proprioceptive and ocular mechanisms, except in the case of nonconcomitant strabismus, these symptoms are not commonly so definite as to be confused with the vertigo or dizziness which occurs with the disturbances in function of the vestibular apparatus.

This discussion will be confined to the treatment of conditions in which the principal complaint, or a main one, is a sensation of unreal movement which appears to be due to irritation of some part of the vestibular system.

If medical treatment is to be effective in controlling the symptom of vertigo, it must be directed at the cause; an etiologic diagnosis must be attempted. As is well known, such differential diagnosis may be difficult or impossible by clinical examination or test. If this proves to be the case, attempts should be made to establish the probable etiology by the results of treatment. If one therapeutic approach proves disappointing, another must be tried in which a different etiologic basis is assumed to be present. If this plan is followed, most patients will receive such effective symptomatic relief that no type of surgical intervention need be considered.

Many of the possible causes of a sensation which a patient might term dizziness are enumerated in Table 1. This should further indicate the difficulty of the diagnostic problem.

TABLE 1. Causes of Dizziness and/or Vertigo

Otologic

1. Impacted cerumen
2. Trauma to the inner ear or eighth cranial nerve (commotio labyrinthi)
3. Dysfunction of the eustachian tube
4. Acute otitis media
5. Labyrinthitis
6. Labyrinthine fistula
7. Bilateral nonfunctioning equilibrial labyrinths
8. Motion sickness
9. Meniere's disease
10. Lermoyez syndrome
11. Vestibular neuronitis
12. Vasculitis involving the internal auditory artery or vestibular emissary veins
13. Tumors of middle ear and inner ear
14. Ototoxic drugs
15. "Focal infection" from tonsils, adenoids, periapical tooth abscesses, and chronically infected sinuses
16. Sinusitis, acute or subacute

Neurologic

1. Degenerating and demyelinating diseases, especially multiple sclerosis
2. Posterior fossa lesions
   a. Fractures, cystic arachnoiditis, syringobulbia, platybasia and Arnold-Chiari malformations
   b. Neoplasms and subdural hematomas
3. Supratentorial lesions with displacement of the brainstem
4. Migraine-like syndromes
5. Convulsive disorders (vestibular epilepsy, vertiginous epilepsy)
6. Temporal lobe lesions with irritation of cortical vestibular areas
7. Toxic-infectious conditions
   a. Aseptic meningencephalitis
   b. Brain abscess
   c. Common viral diseases such as mumps, measles, whooping cough.
8. Vascular, including atherosclerosis, thrombosis, embolic occlusion, and hemorrhage, especially in vessels to the brainstem.

Systemic

1. Allergic reactions involving the inner ear
2. Dizziness of the aged due to indeterminate vascular cause or end-organ degeneration due to aging process
3. Cardiac diseases
4. Hypertension (paroxysmal)
5. Hypotension (syncope)
6. Hyperactive carotid reflex
7. Blood dyscrasias (anemia, leukemia, lymphomas, reticulosis, polyctyhemia, purpura)
8. Cogan's syndrome (nonsyphilitic interstitial keratitis with vestibulocochlear symptoms—panarteritis nodosa)
9. Episodes of hypoglycemia
10. Hypocortoadrenalism
11. Cervical myalgia

Ophthalmologic

1. Nonconcomitant strabismus
2. Refractive errors
3. Optokinetic vertigo

Psychogenic

1. Tension—anxiety state
2. Conversion reactions
3. Neuroses (agaraphobia, claustrophobia)
4. Hyperventilation syndrome

Working Hypotheses as to the Etiology of the Various Kinds of Episodic Vertigo

Failure to obtain consistently favorable clinical results from medical treatment in episodic vertigos probably results from the fact that conditions of diverse etiology are given a stereotyped treatment which in many instances should be considered illogical. In attempting etiologic diagnosis of vertigo, it is necessary to be aware of the various hypotheses as to etiology and some of the more valid objections and criticisms that have been made to them.

Angiospasm Labyrinthique

The first widely accepted hypothesis as to the etiology of episodic vertigo was that offered by Lermoyez for Meniere's disease. His concept was that of vasomotor labyrinthine ischemia, in which he suggested that the internal auditory (labyrinthine) artery or its larger branches might develop intermittent vasospasm. He also described a condition of long-continued spasm of the internal auditory artery in which a gradually increasing hearing loss and progressing unsteadiness over a long period would suddenly change into a violent attack of vertigo. Closely following the vertiginous attack there would be a restitution of hearing to or toward normal. This was subsequently called "Lermoyez syndrome." For this latter condition he advised "proof with amyl nitrite." In patients with Lermoyez syndrome a strong inhalation of amyl nitrite was said to precipitate an attack of vertigo with symptomatic relief.

Thrombosis or Embolism. Owing to mistranslation of Meniere's papers it was also stated that thrombosis or embolism of the labyrinthine artery or its branches could produce Meniere's disease. Included among the objections to this hypothesis are that thrombosis or embolism would not produce repeated episodes of vertigo, the vertigo would be of long duration and slow recovery, and slow fluctuations of hearing such as are characteristic of the early stages of "true" Meniere's disease would not be seen.

The chief objection to both the above hypotheses for Meniere's disease, however, was that following the histologic observations of Hallpike and Cairns, which were rapidly confirmed by so many pathologists in many countries, no one could conceive in what manner spasm of the labyrinthine artery or its branches, or thrombosis or embolism of these vessels, could produce the evidently increased hydrodynamic pressure in scala media. Therefore, the hypotheses that either thrombosis or embolism or spasm of the labyrinthine (internal auditory) artery or its larger branches could cause Meniere's disease was universally abandoned.

There can be little doubt, however, that vasospasms, thrombosis or embolism involving the labyrinthine artery might produce the condition known as sudden deafness and that vasospasm might produce episodes of intermittent vertigo. It is also probable that intermittent spasm of the fine branches of the basilar artery which supply the vestibular nuclei may also be a cause of recurring episodes of vertigo. Houssay stated that intermittent functional disability is a characteristic condition resulting from a local and persistent angiospasm.

Vasospasm labyrinthique may well be the cause of Lermoyez syndrome, a condition of great rarity. Observers who have seen thousands of patients with episodic vertigo have rarely seen more than three or four instances of "le vertique qui fait entendre."

Glaucoma of the Ear

If the structure of the labyrinth is compared to that of the eye, it is possible to point out many analogies. In the inner ear, just as in the eye, a delicate nervous mechanism is enclosed in a rigid capsule of definite volume. An increase in hydrodynamic pressure resulting from an excess of fluid flowing in over that flowing out is a concept for the production of hearing loss and vertigo that has appealed to many observers. House recently suggested that the vertiginous crises of the disorder were produced by the endolymphatic pressure reaching a certain critical level which caused stimulation of macula and cristae. The attack of vertigo produced was then suddenly relieved by rupture of Reissner's membrane or the saccule. The remissions of the disease according to this hypothesis are produced by the formation of a more or less constantly draining fistula or resumption of function by "normal" mechanisms for absorption of endolymph.

Objections to the Knapp-House hypothesis are: (1) There is no obvious mechanism which could interfere with the escape of endolymph, such as is present in the "filtering angle" of the eye, in chronic simple glaucoma; the hearing changes in Meniere's disease usually referred to are not the abrupt losses that occur with the attack, but the slow diurnal changes (described by Lillie, Thornell, and Horton) which have no relation to the vertiginous attacks. The diurnal hearing variation is not explained by the "glaucoma" hypothesis. (2) There is no evidence that "critical pressure" causes stimulation of cristae or macula. (3) The hypothesis allows no explanation for the frequently observed fact that a cholinergic blocking drug such as atropine sulfate or an adrenergic drug such as adrenaline or amphetamine will abort and/or rapidly terminate a vertiginous episode of true Meniere's disease or of vertigo of the autonomic imbalance type. It would seem more reasonable to suppose that the increased hydrodynamic pressure in scala media might result from an excessive production of endolymph rather than failure of absorption.

Brunner described a type of case which he termed "stagnation hydrops," which would seem to fit more closely the symptoms of the patients relieved by the operation of Portman and of House. It would seem justifiable to draw the conclusion that there is a relatively common condition which may produce hearing loss and episodic vertigo on the basis of 'stagnation hydrops," and that it can be relieved by drainage of localized C.F.S. hypertension in the region of the cisterna pontis, but that this condition is not Meniere's disease, but rather "arachnoid vertigo."

Autonomic Dysfunction

Following the reports of the pathologic changes found in Meniere's disease, the rather old hypothesis of autonomic imbalance rapidly gained ascendancy and almost universal acceptance. In his study of disease of the microcirculation Müller found that in certain disorders, which he termed "the vasomotor neuroses," in many isolated areas of the skin there exists a disorder of the capillary beds in which arteriolar spasm is present, associated with a pathologic "varicose" dilation of the subjoined capillary loops. This "spastic-atonic state" of arterioles and muscled venules may occur in response to preferred stimuli which will not produce a similar response in presumably normal arteriolar-capillary combinations in neighboring areas nor produce a response in normal individuals. He pointed out that this same arteriolar-capillary picture is produced in all capillary beds of the normal individual on exposure to extreme and damaging stress. Parresius found that a tendency to develop abnormal areas of arteriolar capillary response on exposure to mild stress was inherited and was present in individuals with migraine, Reynaud's disease, Meniere's disease, and other members of the group of vasomotor neuroses. It can be observed that this definition of "the vasomotor neuroses" is essentially that of allergy, but considered from the standpoint of pathophysiologic effect rather than that of probable cause.

Davis stated, however, that it was not clear to him how arteriolar spasm could produce increased hydrodynamic pressure in scala media. Seymour attempted to answer Davis's implied objection by recalling the hypothesis that the endolymph in Meniere's disease is secreted under decreased hydrodynamic but increased osmotic pressure as was suggested previously by Fowler. Seymour called attention to the pathologic reports of Arnvig and of Berggren of apparently authentic cases of Meniere's disease in which no pathologic evidence of increased hydrodynamic pressure was found in scala media on histologic examination. Seymour suggested that after a time increased osmotic pressure in the endolymph attracts fluid from the neighboring tissue spaces and secondary endolymphatic hydrops is produced. This suggestion has not received confirmation, however.

There can be little doubt that autonomic dysfunction may be the cause of episodic vertigo sometimes associated with hearing loss on the involved side and sometimes without evidence of cochlear involvement. The pathologic changes produced by autonomic dysfunction, however, in many instances do not meet the histologic criteria established by Hallpike and Cairns. The clinical criteria established by the panel on vertigo at the meeting in Madison, Wisconsin of the National Institute of Neurologic Diseases and Blindness are also often not met in vertigo caused by cholinergic overaction. It seems to be, however, a much more frequent cause of episodic vertigo and/or dizziness than "true Meniere's disease.

The Pathologic Release of Induced Histamine

It would seem necessary to propose an entirely new working hypothesis for Meniere's disease if we are to have one that does not conflict with any of the known pathophysiologic facts, the histologic findings of Hallpike and Cairns, and the clinical criteria established for the diagnosis of Meniere's disease. Fortunately, new evidence bearing on the physiology of the microcirculation has recently been furnished by Schayer, and his findings in regard to induced histamine have been confirmed by Kahlson.

Shayer introduced the concept of "induced" histamine, synthesized within cells of the walls of capillary-sized vessels not directly supplied by fibers of the autonomic nervous system. It is believed that induced histamine participates in the normal regulation of local nutritive blood flow, but that after drastic local or systemic stimuli an increased rate of histamine synthesis mediates the gradual opening of the capillary beds characteristic of slowly developing inflammatory or stress states. Shayer presents evidence that the normal antagonist of induced histamine is the glucocorticoids. Antagonism of the basic microcirculatory actions of induced histamine by corticoids could underlie their anti-inflammatory effect, their need in stress, and many of their metabolic consequences.

It does not seem too imaginative to suggest that through the influence of a cholinergic hypothalamic stimulus, induced histamine may be synthesized in the beds of stria vascularis in a quantity greatly in excess of local homeostatic needs — indeed, in toxic concentrations — and result in the histopathologic picture of Hallpike and Cairns and the clinical signs and symptoms established by the panel on vertigo (NIMDB) as necessary for the diagnosis of Meniere's disease. A primary vasodilation in the capillary beds of stria vascularis would be produced with a primary increase in the hydrodynamic pressure of the endolymph.

Gellhorn has pointed out that abnormal stimuli arising in the hypothalamic centers may produce a unilateral discharge and that, furthermore, the unilateral discharge may change sides. Changing of the side involved has been observed in Meniere's disease.

In attempting to separate the etiology of "true" Meniere's disease from episodic vertigo resulting from autonomic dysfunction, it is realized that we are approaching dangerously close to the hypothesis of Atkinson, who suggested that Meniere's disease could be divided into two types on the empiric grounds of response to treatment. Our categorization on the basis of differing etiologies appears to be valid, however, and since "autonomic dysfunction" can produce clinical pictures both relatively easy and extremely difficult to differentiate from the clinical picture produced by "pathologic synthesis of induced histamine," I believe that the term "Meniere's disease" should be reserved for the latter.

Dysfunction of Righting Reflexes

Magnus pointed out that attitudinal reflexes are present in man, although in healthy adult persons under normal conditions they are only exceptionally demonstrable. He found that they could be clearly seen, however, under many pathological conditions. It has been found, for instance, that the dysequilibrium of the inebriate is due to the fact that the attitudinal reflexes are depressed earlier and to a greater degree than the cortical functions by the ingestion of ethyl alcohol.

Pain due to sustained contraction of muscles of the neck and scalp has been well known since the investigations of Lewis and of Kellgren. It has also been recognized that such painful contraction can be initiated by a seemingly trivial focus of irritation.

An occasional patient is seen in whom a sudden jerk of the neck, such as is produced by stepping down unexpectedly from a curb, will produce falling which will be followed by a typical vertiginous attack. Such patients also meet the other criteria for the diagnosis of Meniere's disease. It is possible that in such an instance the sudden activity of the head-on-neck righting reflex precipitated an episode of true vertigo in a hyperirritable labyrinth. Gerlings' observation that the head is often held to one side during an episode of Meniere's disease suggests that the head-on-neck righting reflex may be involved in some cases of Meniere's disease.

It is probable that a stimulus affecting the head-on-neck righting reflex is a common but usually unrecognized cause of the more minor varieties of dizziness and vertigo. It certainly should be suspected as the cause of episodic dizziness far more frequently than it is.

THERAPY IN EPISODIC VERTIGO

Having established a tentative etiologic classification of episodic vertigo of labyrinthine origin, it is possible to proceed to the medical treatment found most effective for each type.

Anxiety

A sudden unexpected attack of vertigo with nausea and vomiting and with maintenance of full consciousness throughout the episode, often in the presence of others, is an embarrassing experience not quickly forgotten. Patients who have experienced such an attack usually continue in a state of apprehension and anxiety, "one of the minor aspects of fear." With repetition of the episodes, the anxiety state may have become so marked that it will have become difficult to make out whether the patient is having continuing episodes of vertigo or anxiety attacks. In most patients with episodic vertigo it is the first duty of the physician to treat the anxiety state by careful examination, discussion, explanation, reassurance, relaxing physical therapy, and, if necessary, by the use of a placebo. Those who decry making use of the placebo effect do not seem to be individuals whose practice has required them to treat many patients who are a prey to worry and self-concern.

The Acute Vertiginous Crisis or Attack

In an initial attack of vertigo it will usually be impossible to make an etiologic diagnosis. In this instance an intramuscular injection of 250 mg. of dimenhydrinate in a suitable solution will usually stop the distressing symptoms rather quickly and throw the patient into a sound sleep from which he often awakens symptom-free.

If the attack is one of a series and a tentative etiologic diagnosis has been made, and if this diagnosis is either autonomic dysfunction or Meniere's disease, a reasonably large dose of atropine sulfate (1/75 grain, 0.00086 Gm.) given subcutaneously will usually terminate even the most severe attack in 15 to 20 minutes. If premonitory symptoms or "aura" give warning to the patient that an attack is imminent, a similar dose will abort its development. This effect of atropine would seem to indicate that "cholinergic overaction" is involved in the production of both types of attacks. Sufferers from recurring episodic vertigo may be instructed in the technic of self-administration of atropine sulfate hypodermically with good effect, not only because the development of acute symptoms will be prevented, but because giving the patient confidence that he can abort an attack will relieve the anxiety state that may have developed because of the fear of having a vertiginous episode in public and away from help.

Conversely, adrenergic drugs can be used to relieve vertiginous attacks of these types, although somewhat less effective than atropine. They are, however, excellent for preventing the development of a "crisis." Amphetamine sulfate or dextro amphetamine sulfate in tablet form, of which 10 mg. should be taken, is usually found an effective dose for abortion of an attack. The long-acting preparations should be avoided, for this use as a prolonged effect is undesirable. Patients should be warned to use these drugs only when necessary, because too frequent repetition will cause them to lose their effectiveness.

No treatment which speeds recovery is known for acute vertigo with symptoms persisting for days to weeks with slow recovery, probably due to thrombosis or embolism of the labyrinthine artery, some of the fine penetrating branches of the basilar artery suppling the brainstem, particularly the vestibular nuclei, or to viral invasion of the labyrinth.

There are two conditions which may produce episodic vertigo which appear somewhat separated from others by the fact that they apparently produce vertigo by stimulating the vestibular receptors by acting through the middle ear and by way of the stapedial footplate and labyrinthine humors. These are cerumen in the external auditory canal impacted against the membrana tensa, and intermittent occlusion of the eustachian tube.

Impacted cerumen may cause true rotatory vertigo and possibly more frequently a less definite hallucination of motion. If impacted cerumen is the cause of the dizziness, it should be easily discovered in the examination of the external auditory canal. Several patients have been seen, however, in whom removal of impacted cerumen relieved episodic vertigo, who after a lapse of years developed Meniere's disease. This also occurred in several patients in whom a simple inflation of the eustachian tube seemed to abolish symptoms of episodic vertigo. These results suggest that if the labyrinthine end-organ is in a hyperirritable condition, minor stimuli will precipitate symptoms.

Dysfunction of the Eustachian Tube

Tubotympanitis may be a cause of recurrent vertigo or dizziness frequently enough so that a patient with severe vertigo or even mild dizziness deserves to have inflation of the apparently affected tube. If a single inflation has not given some relief, however, repetition will not produce added benefit. Tubal occlusion on an inflammatory basis usually has followed an acute inflammation of the upper respiratory tract, either viral or bacterial.

Myxedema or a state of lowered basal metabolism without myxedema, often referred to as a hypometabolic state, may interfere with the function of the eustachian tube by producing swelling of its submucosal and mucosal linings. Several authors have insisted that hypometabolism or tubal dysfunction or both are the principal causes of Meniere's disease, but this cause of episodic vertigo is actually rather uncommon. Treatment of the dizzy patient with desiccated thyroid for a trial period of a week or two, with continuance of low dosage if symptomatic relief is obtained, may be found worthwhile.

One should always keep in mind that in an adult unilateral occlusion of the eustachian tube may be produced by a malignancy of the nasopharynx. In tubal dysfunction nonspecific dizziness is more apt to be the presenting symptom than are recurring episodes of severe rotary vertigo.

Motion Sickness

The sensitivity of the equilibrial labyrinth of normal individuals to stimulation varies widely. In patients with labyrinths in the high normal range of sensitivity a seemingly inadequate stimulus may produce sensations described by the patient as dizziness. A patient has been seen in whom moderately vigorous use of a rocking chair caused dizziness. A history of car or train sickness in childhood is always obtainable from such patients and their descriptions of the sensations they are experiencing are apt to be vague. The symptom of dizziness in such patients is readily controllable by one of the centrally acting drugs, such as a phenothiazine.

PREVENTIVE AND PROPHYLACTIC TREATMENT OF EPISODIC VERTIGO

It is in the prophylactic and preventive treatment of the episodic vertigos originating from irritation of the labyrinthine system that the need for an etiologic diagnosis of the various types is most apparent.

Autonomic Dysfunction

In episodic vertigo on the basis of autonomic dysfunction, as pointed out by Mygind and Dederding, a great many stimuli to the autonomic system may be reflected in a stereotyped reaction of the arteries and arterioles of the labyrinth. It should be recalled that the autonomic nervous system does not produce vasomotion peripheral to the arteriole, the contractile elements of the metarteriole, precapillary sphincters, and muscled venules being under nearly autonomous control by vasoactive chemicals. Autonomic nervous stimuli to the fine branches supplying the longitudinal fasciculi and vestibular nuclei and possibly to cortical areas may also be postulated. The resulting effect is presumed to be anoxia leading to local cellular injury, intravascular agglutination, increased vascular permeability, increase in interstitial fluid, and release of toxic metabolites, such as histamine, serotonin, and bradykinin with capillary dilatation.

In the involvement of the larger vessels vasospasm seems to be the principal precipitating feature and the logical therapy would seem to be the use of vasodilators. Vasodilators have been used for vertigos in which there seemed to be a component of atherosclerosis, such as in the dizziness of the aged, with variable degrees of success. On the other hand, in certain types of sudden deafness in which thrombosis or embolism were presumed to be the cause of an enduring vertigo, no observable effect from the use of vasodilators has been obtained. Those patients whose symptoms seem to respond most favorably to the use of vasodilators alone are in the group in whom an intermittent irritation of the labyrinthine system has occurred at the end-organ or vestibular nuclei with the production of episodic vertigo. On the grounds of intermittency, it is presumed that they can be classified as being due to arterial or arteriolar vasospasm. It has been found that it is possible to achieve a higher percentage of good therapeutic results when the vertiginous attacks are not associated with hearing loss but are of the type once characterized by Lindsay as "pseudo-Meniere's disease."

In his study of the effect of vasoactive chemicals on the inner ear, Seymour found that the greatest degree of vasodilation in this location was secured with nicotinic acid. Histamine was found to be less effective as well as variable in its effect. Nicotonic acid itself is relatively insoluble, and therefore monoethanolamine nicotinate, which is freely soluble, has been found the simplest, easiest, and least time-consuming vasodilator to use from the standpoint of both patient and physician. When given subcutaneously this drug has the additional advantage of being given under the supervision of the physician. This allows him to observe the progress of the patient and to give helpful advice and/or make additions and alterations to vasodilating treatment if this seems necessary. With monoethanole amine nicotinate (Nicamin), 25 mg. is given subcutaneously as the initial dose. If this dose is well tolerated, the quantity injected is increased by an equal amount (25 mg.) at one or twice daily injections until the symptoms are relieved. The dose given at this time is termed the optimum dose and it is not further increased. It is given daily, preferably as early in the morning as possible, and is continued under the physician's supervision for 1 or 2 weeks. If the optimal dose is much exceeded, symptoms will be again precipitated.

Some individuals are unable to tolerate an initial dose of 25 mg. For them the dose is successively halved until one which will not produce an excessive general vasodilation of the skin capillaries is found. The dose can then be increased by small increments. What appears to be a specific hypersensitivity to Nicamin will occasionally develop. The drug then produces urticarial lesions and dermatitis. For such individuals it is advisable to substitute another vasodilator. If good therapeutic results are obtained in the 2-week trial period, the patient may be instructed in the technique of self-medication and told to continue treatment at home. The real test of the effectiveness of any treatment has been found to be its effectiveness under the individual's normal living condition. The injections are continued by the patient at home for 2 months and then dosage is decreased by increasing the interval between injections, being given every other day for a week, 3 times a week for another week, and twice a week for a final week. If there has been no evidence of a return of symptoms, medication is stopped. It has been observed that patients tend to remain symptom-free for from 3 months to a year, and then often gradually develop a return of symptoms. The patient should be warned of this possibility so that he will return to his physician at the first sign of symptomatic return. Nicamin is again started at the initial 25 mg. dosage and built up again to the "optimal dose." This dose is continued daily for a week and then stopped. The patient should then experience another long remission of symptoms. Such booster courses are required by the average patient 2 or 3 times a year.

Autonomic Dysfunction with Cochlear Involvement

On the basis of histologic investigation Brunner stated that as a result of "vasomotor labyrinthitis" a "hydrolabyrinth" could be produced in which the scala tympani and scala vestibule showed equal or greater evidence of fluid accumulation than did the scala media. He found that this condition might, or might not, result in the combined symptoms of pressure, tinnitus, deafness, and vertigo, and he was at a loss for an explanation of the variability of the symptoms. The group of patients described as being subject to generalized edema of the labyrinth may well be a large one. The differentiation of this condition from Meniere's disease would obviously present great difficulty in certain instances. It seems highly probable that in the past most of this group of patients have been diagnosed as having Meniere's disease. This confusion of two conditions of different etiologies has had a great deal to do with the bad reputation of treatment for Meniere's disease.

Labyrinthine Hydrops

Lindsay's term "labyrinthine hydrops" would seem the best term for the condition described by Brunner and will be adopted here for episodic vertigo with the etiologic basis of cholinergic preponderance with vasospasm of the labyrinthine arterioles and combined hearing loss and vertigo. In these instances the cochlea is involved in addition to the semicircular canals with a relatively massive collection of what is essentially interstitial fluid in the scalae. Here, producing vasodilation without at the same time increasing the elimination of extracellular fluid would tend to make a bad matter worse.

In a series of controlled studies on patients with episodic vertigo, Furstenberg and his associates found that retention of sodium was more important in precipitating vertiginous attacks than any other factor. They advocated 0.5 Gm. sodium diet plus the elimination of fluid by the use of ammonium chloride given in doses of 3 Gm. 3 times a day with meals for 3 days. The ammonium chloride was then omitted for 2 days to avoid gastric irritation and the process was repeated. Perlman, et al. criticized this treatment on the grounds that they were not able to precipitate attacks of vertigo by sodium retention produced by cortisone. No attempt was made to control the hypokalemia produced by the cortisone. What effect this might have had is unknown. In addition, most of the patients were instances of "bilateral Meniere's disease" and what the actual etiology of their attacks may have been cannot be ascertained at this time. The Furstenberg regimen seemed to give good results in our hands as long as the patients could be kept on the diet. This proved impossible on their return to home surroundings.

Schemm found that interstitial collections of fluid tend to be maintained by the sodium in the solution, a sodium brine being formed. Without elimination of the sodium he found it impossible to eliminate the fluid. If, however, the patients were put on a diet only moderately low in sodium but one which gave an acid to neutral ash residue, and given an unlimited supply of "pure water," excessive interstitial fluid would be rapidly eliminated. Hydration in this instance tended to reduce the collection of interstitial fluid. A modified Schemm diet will achieve the results of the Furstenberg regime, and patients can be persuaded to stay on it with relative ease (Table 2).

Meniere's Disease

True Meniere's disease, if selected according to the criteria suggested by the panel on vertigo of the NINDB, is a relatively rare condition and not often seen even in a large outpatient service. If the hypothesis presented as to etiology is valid, it would suggest that a new method of approach to treatment should be sought. The new hypothesis would explain the observation that while vasodilators, such as nicotinic acid, and low sodium diets, such as those suggested by Furstenberg, Schemm, and Beckman, produce considerable symptomatic relief in instances which seem to be on the etiologic basis of autonomic dysfunction, they give such disappointing results in the treatment of a "true" Meniere's disease. It would also explain the failure of diets low in sodium, either with or without diuretics, such as ammonium chloride or azetolamide (Diamox), to produce significant symptomatic relief.

If an ictal type of reaction in the cells in the region of the "hypothalamic centers" in the hypothalamus is the cause of the stimulus triggering Meniere's disease, anticonvulsant drugs should produce relief. Indeed, such drugs as diphenylhydantoin (Dilantin) seem to have done so, although this observation needs confirmation.

Recently, one of the bioflavinoids, eriodictyol glycoside, has produced relief to the symptoms of nausea and vomiting in most cases of Meniere's disease and has produced restoration of hearing in some. This is one of the two bioflavonoids which Szent-Györgyi thought had biologic activity by virtue of the OH groups at positions 3′ and 4′ of the phenol radical. It is thought possible that eriodictyol glycoside might act as a blocking agent to histidine decarboxylase. That eriodictyol glycoside does not reverse a fundamental pathophysiologic fault is indicated by the fact that when medication with this substance is stopped, the symptoms and signs often return in 1 to 2 weeks.

Allergic Vertigo. The autonomic dysfunction type of vertigo which is thought to have an antigen-antibody etiology has been considered in detail in Chapter 22, "Allergic Aspects of Vertigo."

Hypometabolism

[See also pp. 000-000.] Rawlins suggested that there was a group of patients with poor stress mechanisms who reacted to stimuli such as exposure to drafts, smog, emotional disturbances, and the like with vasomotor symptoms such as headache, vasomotor rhinitis, and dizziness or vertigo. He recommended the use of glucocorticoid preparations in this condition. He called attention to a paper of Tintera on "The Hypoadrenal State and Its Management," and stated that he was able to get encouraging results by following Tintera's suggested regimen in some patients with a major complaint of dizziness or vertigo.

Goldman has become rather enthusiastic in

Table 2. Low Sodium Acid or Neutral Ash Diet as Modified from Schemm

Maximal Intake in 24 Hours		Minimal Intake in 24 Hours	
Food	*Amount*	*Food*	*Amount*
Milk	1 pint	Eggs	2
Vegetables	2 servings	Meat, fowl, fish	2 servings
		Cereal foods	Equivalent to 6 slices of bread
Fruit (except for plums)	2 servings prunes, plums, cranberries. As desired.		

1. Avoid soda, such as baking soda, soda biscuits, soda drinks, and artificially softened water.
2. Avoid adding salt to food and avoid foods prepared with salt, such as sauerkraut.
3. Avoid salty broths and soups.

regard to the hypothesis that the hypometabolic state is responsible for the symptoms of dizziness, vertigo, or syncope. He prefers the term "hypocortoadrenalism," suggesting that a relative deficiency in the production of the steroid hormones of the adrenal cortex, either on a genetic basis or acquired, exists in certain patients.

Goldman's papers are difficult to evaluate because he makes no attempt to differentiate between the various sensations which patients usually describe with the terms "dizziness or vertigo"; he also uses the terms "Meniere's syndrome" and "Meniere's disease" interchangeably as synonyms. It therefore becomes impossible to tell whether one of his patients is being treated for a sensation arising by virtue of irritation of the labyrinthine system or for a different sensation lumped with vertigo by the patient under the term "dizziness."

Thorn suggested the concept of a genetically propelled hypofunction of the adrenal cortex but has been unable to discover substantiating evidence. He found the fasting blood sugar level in most instances of Addison's disease to be in the low normal range (less than 80 mg. per cent). The oral glucose tolerance curve in patients with adrenal cortical insufficiency usually yielded a typical pattern characterized by a fairly low or normal fasting blood sugar level, a flat type of curve, and a considerable degree of hypoglycemia several hours after the ingestion of glucose. This finding appears to be identical to the results of the oral glucose tolerance test obtained by Tintera and by Goldman in their groups of patients. The intravenous glucose tolerance test, on the other hand, according to Thorn, produced a "normal height" curve but with severe hypoglycemic reactions several hours later from which spontaneous recovery was difficult. Thorn stated that the difference in behavior in response to the oral and the intravenous glucose tolerance test would suggest that the flat curve in the former is due to poor intestinal absorption of glucose.

Sofer et al. called attention to the fact that with atrophy of the anterior lobe of the hypophysis there occurs actual atrophy of the adrenal cortex with some symptoms of adrenal cortical hypofunction. It is therefore conceivable that Goldman's patients might be characterized as suffering from hypopituitarism rather than hypocorticoadrenalism. Sofer et al. also pointed out that neurasthenia may be difficult to differentiate from Addison's disease. These patients complain of marked weakness and anorexia; they will frequently have a low blood pressure and low basal metabolic rate; they may have a flat glucose tolerance curve with episodes of hypoglycemia and dizziness as a frequent complaint. It appears reasonable to suppose that the neurasthenia described by Sofer and the "hypocorticoadrenalism" described by Goldman are actually the same condition. The "dizziness" of which the neurasthenic group complains seems related to emotional and environmental stress in nearly every instance. They give evidence of inefficient maintenance of physiologic equilibrium or homeostasis, but this is not quite the same as stating that they have a congenital deficiency in adrenal cortical steroids. If a deficiency is present, it should lie in the hypophysis.

Vertigo of Vestibular Paralysis

This term was introduced by Kerrison in 1910 and has not since been improved on. Kerrison stated: "If the faculty of orientation is suddenly ablated, the individual at once loses his sense of stability in space or, in other words, experiences vertigo. The opposing labyrinth must become accustomed to unopposed unilateral activity and the muscular, arthrodial, and tactile impression of space and position must be immensely increased."

McCabe and Gillingham, in reporting on suppression of reaction to repeated labyrinthine stimulation, stated that this is probably a central process. It appears likely that the mechanism is very similar, if not the same, if the stimulus producing the symptomatic response is destruction of an end-organ.

Cawthorne reported that the process of "compensation" following a destructive labyrinthotomy was markedly speeded up by a series of graduated exercises. These should be started as soon as possible following operation. The first or second day following the day of operation is best, even if the patient feels sure the dizziness or vertigo is too severe to permit any head movement. On the first day the patient should sit up in bed and turn his head from side to side and up and down for 5 minutes. The periods of exercise should be lengthened by 5 minutes each day for 3 days. On the fourth day the patient should go through the same series of exercises while "dangling," and in another day or two while standing on the floor. In another day or two bending forward and from side to side should be added to the routine. Then a ball should be introduced which may be tossed from hand to hand and bounced on the floor. Following this the patient should add leaning forward and passing the ball between the legs. Finally, a friend or attendant should be added who is to toss the ball back and forth with the patient and who, after a day or two, is to circle around the patient, continuing to toss the ball back and forth. Each day the exercise period should start with the head movement and progress through the entire series of exercises.

At the end of 2 weeks the patient should have achieved nearly complete compensation. The patient should be encouraged to go about his daily routine and to practice physical exercises requiring active movement of the head and body, such as golf or bowling. In a short time (2 weeks to a month) a patient should be completely free of symptoms except when subject to extreme physical fatigue or encountering a new physical situation, when short-lived dizziness may be experienced.

Cervical Vertigo

Travell stated that disturbances of the head-on-neck righting reflex secondary to "trigger areas" in the sternomastoid are of two kinds: (1) sudden falls without warning, especially when the patient stoops over, and (2) veering toward the affected side when walking with head erect. I have found that such patients may complain of a swaying motion which may last from one-half to 1 or 2 hours. This is especially noted if the patient lies flat on the back with the neck extended. Supplying 1 or 2 pillows will sometimes terminate this sensation. These patients may sometimes show a benign positional vertigo and nystagmus. It is probable that the sensations of veering, lateral pulsion swaying, and so forth, are all on the basis of stimulation of the utricular macula. Such stimulation may frequently be on the basis of signals from the head-on-neck righting reflex. Myalgic areas in skeletal muscle have seemed to be frequently on the basis of sensitization to physical agents.

Among the conditions which seem to predispose to development of trigger mechanisms in skeletal muscle, Travell lists (1) acute upper respiratory infections, especially of viral etiology; (2) chronic foci of infection; (3) nutritional deficiencies, especially avitaminosis; (4) syndromes of the menopause and male climacteric; (5) hypometabolism; (6) chronic muscular strain; (7) whiplash injuries to the cervical region; and (8) osteoarthritis of the cervical spine. Precipitating causes are listed as (1) poor posture with drooping shoulders, which may put excessive strain on the scalenus anticus and medius muscles and on the sternocleidomastoid muscle; (2) unusual or excessive exercise, especially with exposure to sudden temperature change; (3) sudden trauma to the fibroskeletal structures of the neck; (4) prolonged immobilization of the head and neck; (5) vascular disturbances; (6) rupture of an intervertebral disk with nerve root pressure; and (7) acute emotional stress. Travell found that headache usually is present in patients with this type of dizziness but vertigo, nearly always "false vertigo" or dizziness, may be the only symptom.

Travell pointed out that a trigger area in a muscle is a physical sign discovered on physical examination. When the examiner sustains pressure on the tender spot, pain is usually induced in an area of reference. An investigation of the sternomastoids and other muscles about the head and neck and a detailed history as to possible predisposing and precipitating causes of cervical vertigo should certainly be the first step in the treatment of a patient with a chief complaint of dizziness, dysequilibrium, or vertigo.

Cope and Ryan state that cervical vertigo is self-limited and will disappear spontaneously in a few months. This has not been true in my experience, although remissions of considerable duration are usually seen. The vertigo will usually be precipitated again by a mild injury or an emotional stress. Cope and Ryan state that a well-fitting cervical collar will give marked symptomatic relief.

When a trigger area is found in the sternomastoid, Travell advises putting the muscle under tension by rotating the chin strongly toward the shoulder of the affected side and then spraying the skin over the tender area with an ethyl chloride spray. This should be repeated on several successive days. If sufficient relief is not secured by spraying, the tender area in the muscle may be infiltrated by a suitable anesthetic. For infiltration, the muscle is put on a slack by rotating the chin toward the opposite shoulder. The muscle is then encompassed by the fingers to lift it off the deeper structures and the hypodermic needle is then inserted into the area of maximum tenderness and the area infiltrated. Occasionally, "trigger areas" are found on both sides. Travell states that although infiltration with procaine is assumed to have only a transitory effect, the infiltration may permanently relieve dizziness of long duration. In my experience, however, the symptom is apt to be precipitated again by one of the factors mentioned previously.

Lewis believed myalgia to be a functional disorder in muscle due to sensitization to an unknown physicochemical agent. Based on this assumption, the physical therapeutic measures of heat and massage have been advised for the localized tender areas in muscle producing referred pain and reflex involvement of the vagotonic type.

In cervical myalgias tinnitus is not infrequently produced, and Decker et al. state that they have observed sensorineural hearing loss on the basis of a cervical myalgia, presumably due to vasospasm anoxia and interference with the oxidative phosphorylation of glucose which furnishes the energy for the conversion of the sound force waves entering the cochlea into the electrical impulses of the fibers of the auditory nerve.

Some of the physiologic effects of heat which may be of benefit in relation to myalgia of the sternomastoid and other cervical muscles are (1) increased circulation to the area, (2) increase in the flow of lymph, and (3) relaxation of the muscles. Luminous heat lamps which produce short infrared rays may be used effectively. These lamps possess a voltage varying from 250 to 1000 watts and may be applied easily over the involved sternomastoid muscle. The lamp should be used at a distance which will produce a comfortable warmth without a burning sensation. It is considered that this form of heat should be applied for 20 to 40 minutes daily over a period of one to several weeks. Shortwave diathermy is effective in producing a more penetrating heat. In the case of myalgia involving the sternomastoid it may be employed by having the patient lie on a coiled induction cable. Air spacing by means of a felt pad or Turkish toweling must be used. If air-spaced electrodes are used, spacing by means of pads or toweling is unnecessary. In certain instances in which general relaxation is desired in patients who have so-called vasomotor instability and/or tension state, hot tub baths may be of benefit. These baths should be given at a temperature of 102° to 104° F. for 15 to 20 minutes. The hot bath can be used readily in home treatment.

Massage seems to be an effective single treatment in myalgia involving the sternomastoid muscle. Massage alone is more effective than heat alone, and a firm, heavy, friction type of massage is more effective than the stroking or kneading types of massage. If the area is very tender, manipulation must be begun gently and applied in a manner to "get rid of the exudation and relieve tension." Then gradually, much firmer pressure should be used. The exact number of treatments necessary to relieve a "cervical" dizziness or vertigo is somewhat indefinite, but usually a period of 1 to 3 weeks of daily treatment will effect considerable relief or complete remission of the myalgia and its attendant dysequilibrium. How long such a remission will last cannot be stated, but usually if the dizziness does recur, the patient can control the symptom readily by resuming either professional or home treatment. In some instances additional benefit can be obtained by exercises which stretch the muscles and ligaments of the neck. Cervical traction has also been found to be of considerable benefit.

It is quite possible that cervical "dizziness" is the most common cause of this complaint when it is not associated with hearing loss and is not of a severe type. Treatment should also be directed against the underlying or predisposing causes of cervical myalgia, such as hypoglycemia, hypothyroidism, ovarian dysfunction, and the like.

CONCLUSION

The medical treatment of the episodic vertigos is not apt to be often successful if a single standard therapeutic program is applied to them under some such meaningless cognomen as "Meniere's syndrome." It must be realized that intermittent stimulation of the labyrinthine system may result from a variety of causes. An etiologic diagnosis should be attempted. If this proves extremely difficult or even impossible, an attempt at differential diagnosis by the effect of treatment should be attempted. If one plan of treatment does not give relief, it should not be too long continued, but another should be substituted. If this is done, there will be few patients whose symptoms will be so poorly controlled that surgery of any type will be considered.

REFERENCES

1. Aboulker, E.: Pathogenic et traitement cherurgical du vertige de Meniere. Presse Med. 35: 1412-1413, 1927.
2. Adam, J.: A case of Menierism and migraine: Recovery. J. Laryng. 55:224-225, 1940.
3. Alexander, L.: Die Anatomic der Sautentaschen der vierten Hernkammer. Z. Anat. Entwicklungsgesch. 95:531-707, 1931.
4. Alfaro, V. R.: Diagnostic significance of fullness in the ear. J.A.M.A. 166:239-245, 1958.
5. Aring, C. D.: Vascular diseases of the nervous system. Brain 68:28-55, 1945.
6. Altman, F., and Fowler, E. P., Jr.: Histological findings in Meniere's disease. Ann. Otol. 56:684-708, 1947.
7. Askerson, N.: The cochlear nerve and the vascular theory of nerve deafness. J. Laryng. 55:531-545, 1940.
8. Biancalana, L.: Arachnoidite cistica dell'angolo ponto-cerebellare. Boll. Mem. Soc. Piemontese Cher. 8:675-680, 1938.
9. Beckman, H.: Allergy considered as a special type of alkalosis. J. Allergy 1:496-500, 1930.
10. Behrman, S.: Vestibular epilepsy. Brain 78:471-486, 1955.
11. Alpers, B. J.: Vertiginous epilepsy. Laryngoscope 70:631-637, 1960.
12. Athens, A. G.: Vertigo in hypothyroidism. Minnesota Med. 29:562-567, 1946.
13. Crow, S. J.: Meniere's disease. Study based on examinations made before and after intracranial division of the vestibular nerve. Medicine 17:1-36, 1938.
14. Dean, L. W., Jr.: Meniere's syndrome and allergy. Int. Clin. 3:231-234, 1941.
15. Droller, H., and Pemberton, J.: Vertigo in a random sample of elderly people living in their homes. J. Laryng. 67:689-694, 1953.
16. Barany, R.: Der Baranysche Symptomenkomplex: Seine Diagnose und Therapie, Aetiologic und Prognose. Verh. Deutsch. Otolog. Ges. 21:108-132, 1912.
17. Brown, M. R.: The factor of heredity in labyrinthine, deafness and paroxysmal vertigo (Meniere's syndrome). Ann. Otol. 58:665-670, 1949.
18. Brown, M. D.: Meniere's syndrome. Report of three cases. Arch. Neurol. Psychiat. 46:561, 1947.
19. Brunner, H.: Serous effusions in the inner ear and in the cisterna pontis. J. Laryng. 68: 378-400, 1954.
20. Cawthorne, T., and Fawcett, M. N.: Fluid balance in Meniere's disease. Lancet 2:1404-1408, 1938.
21. Conn, J. W.: Spontaneous hypoglycaemias. J.A.M.A. 115:1669-1675, 1940.
22. Cope, S., and Ryan, G. N. S.: Cervical and otolith vertigo. J. Laryng. 73: 113-120, 1959.
23. Davis, H.: A functional classification of auditory defects. Trans. Amer. Otol. Soc. 50:98-111, 1952.

24. Davis, D.: Common type of vertigo relieved by cervical traction. Ann. Intern. Med. 38:778-786, 1953.
25. Decher H., Unterharnscheidt F., and Rohr, H.: Further otological contribution on the syncopal vertebral syndrome, Hals-, Nasen-, Ohrenheilkunde 7:321-324, 1959.
26. Demetriades, T. D.: Die Wechselbeziehungen zwischen Labyrinth und vegetativen Nervensystem. Wien. Klin. Wschr. 40:1471, 1514, 1544. 1927.
27. Dohlman, G.: Meniersche Krankheit auf allergische basis. Acta Otolaryng. 27:245, 1939.
28. Duke, W. W.: Allergy, Asthma, Hayfever, Urticaria and Allied Manifestation of Reaction. St. Louis, C. V. Mosby Co., 1925.
29. Flett, R. L.: The success and failure of the Portmann operation. Ohio Med. J. 48:11, 1952.
30. Goldman, H. B.: Hypoadrenocorticism and Endocrinologic Treatment of Meniere's Disease. New York. J. Med. 62:377-381, 1962.
31. Guilford, F. R., Fields, W. S., and Alford, B. R.: Treatment of Meniere's disease. *In:* Neurological Aspects of Auditory and Vestibular Disorders. Springfield, Ill., Charles C Thomas, 1965.
32. Gerlings, P. G.: Peripheral positional nystagmus. J. Laryng. 62:147-162, 1948.
33. Hallpike, C. S., and Cairns, H.: Observations on the pathology of Meniere's syndrome. J. Laryng. 53:625-655, 1938.
34. House, W. F.: Subarachnoid shunt for drainage of endolymphatic hydrops. Laryngoscope 72: 713-728, 1962.
35. House, W. F.: Subarachnoid shunt for drainage of hydrops. A report of 68 cases. Arch. Otolaryng. 79:338-354, 1964.
36. Ireland, P. E., and Farkashidy, J.: Electron microscopic studies of Meniere's disease. Twelve fresh specimens taken at operation. Trans. Amer. Acad. Ophthal. Otolaryng. 67: 28-36, 1963.
37. Jorgensen, M. B.: Changes of aging in the inner ear. Arch. Otolaryng. 74:164-177, 1961.
38. Kerrison, P. D.: Vertigo of Vestibular Paralysis. Trans. Amer. Otol. Soc. 12:367-378; also Laryngoscope 21:978-985, 1911.
39. Kjaer, M.: Meniere's disease and allergy. Acta Otolaryng. 35:390-403, 1947.
40. Knapp, H.: A clinical analysis of the inflammatory affections of the inner ear. Arch. Ophthal. Otol. 2:204-238, 1871.
41. Kuntz, A.: The Autonomic Nervous System. Philadelphia, Lea & Febiger, 1953.
42. Lawrence, M., and McCabe, B. F.: Inner ear mechanisms and deafness. J.A.M.A. 171: 1929-1932, 1959.
43. Lindsay, J. R.: Vertigo. Differential diagnosis and treatment. J. Minnesotta Med. Soc. 47: 632-636, 1948.
44. Magnus, R.: Animal posture. Proc. Roy. Soc. London S.B. 98:339-353, 1925.
45. Magnus, R.: Cooperation and interference of reflexes from other sense organs with those of labyrinths. Laryngoscope 36:701-712, 1926.
46. Mayoux, R., and Chossegros, H.: Le vertigue de origine cervicale. J. Med. Lyon 31:793-798, 1950.
47. McLaurin, J. W.: Dizziness and vertigo. Etiologic diagnosis the essence of the problem. Med. Times (Apr.) 1955.
48. Myrhaug, H.: Functional diseases of the jaws with ear symptoms. Nord. Med. 50:1107-1110, 1953.
49. Petersen, W. F.: The Patient and the Weather; Autonomic Disintegration. Vol. 2. Ann Arbor, Mich., Edwards Bros., 1934, p. 530.
50. Parresius, W.: Kapillarstudien bei vasoneurosen. Deutsch. Festschr. Nervenheil. 72:310-358, 1921.
51. Portmann, M.: Decompressive opening of the endolymphatic sac. Arch. Otolaryng. 79:328-337, 1964.
52. Rawlins, A. G.: Review of the corticosteriods. Their application to otolaryngology. Laryngoscope 66:674-686, 1956.
53. Shuknecht, H. F., Bentley, J. R., and Beckhuis, J.: Further observations on the pathology of Meniere's disease.
54. Rostenberg, A., Jr.: Some speculations concerning allergy. J. Asthma Res. 2:25-32, 1964.
55. Seymour, J. C.: Observations on the circulation in the cochlea. J. Laryng. 68:689-711, 1954.
56. Schayer, R.W.: Significance of induced synthesis of histamine. Physiol. Path. Chemotherapia (Basel) 3:128-136, 1961.
57. Schayer, R. W.: A unified theory of glucocorticoid action. Perspect. Biol. Med. 7:71-84, 1964.
58. Szent-Györgyi, A.: Studies on Biological Oxidation and Some of Its Catalysts. Budapest, Karl Renyi, 1937.
59. Thorn, C. W., Koept, G. F., Lewis, R. A., and Olsen, E. F.: Carbohydrate metabolism in Addison's disease. J. Clin. Invest. 19:813, 1940.
60. Soffer, L. J., Dorfman, R. I., and Gabrihove, J. L.: The Human Adrenal Gland. Philadelphia, Lea & Febiger, 1961.
61. Tintera, J. W.: The hypoadrenocortical state

and its management. New Jersey Med. 55: 1869-1876, 1955.

62. Travell, J.: Referred pain from skeletal muscle. New York J. Med. 53:331-340, 1955.

63. Jorgensen, M. B.: Changes of aging in the inner ear. Arch. Otolaryng. 74:56-62, 1961.

64. Wullstein, H., and Rauch, S.: Endolymph and perilymph in Meniere's disease. A report of biochemical findings in three cases. Arch. Otolaryng. 73:262-267, 1961.

65. Weiss, S.: The pharmaceopeia and the physician. Treatment of vertigo and syncope. J.A.M.A. 118:529-553, 1942.

66. Wright, Sir A. J.: Aural vertigo. J. Laryng. 53: 97-112, 1938.

67. Williams, D.: Central vertigo. Trans. Med. Soc. London 74:15-19, 1957.

68. Williams, H. L.: Meniere's Disease. Springfield, Ill., Charles C Thomas, 1952.

69. Williams, H. L.: Allergy of the inner ear. (Meniere's disease). Trans. Amer. Acad. Ophthal. Otolaryng. 56:176-195, 1952.

70. Williams, H. L.: Meniere's disease. Etiology Trans. Amer. Acad. Ophthal. Otolaryng. 60:167-171, 1956.

71. Williams, H. L., and Corbin, K. B.: The differential diagnosis of vertigo. Ann. Otol. 67: 869-889, 1958.

72. Williams, H. L., and Corbin, K. B.: The dizzy patient. Med. Clin. N. Amer. 46:669-688, 1962.

73. Williams, H. L.: A new hypothesis of vascular dysfunction, linking certain pain syndromes of the head and neck with Meniere's disease. J. Lancet 84:344-349, 1964.

74. Williams, H. L., Maher, F. T., Corbin, K. B., Brown, J. R., Brown, H. A., and Hedgecock, L. D.: Eriodictyol glycoside in the treatment of Meniere's disease. Ann. Otol. 72: 1082-1102, 1963.

75. Williams, H. L.: Eriodictyol glycoside in Meniere's disease. Trans. Amer. Acad. Ophthal. Otolaryng. 68:45-59, 1964.

Dizziness in Hypoadrenocorticalism

Herbert Goldman

There is no doubt that Meniere's disease is a general condition whose local manifestations (vertigo, tinnitus, and deafness) are more dynamic and outstanding.

We have found that these patients have a hypoglycemic tendency. A 4-hour glucose tolerance test reveals (1) a continued gradual drop in blood sugar, instead of any leveling off; (2) a blood sugar level which stays flat and never rises; or (3) a rather high rise in blood sugar level, especially in the older patients, with a marked drop after 2-3 hours. It seems to be due to some defect in metabolism of carbohydrates. These patients also show many clinical symptoms of lowered function of the adrenal cortex. They have an allergic background, a marked asthenia, and many anxieties, and they respond poorly to different varieties of stress. Every patient has had an unusual accumulation of stresses 1 to 2 years before his first attack of vertigo.

The recent work of Vosteen in Germany, and Koide in Japan, has shown that the amount of energy leaving the inner ear is more than that which enters it. This energy is provided by a glucose catabolism which depends on the necessary amounts of oxygen, glucose, and enzyme supplied to the inner ear.

Treatment based on this reasoning has given uniformly good results which continue to stand up after 10 years. We have statistics collected on 250 cases. However, in view of the periodicity of Meniere's disease in many patients, it is admittedly difficult to evaluate results unless on a large scale over a long time.

We find that the diet is more than 50 per cent of the treatment. It must be continued over several or many years, depending on the particular condition of each patient. Treatment must be individualized. A rigid diet low in carbohydrates, moderate in fats, and high in proteins is used. Feedings must be given between meals to keep the blood sugar fairly steady. It is important to have a snack every 2 hours after dinner, for the patient goes all night without any food. New patients must have fresh unsweetened juice ready on awakening. Mimeographed copies of the diet are given to the patient. Constant reviews of the diet are in order, by having the patients regularly keep a food diary. The patients are warned to keep away from readily absorbable carbohydrates (such as sweets, starches, alcohols, etc.); any foods having more than 15 per cent carbohydrates; caffeine and cola foods, which stimulate the liver to send sudden amounts of glucose into the blood stream; and all wheat flours. The patients are taught how to interpret labels on packaged and canned foods.

Whole adrenal cortex extract medication helps the response to stress and the proper metabolism of carbohydrates. The change in general body metabolism effectuates a local improvement in symptoms. Vertigo is the first symptom to go. Better results are obtained here rather than for the tinnitus and deafness. The extracts can be given intravenously or in an intramuscular form. They have been in existence a long time. There are absolutely no side effects, since the whole balanced extract is used. The aqueous extract* is given intravenously in 10 cc. doses slowly, at daily to weekly intervals, depending upon the severity of the disease. The extract in oil† is given intramuscularly when injections can be given at 2-4 week intervals, as the patient's condition improves. Salt is taken without restrictions.

Other endocrine therapy is frequently necessary, more in women than in men. The younger woman has a lowered ovarian function. The majority of the women are just commencing their menopause. This upsets the balance. The men need some testosterone.

Although a lowered metabolic activity is generally present, this is on an adrenal cortex basis and not thyroid in origin. The basal metabolic rate is usually slightly lowered but tests for thyroid function show normal results. Occasionally, small doses of whole thyroid extract (proloid gr. ¼) are used for about 3-4 months until the thyropituitary axis is reestablished.

Because the autonomic nervous system is so deranged, Bellergal (a combination of belladonna, ergotrate, and phenobarbitol) is given for a few months.

The most striking change noticed in these patients is their general physical improvement and their changed outlook on life. They themselves notice how much more easily they can meet the various different stresses of life.

*Parke Davis & Co.—Eschatin.

†Upjohn & Company—Lipoadrenal Cortex Extract.

CHAPTER 25

Histamine Therapy in Episodic Vertigo

WILLIAM H. WILSON

Histamine therapy offers a therapeutic tool which warrants consideration in selected cases of episodic vertigo. The role of histamine in arteriolar vasodilatation and anaphylactic shock was first suggested by Dale and Laidlaw[1] in 1910. The following year Barger and Dale[2] demonstrated its presence as a normal constituent of several body tissues. A decade passed before the work of these and other physiologists found clinical application. In 1924 Ramirez and St. George[3] reported a technique for performing dermal scratch tests for histamine tolerance and described a method by which asthmatics were treated by hypodermic injections of histamine.

The successful treatment of a cold-sensitive patient by injecting progressively increasing amounts of histamine subcutaneously was reported by Bray[4] in 1931. Eight years later Horton et al.[5] described a vascular headache syndrome which he termed "erythromelalgia of the head" and attributed to an abnormal release of histamine. While treating a woman so afflicted, Horton[6] observed that following a course of subcutaneous injection of histamine, her Meniere's disease, of over 4 years duration, was greatly improved. He reported 3 additional cases of Meniere's disease successfully treated by the same technique. Shelden and Horton[7] first used intravenous histamine in the treatment of Meniere's disease in 1939.

Alexander[8] offered an explanation for the therapeutic effect of histamine therapy by citing the observation of Grant et al.[9] that once the H-substance is released by the cells of the skin, a refractory period of less than 48 hours develops when no further H-substance appears. Alexander considered the possibility that daily doses of histamine might gradually induce such refractoriness. He felt that such a tolerance buildup resembles, but actually is not, an immunization, and he suggested that histamine therapy operates through the production of histaminase.

Brown[10] emphasized that histaminase is not the only enzyme which inactivates histamine and listed the methylating enzymes as additional factors.

Atkinson[11] presented a classification of Meniere's disease which divided patients into two groups, depending upon the degree of the skin whealing response obtained with an intracutaneous injection of histamine. He found a small group to be histamine-sensitive and a larger group to be histamine-insensitive. In discussing the pharmacologic actions of histamine, Code[12] noted that its presence, in quantities in excess of those required for physiologic processes, soon resulted in many abnormalities.

A dual source of histamine availability has been demonstrated by Schayer.[13,14] In addition to its being synthesized and stored in tissue for subsequent release, it may be newly synthesized in response to local or systemic stress. Stress-induced synthesis occurs in or near vascular endothelial cells to regulate the response of small blood vessels to environmental change as the requirements of the tissue for blood vary. He further indicated that although induced histamine is a useful agent, excessive formation may cause damaging local inflammation or systemic shock. The various clinical manifestations of this abnormal state have been referred to as the vasometer neuroses. The potency of induced histamine was felt to be much greater than that of released, bound histamine because of the strategic point of synthesis. A state of local hypersensitivity is thought to develop, possibly due to the tendency toward a prolonged synthesis of induced histamine, once the process is initiated.

Modifications of the histamine therapy techniques of Horton and of Atkinson fall under the category of optimal dose therapy. Hansel[15] found that smaller doses of histamine, given every 2 to 3 days, were effective in maintaining relief in cases of histamine cephalgia. His injections varied from 0.10 cc. of a 1:1,000,000 solution to 0.50 cc. of a 1:100,000 solution. This was supplemented with sublingual administration, using 1 to 2 drops of a 1:10,000 or 1:1000 solution once or twice a day.

Shambaugh[16] adapted the technique of Hansel to the treatment of postfenestration labyrinthine hydrops, which he felt closely resembled Meniere's disease. In treating postoperative hydrops and Meniere's disease, the most effective dilution was determined by the clinical response of the patient.[17]

The "low dose" techniques of Hansel used in antigen hyposensitization were practiced and modified by Rinkel.[18] He also found smaller doses of histamine more effective and reported successful treatment of cold-sensitive patients by the optimal-dose technique.[19] Details of the serial dilution method of intracutaneous testing have appeared in the literature on several occasions.[18,20]

METHOD

Rinkel's solutions were diluted* in a ratio of 1:5 instead of 1:10 as employed by Hansel. In his later papers he designated the commercially prepared 1:10,000 dilution of histamine, which contained 0.275 mg. of histamine diphosphate per cc., as the stock or concentrated solution. The first 1:5 dilution of the stock solution was designated as #1. A 1:5 dilution of the #1 solution was designated as #2. Solution preparation was continued in this manner through #7.

This designation and diluting procedure is currently employed by the author, who has used serially diluted intradermal skin tests for determining histamine sensitivity in episodic vertigo for many years. It is felt that a therapeutically effective dose, both from the standpoint of amount and strength of the solution, can be ascertained more accurately and rapidly by this technique.

The method, basically Rinkel's, is as follows: An intracutaneous wheal, 4 mm. in diameter, is made with each of the 5 solutions from #7 through #3. These are placed as superficially as possible, in a vertical line. The

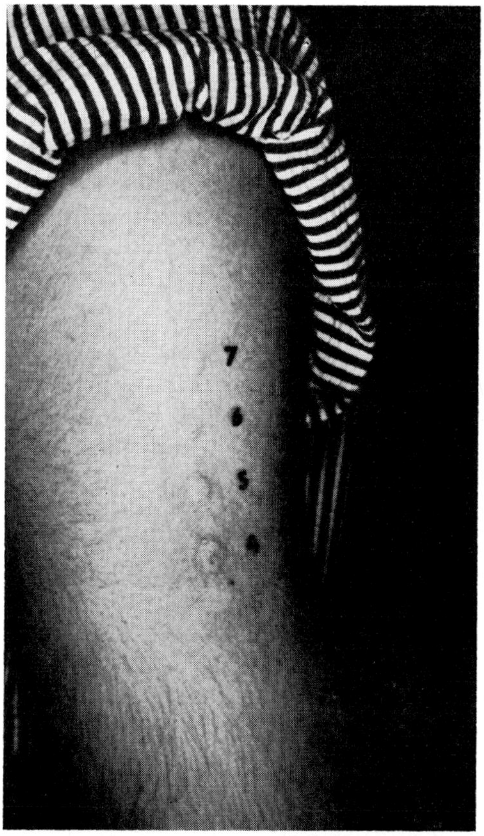

FIG. 1. Serially diluted intracutaneous tests for histamine. Number 5 was the most dilute solution to show an increase in whealing response 10 minutes after the initial wheals were made.

*Diluent = 0.4 per cent phenol in normal saline.

more dilute solutions are not expected to react, but rather to serve as a basis for comparison in evaluating the point of the first reaction. A reading is made in 10 minutes. The most dilute solution capable of producing a definite increase in the size of the initially injected wheals is considered the most effective solution for beginning therapy. This wheal will frequently be accompanied by a peripheral erythema. Intracutaneous tests which do not show a whealing response will be less discrete at the end of 10 minutes, but may increase in size from 4 to 5 millimeters.

Serial dilution intracutaneous tests are recorded by indicating the numbers of the solutions tested. Starting with the most dilute, the size of the wheal for each dilution is noted as read after 10 minutes. For example, a test which first reacts at a #4 solution may be recorded thus: #7=5 mm., #6=5 mm., #5=5 mm., #4=7 mm., #3=8 mm. Solutions more dilute than the one to first react may produce wheals up to 6 millimeters in diameter, but will not be discrete and rarely produce an erythema. Such a test, reacting first at a #3 solution may be recorded thus: #7=6 mm., #6=6 mm., #5=6 mm., #4 =6 mm., #3=7 mm.

The first injection given is 0.05 cc. of the solution, which shows an increased whealing response. The second is 0.07 cc. of the same solution and is given 24 to 48 hour hours later. The third dose is 0.10 cc. and the fourth 0.15 cc. Patients are instructed in giving their own injections and are told not to increase the dosage level above the amount that affords relief from vertigo or, if present, from fullness of the ears and pitch dysacusis. This determined quantity of the optimal solution is injected every 2 days until the patient is seen 7 days after the previous visit.

If the patient reports a definite improvement in vertigo or, in the case of associated cochlear involvement, if the pure tone audiogram, diplacusigram, or discrimination score show improvement, the optimal dose, as previously determined, is maintained every 2 days for at least 2 weeks. An attempt is then made to increase the interval between doses to every 3 days. Many patients find that they experience a return of symptoms when the interval between injections is extended beyond 48 hours. A return to an interval of 2 days is then essential. Several weeks later the timing may be successfully extended. Lengthening the injection interval to once a week is a distinct possibility, after 6 to 8 weeks of therapy.

Patients who do not show improvement during the first week of treatment are retested, using the same solutions of histamine. An error may be disclosed in the initial reading of the first reaction point of the whealing response, or an actual change in sensitivity response may be found due to the recent histamine therapy. If there is a change, the patient is given a vial of the newly selected solution and instructed to follow the same dosage schedule as for the previous week.

Patients who have not improved on the therapy of the first week, and do not show a change in the serial dilution testing, are instructed to increase the dosage above 0.15 cc., using the same strength solution. The amounts suggested are 0.25 cc., 0.35 cc., 0.50 cc., and 0.75 cc. The dose which affords relief is maintained according to the schedule previously outlined. Patients who do not improve are again retested. Those showing a change are given a new solution for treatment. Histamine therapy is discontinued in those who still maintain the same point of initial whealing response.

The most effective dose is frequently 0.10 cc. or 0.15 cc. of the first reacting solution. Patients may be symptom-free on the same dose for months and then experience an exacerbation. This may be an expression of the episodic nature of their vertigo or it may be due to an increase in their exposure to stress. Retesting may show a change in the whealing response. If there is a change, the new solution is scheduled. If the test is the same, the dosage schedule is dropped back to

0.05 cc. and increased every 2 days until a therapeutically effective amount is again found. This may vary from the previous satisfactory dose.

Due to the episodic nature of vertigo of end-organ origin, coincident factors must always be taken into consideration in evaluating results in histamine therapy. Experience with dosage requirements and interval timing, in the treatment of histamine cephalgia (erythromelalgia of the head), has been of great value in regulating histamine therapy in episodic vertigo.

The treatment of women with histamine cephalgia has shown that many patients experience a "breakthrough" of symptoms a few days before a menstrual period. Reducing the previously effective dose by one-third during the premenstrual interval will, in most instances, prevent the cephalgia from developing at this time. Women on histamine therapy for episodic vertigo may also experience a return of symptoms during premenstrual periods. Reducing the previously effective dose by one-third just prior to their menses will frequently prevent a recurrence of vertigo at this time.

The treatment of histamine cephalgia has shown that many patients will find an effective dose, but that they experience a return of pain 36 to 48 hours after each injection. If injections are given every 36 hours, they remain free of symptoms. If the dose is lowered below or raised above the proved optimum, the cephalgia again reaches its pretreatment proportion. An increase in dose may precipitate an attack. Most patients with histamine cephalgia who are relieved for only 36 hours with an injection are able to lengthen the interval after 2 or 3 weeks of treatment. These observations are occasionally applicable in the histamine therapy of episodic vertigo.

The intravenous administration of histamine in the treatment of Meniere's disease and episodic vertigo is frequently described under the category of vasodilator drugs. The arrest of an acute episode of vertigo by this means, when achieved, must certainly be attributed to the vasodilating effect of histamine. The possibility that the production of histaminase may be stimulated also by this method is a matter of conjecture.

The technique of injecting histamine intravenously has varied little from the method as originally described by Shelden and Horton.[7] The equivalent of 2.75 mg. of histamine diphosphate is diluted in 250 cc. of an isotonic solution of sodium chloride. If the administration of sodium is of concern, the histamine may be diluted in an 0.8 per cent solution of potassium chloride or in a 5 per cent solution of dextrose.

The rate of intravenous administration should vary between 30 and 45 drops per minute. The flow is altered according to the patient's response. General flushing of the face and neck is desirable, but extension onto the thorax is indicative of a too rapid rate. The flow should be kept below that which produces head pain. One and a half to 2 hours is the usual time required for administration of 250 cc.

Three to 4 intravenous injections on successive days are generally considered adequate for the initial course of treatment. The procedure is frequently continued twice a week for another 3 weeks.

Acceptance of William's theory, that the pathologic neosynthesis of induced histamine in stria vascularis is responsible for true Meniere's disease, requires reevaluation of previous indications for intravenous histamine therapy. With the resulting pathologic picture one of dilatation of terminal arterioles and precapillary loop sphincters, the reasoning behind the use of intravenous histamine as a vasodilating agent in the treatment of Meniere's disease demands reexamination.

The selection of patients for subcutaneous histamine therapy necessitates ruling out possible systemic factors and antigenic excitants. Vertiginous patients who fall into the classification of the vasomotor neuroses are to be considered as candidates for histamine therapy only after potential endocrine and antigenic factors have been eliminated.

Histamine therapy has been enthusiastically endorsed by several authors, but many clinicians have become discouraged with its use. Failure to obtain satisfactory results may be attributed largely to improper screening of candidates for treatment. Patients who are vertiginous because of a hypoglycemia, hypothyroidism, adrenal insufficiency, or ovarian dysfunction cannot be expected to respond to histamine therapy, but must receive treatment for the basic pathologic problem responsible for labyrinthine involvement. The use of commercially prepared concentrates of histamine for injection, without thought of individual tolerance, is an additional cause of failure.

SUMMARY

A selective review of the literature on histamine therapy with an examination of the evolution of various techniques employed in its use has been presented. Histamine dosage determination, through use of Rinkel's serial dilution testing techniques, is outlined as a method for planning histamine therapy in selected cases of episodic vertigo.

REFERENCES

1. Dale, H. H., and Laidlaw, P. P.: The physiological action of B-iminazolylethylamine J. Physiol. 41:318, 1910.
2. Barger, G., and Dale, H. H.: B-iminazolylethylamine, a depressor constituent of intestinal mucosa J. Physiol. 41:499-503, 1911.
3. Ramirez, M. A., and St. George, A. V.: A contribution to the etiology of asthma. Med. J. Rec. 119:71-72. 1924.
4. Bray, G. W.: A case of physical allergy: a localized and generalized allergic type of reaction to cold. J. Allergy 3:367-374, 1931-1932.
5. Horton, B. T., MacLean, A. R., and Craig, W. M.: A new syndrome of vascular headache: results of treatment with histamine: a preliminary report. Proc. Mayo Clin. 14:157-260, 1939.
6. Horton, B. T.: The use of histamine in Meniere's disease. Surg. Gynec. Obst. 72: 417-420, 1941.
7. Shelden, C. H., and Horton, B. T.: Treatment of Meniere's disease with histamine administered intravenously. Proc. Mayo Clin. 15: 17-21, 1940.
8. Alexander, H. L.: Treatment of allergic disorders with histamine and histaminase. J. Lab. Clin. Med. 26:110-116, 1940.
9. Grant, R. T., Oearson, D., and Comeau, W. S.: Observations on urticaria provoked by exercise and by warming the body. Clin. Sci. 2:253, 1935.
10. Brown, E. A.: Enzymes and allergy. Ann. Allergy 22:611-631, 1964.
11. Atkinson, M.: Observations on the etiology and treatment of Meniere's syndrome. J.A.M.A. 116:1753-1760, 1941.
12. Code, C. F.: Histamine in human disease. Proc. Mayo Clin. 39:715-737, 1964.
13. Schayer, R. W.: The Normal Cell and its Response to Allergic Stimuli, Report of the Thirty-Eighth Ross Conference on Pediatric Research. Columbus, Ohio, Ross Laboratories, 1961, pp. 52-57.
14. Schayer, R. W.: Evidence that induced histamine is an intrinsic regulator of the microcirculation system. Amer. J. Physiol. 202: 66-72, 1962.
15. Hansel, F. K.: Treatment of certain specific types of headache with histamine. Ann. Otol. 56:152-160, 1947.
16. Shambaugh, G. E., Jr.: Histamine in treatment of certain types of headache and vertigo following the fenestration operation. Arch. Otolaryng. 51:781-785, 1950.
17. Shambaugh, G. E., Jr.: Surgery of the Ear. Philadelphia, W. B. Saunders Co., 1959, pp. 524-526, 586.
18. Rinkel, H. J.: Inhalant allergy. III. The coseasonal application of serial dilution testing (titration). Ann. Allergy 7:693-645, 1949.
19. Rinkel, H. J.: Thermal allergy. Clinical evaluation and management. South. Med. J. 44: 1067-1073, 1951.
20. Rinkel, H. J.: The management of clinical allergy. Part II. Etiologic factors and skin titration. Arch. Otolaryng. 77:42-75, 1963.

CHAPTER 26

Surgery for Vertigo

MARTIN SPECTOR

The primary indication for labyrinthine surgery is intractable, incapacitating episodes of vertigo in a patient for whom medical treatment has failed to give sufficient relief. Six weeks loss of time from work may cause an economic problem for a laborer, although this might not be a hardship to some people. The attacks may produce such severe anxiety that it may be feared that a psychosis will be precipitated or the patient may threaten suicide. In such cases, surgical intervention should be considered much sooner. In special occupations, such as working at heights or driving a truck, vertiginous attacks may lead to physical injury and may even be dangerous to life.

The incidence of surgical intervention is reported to be from 25 per cent to 0 per cent in various series. Meniere's disease has been the main diagnosis in patients in whom vertigo has become so incapacitating that surgery has been required. However, occasionally following trauma to the ear and in rare cases of positional vertigo, vertigo has been so severe that surgical measures for relief have been required. The criteria for ablation had been a discrimination score of 40 per cent or worse and a speech reception threshold of 60 decibels or worse plus incapacitating vertigo. It is particularly pertinent that when surgery is considered, the diagnosis must be established as certainly as possible. Bilateral Meniere's disease is often considered an indication for surgical intervention. Some observers report that about 10 per cent of cases of endolymphatic hydrops are bilateral. Usually the second ear is affected within a few months after the first, but sometimes the second ear is not involved for years.

The *theoretically ideal objectives of surgery* are (1) to eliminate vertigo, (2) to restore or to maintain hearing, if possible, and (3) to eliminate or ameliorate the tinnitus. The ideal surgical procedure should have a simple approach, low morbidity, and no mortality. These ideal objectives cannot be attained at the present time in every case.

The surgical procedures suggested for the relief of intractable episodic vertigo follow.

FENESTRATION

It was thought that making an opening in the bony lateral semicircular canal in endolymphatic hydrops without disturbing the membranous tube would release the pressure and preserve the hearing. However, in the majority of patients, the procedure caused further loss of hearing. There seems to be a special factor in endolymphatic hydrops which makes the cochlea susceptible to deterioration after surgical exposure. The principal cause for failure of destructive labyrinthotomy to relieve symptoms has been an incomplete destruction of the vestibular sense organs. In Meniere's disease, often it has only been necessary to tear into the endolymphatic system for all eighth nerve function to be lost, but this simple approach has failed to give relief in many instances. The mixing of endolymph and perilymph does not appear to be catastrophic in itself.

If the stapes is freely movable and an additional mobile window is made on the vestibular side of the membrane, such as in the lateral semicircular canal, a disturbing condition may follow in which a loud sound may cause vertigo. This is the Tullio phenomenon.

The fenestration operation is not advised for the relief of episodic vertigo of any type.

Fick reported a procedure through a transmeatal approach in which footplate fenestration and puncture of the saccule is done: "In endolymphatic hydrops, the saccule is usually distended so that it presses against the medial side of the stapes footplate. After the standard meatal approach, the stapedial footplate is opened. The patient is now warned of a sudden loud sound in the ear and also that vertigo may occur. With a very fine needle, a perforation is made through the footplate to a depth of approximately 2 mm. After the perforation is made, if the saccule is punctured there is usually marked and rapid escape of fluid through the opening, which seems to indicate an increased hydrodynamic pressure of the endolymph. A fenestra in the footplate, 1 mm. in diameter, is then made, and with a fine suction cannula more fluid is drawn from the labyrinth; this sometimes causes vertigo. The mucosa which was teased toward the promontory is put back in place across the fenestra." Reports of the Fick procedure indicate that hearing has often been destroyed. Schuknecht has confirmed Fick's contention that introducing a needle through the footplate so as to rupture the saccule usually leaves a large fistula in the footplate.

SYMPATHECTOMY

The rationale of sympathectomy, cervical or dorsal, is based on the concept that interruption of the sympathetic chain on the involved side will relieve vasospasm and restore normal blood and endolymphatic circulation of the labyrinth and relieve anoxia and will, eventually, relieve increased hydrodynamic pressure in the scala media.

Passe performed a dorsal sympathectomy, a modification of the Smithwick operation which is, essentially, a preganglionic section of the sympathetic nerves. Sympathectomy did not produce regular symptomatic relief and few of these operations are now performed.

Sellers advised alcohol block of the cervical ganglion. A needle is introduced 4 cm. above the clavicle midway between the anterior and posterior borders of the sternomastoid muscle, with the head turned partly away. Procaine is then injected to make sure that a Horner's syndrome is produced. There may also be slight hoarseness and some nasal stuffiness. If signs are produced, and the patient is willing to bear the side effects, then alcohol and phenol are injected. The results of this procedure have been found somewhat unpredictable and injuries to the cervical plexus have been produced. This procedure has achieved little popularity.

DESTRUCTIVE LABYRINTHOTOMY THROUGH A FISTULA IN THE LATERAL SEMICIRCULAR CANAL

Destructive labyrinthotomy was first done by Day through the horizontal semicircular canal by way of a mastoidectomy approach. In 1938, Cawthorne and Hallpike stated that by simply removing the membranous external semicircular canal with fine watchmakers forceps in cases of Meniere's disease, all cochlear and vestibular function was destroyed in the operated labyrinth. Later, it was noted that this procedure's destructive effect upon the labyrinth was not dependable and that reoperation was frequently required.

Fernandez, Ludwig, and McAuliffe demonstrated that the structures of the normal vestibule could not be completely destroyed by surgical injury, by a dental broach, or even by electrocoagulation. The crista of the posterior semicircular canal and the macula of the saccule often persisted. They found that if roaring tinnitus persisted, it usually meant that there had been an incomplete destruction of the cochlea.

In episodic vertigo associated with chronic suppurative otitis media, mastoidectomy is, of course, indicated. Cawthorne has reported that in patients with disabling vertigo and an active fistula sign, despite a radical mastoidectomy, overlooked latent disease in the perilabyrinthine cell tracts may be the cause.

If disease is eradicated, the vertigo usually disappears. He reports a rare instance in which a superior and inferior vestibulotomy, with particular attention to removal of the utricle, may be required.

Although the lateral semicircular canal approach with fenestration can be favorably compared with any other, it now seems somewhat unfashionable.

TRANSCANAL LABYRINTHOTOMY

This method is more fashionable today for complete destruction of the labyrinth. The approach is the one used for stapedectomy, the operation being performed through the external auditory canal. After a Rosen or Shea incision, the posterior part of the tympanic membrane is folded anteriorly. The stapes is extracted and moved onto the promontory to provide easy access and good vision into the vestibule. The normal stapes without otosclerosis is easily lifted out of the niche without breaking the crura or footplate. The stapes tendon should be preserved for easy reinsertion later. The perilymph is sucked out by suction cannulas, and then with right-angled hooks the utricle, saccule, and the various semicircular canals in turn are disrupted. One must destroy the entire vestibule as well as tear out the horizontal canal. Some operators use a dental broach. It has been suggested by Fernandez that in those cases which fail, the crista of the posterior semicircular canal and the macula of the saccule are most likely to survive. The posterior semicircular canal is most distant from the oval window, posteriorly and inferiorly. It is well to scrape the endosteum, since this causes fibrosis and bony growth. Pushing should be avoided, for it is possible to break into the internal auditory meatus through the thin perforated lamina with production of a leak of spinal fluid. Concentrated streptomycin solution instilled into the vestibule with pledgets of gelfoam helps destruction. Schuknecht reports that one of the effects of the various labyrinthotomy operations is to compromise the blood supply. When the blood supply is

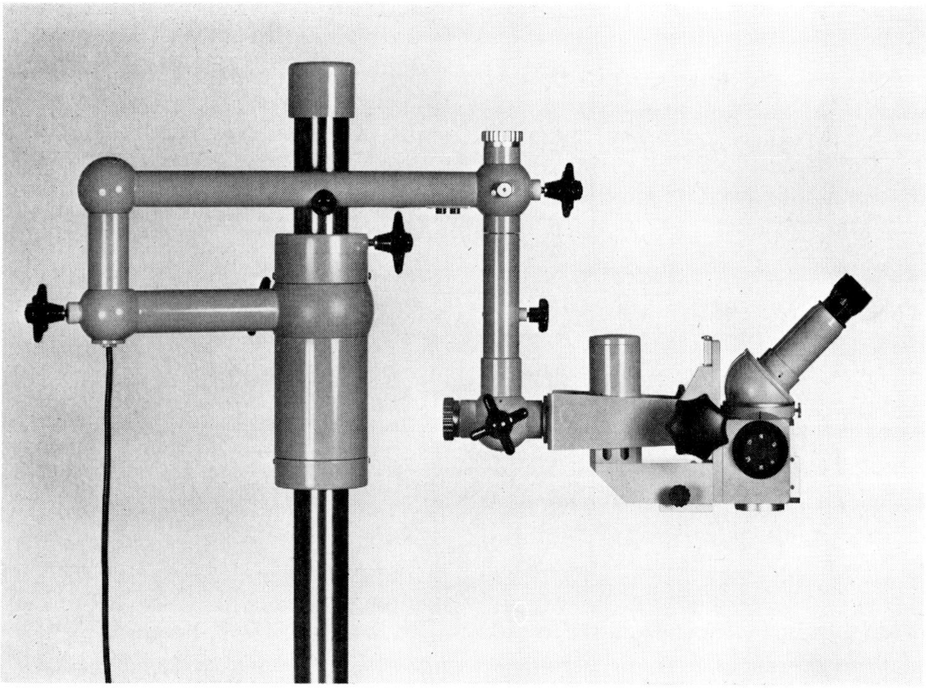

FIG. 1. Zeiss surgical microscope as used in transcanal labyrinthectomy.

compromised, there is proliferation of the endosteum.

Many operators prefer general anesthesia for destructive labyrinthotomy, since there may be a good deal of vomiting and vertigo once the labyrinth is disturbed. Williams reported the wisdom of closing any opening in the labyrinth to prevent the possibility of future meningitis. The stapes itself is the best cover, but if this is not feasible, bone chips can be used to fill the vestibule. Some men (Lempert, Ariagno, Armstrong) have advised connecting the oval window and the round window to insure access for better destruction of the neuroepithelium. The membranous labyrinth is completely destroyed with hooks and suction tip. Special 3 and 4 mm. right-angled hooks are manipulated superiorly beneath the facial nerve to engage the utricle and ampullae of the semicircular canals and draw them down to the operated area. A 5 mm. reamer has been designed by Ariagno to probe the bony semicircular canals. The incus and stapes can be broken and packed into the cavity to stimulate an obliterative osteitis. The tympanic membrane is replaced at the end of the procedure.

PROGNOSIS

Simonton and Sciara reported the prognosis and postoperative disability in cases of surgical labyrinthectomy via the lateral semicircular canal. They reported that the hospital stay of the average patient was 8 days and that one-third of the patients returned to work within a month, but one-third were disabled for 2 months or more. In 5 per cent there was disequilibrium, and in another 31 per cent there was dizziness on quick movements. They reported several cases in which meningitis developed after operation, before the technique of filling the fenestra with bone chips was adopted. They felt that the prognosis for complete compensation depended upon the nervous stability, ambition, and economic necessity in the individual patient. Mild degrees of disequilibrium persisted in 71 per cent of cases. Cawthorne stated that after surgery, patients may have some residual dizziness provoked by sudden head movements and may also tire easily. Jordan suggested that a 5-year period be used to judge results of labyrinthine treatment. Schuknecht reported that in 2 out of 4 patients in whom only the round window membrane was ruptured and the stapes removed without probing and aspiration, there was recurrence of dizzy spells, although the attacks were less frequent and less severe than before surgery. The attacks recurred 7 months after operation in one case and 12 months in the other. He stated that it is surprising that so few patients experience improvement in tinnitus following cochlear ablation.

The chief concern in regard to the destructive operation is the possibility of future in-

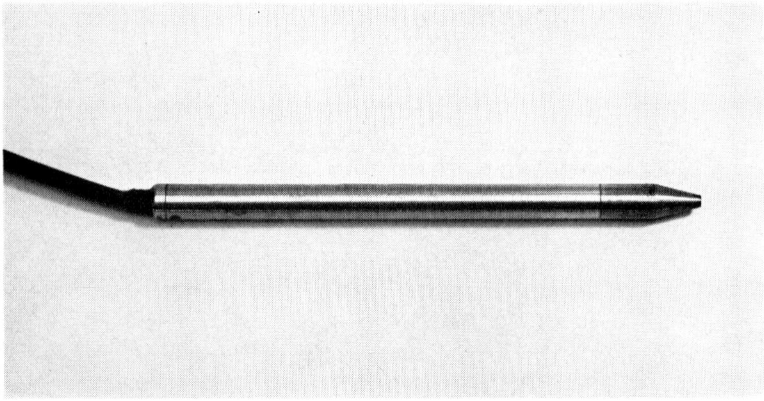

FIG. 2. Applicator (or transducer) of Australian ultrasound apparatus.

volvement of the opposite ear, since the operation completely destroys the residual hearing in the involved ear. Cawthorne reported that 8 per cent of his operated cases developed hydrops in the other ear. Although this is indeed a cause for concern, careful selection of patients for the destructive procedure with choice only of those whose hearing is irretrievably lost tends, to some extent, to minimize this danger. The operation is, however, performed with some reluctance for this reason.

METHODS TO ATTEMPT HEARING PRESERVATION

Ultrasonic Destruction of the Labyrinth

Ultrasound was first used in episodic labyrinthine vertigo by Arslan of Padua in 1952 to attempt destruction of the labyrinth while sparing the cochlea. The labyrinth is approached through the mastoid process by the usual mastoidectomy route. The operation is performed under local anesthesia so that the reactions of eye nystagmus may be observed. By observation of the nystagmus, it is stated that it is possible to know when the labyrinth has been paralyzed and the object of the application achieved. The steps of the operation are as follows: light premedication is given prior to operation; local anesthesia is induced by the infiltration of xylocaine, 1 per cent, and epinephrine, 1:100,000, over the mastoid process and into the wall of the external auditory canal. A postauricular incision is made. The mastoid antrum is opened. After opening the mastoid process, the cavity is enlarged in order to give free access for the application of the tip of the transducer to the posterior part of the lateral semicircular canal. The bone over the lateral semicircular canal is burred down until a wide blue line is clearly visible and the surface is flattened so that the tip of the transducer rod may sit as accurately as possible on the bone. Ultra-

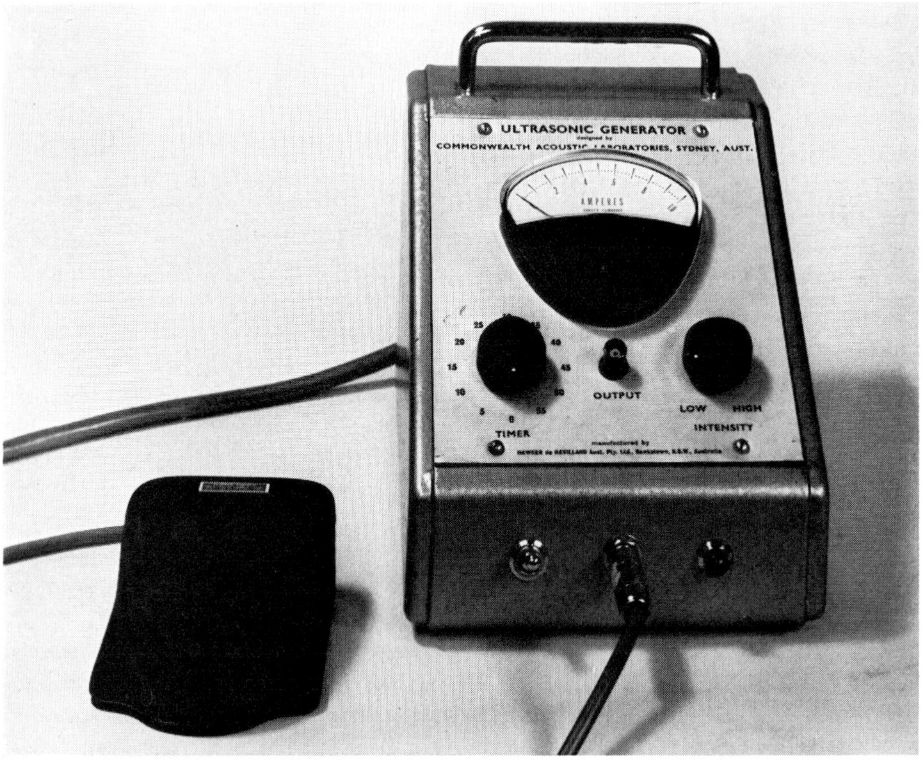

Fig. 3. Australian ultrasound generator with attached foot pedal.

sound is not transmitted freely by bone; the half-intensity power distance is only ½ mm. at one million cycles per second. Fortunately, ultrasonic vibrations are transmitted very freely by liquids, and therefore once the vibrations have reached the labyrinthine fluids, they are transmitted to all parts of the labyrinth with very little loss of power. The half-intensity power distance in liquid is 15 meters. Inside the labyrinth the sound vibrations are reflected from the bony surfaces of the canals and vestibule in the same way as audible sound vibrations are reflected from the walls of a speaking tube. Thus, nodes and antinodes, where the waves interfere with or supplement wave motion, produce zones of extremely high and very low pressures. The mechanical effects of these alternating pressures on the cell walls and contents are responsible for the damage to the cell and for its ultimate death. Animal experiments show that ultrasound does have a destructive effect on the neuroepithelium and the secretory epithelium in the ampullae.

Very shortly after the first application of the ultrasound over the lateral semicircular canal, the patient complains of rotatory vertigo, and this is accompanied by nystagmus beating toward the operated side. After some minutes, the irritative nystagmus gradually fades away and is replaced by a paralytic nystagmus beating away from the operated side. The application of ultrasound is continued until there is no further irritative nystagmus visible after a rest period of approximately 15 seconds. The ultrasound is usually applied for from 20 to 30 minutes. At the end of the operation the wound is sutured without drainage. For the first few days after the operation, the patient is very giddy and exhibits a paralytic nystagmus, but this rapidly subsides. Patients are allowed to walk as soon as they are able to balance with assistance. They are usually ready to leave the hospital after 7 days. The final degeneration of the labyrinth, with complete loss of function, seems to take some weeks or months, and after an ultrasonic treatment patients may still have minor attacks of vertigo during the next 3 months.

The special indications for ultrasound are:

1. Incapacitating unilateral Meniere's disease with good hearing.
2. Bilateral Meniere's disease.
3. Persistent vertigo after a mastoidectomy or tympanoplasty where hearing is good.
4. Severe intractable positional vertigo which can be localized to one ear.
5. Vertigo after stapedectomy which has not responded to revision but where good hearing has been retained.
6. Certain cases of unilateral central vertigo.

Results of the Ultrasound Operation

Hearing. It is a remarkable thing that the organ of Corti in the human being escapes serious damage in the majority of cases. This is probably because the cochlear duct opens into the vestibule at an oblique angle, and therefore very little of the reflected ultrasonic vibrations are traveling in the direction necessary to enter the cochlea itself. That some of these vibrations enter is quite certain, however, as shown by the temporary increase in perceptive deafness that follows immediately after the operation. This usually recovers during the first 2 or 3 weeks but it may take longer, and in 10 per cent of cases a permanent reduction occurs.

Improvement in Vertigo. The improvement rate was about 80 per cent according to most participants in the Padua conference (1963). With failure ultrasound may be administered again. If definite improvement does not arise in 6 to 12 weeks, further therapy should be considered.

Tinnitus. The improvement in tinnitus averages about 35 per cent, which may be the natural improvement rate in Meniere's disease (many different forms of treatment give the same figure).

Facial Palsy. Since the facial nerve is only a millimeter or so from the lateral semicircular canal, there is a risk of causing facial paralysis. Facial palsy has been reported in approximately 10 per cent of cases. The facial palsy is temporary, often lasting only days. The onset of facial palsy may be immediate, but more commonly, it begins a week after operation. It seems that application of ultrasound far from the facial nerve, either through the superior part of the vestibule or more easily through the superior crus of the posterior semicircular canal, may eliminate facial palsy entirely. Improved apparatus with less emission of heat, less dispersion of ultrasound, and narrower transducers also help in the elimination of facial palsy.

Apparatus

The Federici apparatus had a transducer head which was rather bulky, with a diameter at the tip of 5 mm. Mechanical difficulties were common. The low efficiency of conversion of electrical energy to ultrasound caused the transducer head to emit a considerable quantity of undesirable heat. There was, likewise, significant side lobe radiation from this emitting tip, and frequent tuning of the apparatus was required throughout the procedure. Several improved ultrasound generators have been made: an Australian apparatus (Kossof), English models (Angell James and Douglas Gordon), and Swedish model (Sjoberg). Improvements are illustrated by those in the Angell James model: ultrasound of three million cycles per second instead of one million cycles; lead zirconate titanate crystal; efficiency of 38 per cent, compared to 2 per cent in the Federici apparatus, with production of much less heat; finer applicator tips; and greater stability in emission of ultrasound.

Systemic Injection of Streptomycin

The injection of streptomycin sulfate is a method of medical labyrinthotomy which tends to preserve hearing. Streptomycin has a remarkable selectivity for the vestibular system. It is not necessary that the patient have a good auditory function. Baseline audiograms and caloric tests are made on different days before treatment is started. After the first 10 days of treatment, caloric tests are done every day and audiograms every second day. The treatment may be given for 10 days on an outpatient basis, and afterwards the patients are admitted to the hospital. Two grams are given per day in 2 equally divided doses for 2 to 3 weeks or more. The end-point is that at which the caloric response to ice water has almost disappeared. The optimum endpoint is that just short of total destruction of the vestibular system. The first adverse symptom is a feeling of unsteadiness, which is followed by ataxia, loss of appetite, and nausea. Spontaneous nystagmus develops about this time. The ataxia lasts for about 6 months up to a year. The patient also often complains of difficulty in judging the speed of moving objects as well as difficulty in watching them. Streptomycin should be avoided in cases in which there is impaired kidney function. The object of treatment is to create a severe but not total loss of vestibular function of both ears. Hanson was an early pioneer in this treatment. Schuknecht does not recommend this parenteral streptomycin for unilateral Meniere's disease because an operation is preferred here. Since ataxia is a more common complication among the elderly, streptomycin should not be administered to patients older than 50 years of age.

Drainage of the Saccus Endolymphaticus

The operation was first described by Portmann in 1927 and was designed to relieve the pressure in the endolymphatic system. The endolymphatic sac was identified by way of the postauricular mastoid approach and a drainage incision was made in the lateral surface of the sac. He reported good results in 60 per cent of cases. Flett later used the Portmann procedure in 73 cases. He stated that the procedure offered 25 per cent chance of retaining the patient's hearing and 61 per cent improvement of the vertigo. This operation has been given a great boost by the improvement in vision rendered by the Zeiss microscope. The endolymphatic sac may be found in the dura posterior to the dome and inferior crus of the posterior semicircular canal. It is in the dura anterior to the lateral sinus where the lateral sinus swerves down toward the jugular fossa. The endolymphatic sac lies in the dura between the lateral sinus and the posterior semicircular canal. House has recently modified the Portmann operation by draining the endolymphatic sac into the subarachnoid space by the use of a silicone rubber tube inserted through the medial wall of the sac. The lateral wall of the sac is first incised and the sac entered. The medial wall is then incised and a tube inserted into the subarachnoid space connecting the endolymph to the spinal fluid. A shunt for the release of pressure in the sac is thus created after the healing of the lateral wall of the sac. A potential hazard with this operation is subsequent meningitis.

Hemisection of the Eighth Cranial Nerve

Intracranial hemisection of the eighth nerve was suggested by Dandy, sparing enough fibers of the auditory division so that the cochlear function could be preserved. However, this preserved hearing in only 22 per cent of Dandy's cases. In the remaining cases, hearing was lost immediately after the operation or rapidly deteriorated. The reason for this was that it was difficult to separate the eighth nerve into grossly distinct trunks. In the area exposed by the posterior fossa approach, according to Rasmussen, there is an intermingling of the vestibular and cochlear fibers in each division so that separate nerve bundles are seldom found. Often when hearing was preserved, vertigo was not abolished, and when vertigo was abolished the hearing was not preserved. Furthermore, the morbidity and mortality from this operation are relatively high.

Recently, House divided the branches of the vestibular nerve in the internal auditory meatus by the temporal approach to the middle cranial fossa for relief of vertigo and preservation of hearing in endolymphatic hydrops. If an intracranial neoplasm cannot be completely ruled out, then the intracranial approach is the procedure of choice.

SUMMARY

The most effective operation for relief of episodic vertigo resulting from irritation of the labyrinthine system appears to be complete destruction of the labyrinth. Conservative measures which attempt to preserve hearing while eliminating vertigo include ultrasound, systemic streptomycin, drainage of the saccus endolymphaticus, and hemisection of the eighth cranial nerve.

REFERENCES

1. Altman, F., and Waltner, J. G.: The present status of the treatment of Meniere's disease with ultrasound. Bull. N.Y. Acad. Med. 37: 621, 1961.
2. Ariagno, R.: Trans tympanic labyrinthectomy. Arch. Otolaryng. 80:282, 1964.
3. Arslan, M.: An improved technique of the ultrasonic irradiation of the vestibular apparatus by Meniere's disease. Acta Otolaryng. 55:467, 1962.
4. Cawthorne, T.: Surgical treatment of Meniere's disease. Laryngoscope 73:1016, 1963.
5. Fernandez, C., Ludwig, H., and McAuliffe, D.: Electrocoagulation of the vestibule in guinea pigs. Laryngoscope 62:1159, 1952.
6. Van Fick, I.: Decompression of the labyrinth. Arch. Otolaryng. 79:447, 1964.
7. Guilford, F.: Surgery of labyrinth. *In:* Neurological Aspects of Auditory and Vestibular Disorders (W. S. Fields and B. R. Alford, Eds.). Springfield, Ill., Charles C Thomas Co., 1964.
8. House, W. F.: Subarachnoid shunt for drainage of endolymphatic hydrops, a preliminary report. Laryngoscope 72:713, 1962.
9. James, J. A., Dalton, M. M., Bullen, H. F., Freundlich, H. F., and Hopkins, J. C.: The ultrasonic treatment of Meniere's disease. J. Laryng. 74:730, 1960.
10. Lumsden, R. B.: Treatment of Meniere's Disease with ultrasound. Proc. Roy. Soc. Med. 51: 617, 1958.
11. Meurman, Y.: The effect of conventional fenestration on Meniere's disease. Arch. Otolaryng. 70:169, 1959.
12. McKenzie, K. G.: Intracranial division of vestibular portion of auditory nerve for Meniere's disease. Canad. Med. Ass. J. 34:369, 1936.
13. Passe, E. R. G.: Sympathectomy in relation to Meniere's disease, tinnitus and deafness. A.M.A. Arch. Otolaryng. 57:257, 1953.
14. Schuknecht, H.: Ablation therapy and the management of Meniere's disease. Acta Otolaryng. Supp. 132, 1957.

Index